On the market today there is an abundance of books addressing grief and loss. Some focus on assisting mental health counselors in their practices and others are self-help focused. Grief Work in Addictions Counseling *is unique. It focuses on grief work applied to addiction counseling, a focus that has long been needed. It is a valuable tool for both addiction professionals and individuals in addiction recovery.*

—Kirk Bowden, *PhD, chair of the Addiction and Substance Use Disorders Program at Rio Salado College, president of the International Association of Addictions and Offender Counselors, and past president of NAADAC, the Association of Addiction Professionals*

Grief Work in Addictions Counseling

Grief Work in Addictions Counseling is a book for practitioners and students in the field of substance abuse counseling who encounter grief and loss issues with clients recovering from addiction.

Enlightening the reader about loss, its relation to addiction, and the need to grieve these losses, this book provides specific strategies and techniques that readers can apply to both individual clients and counseling groups. Chapters address multicultural themes to help clinicians design treatments that will meet the needs of diverse genders, sexual orientations, cultures, ages, and spiritual orientations.

This book is useful both for professionals and as a supplemental textbook for students preparing to become addictions counselors.

Susan R. Furr is a professor in the Department of Counseling at the University of North Carolina at Charlotte and a licensed psychologist with over 20 years of full-time practice as a counselor. Her areas of interest include suicide and crisis intervention as well as grief counseling, where she has published research on losses related to addictions.

Kathryn Hunsucker is a licensed clinical mental health counselor and supervisor and licensed clinical addictions specialist who has worked in outpatient treatment programs, hospitals, disaster services, and state/local government with children, youth, families, adults, and geriatrics with mental health, substance abuse, and developmental disabilities.

Grief Work in Addictions Counseling

Edited by Susan R. Furr and Kathryn Hunsucker

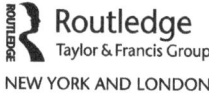
Routledge
Taylor & Francis Group

NEW YORK AND LONDON

First published 2022
by Routledge
605 Third Avenue, New York, NY 10158

and by Routledge
4 Park Square, Milton Park, Abingdon, Oxon, OX14 4RN

Routledge is an imprint of the Taylor & Francis Group, an informa business

Library of Congress Cataloging-in-Publication Data
Names: Furr, Susan R., editor. | Hunsucker, Kathryn, editor.
Title: Grief work in addictions counseling / edited by Susan R. Furr and Kathryn Hunsucker.
Description: New York, NY : Routledge, 2022. | Includes bibliographical references and index.
Identifiers: LCCN 2021046549 (print) | LCCN 2021046550 (ebook) | ISBN 9780367538576 (hardback) | ISBN 9780367538569 (paperback) | ISBN 9781003106906 (ebook)
Subjects: LCSH: Substance abuse—Treatment. | Drug abuse counseling. | Addicts—Rehabilitation. | Grief.
Classification: LCC RC564 .G74 42022 (print) | LCC RC564 (ebook) | DDC 362.29—dc23/eng/20211220
LC record available at https://lccn.loc.gov/2021046549
LC ebook record available at https://lccn.loc.gov/2021046550

ISBN: 978-0-367-53857-6 (hbk)
ISBN: 978-0-367-53856-9 (pbk)
ISBN: 978-1-003-10690-6 (ebk)

DOI: 10.4324/9781003106906

Typeset in Times New Roman
by Apex CoVantage, LLC

Ted—Thank you for your continuous support and encouragement. You enrich my life and help me find balance.

Kasey and James—You continue to amaze me with your sense of curiosity and adventure. Thank you for inspiring me to take risks and journey to new places. Being your mom has been the best adventure ever. Susan

To Dr. Furr—Thanks for making this book happen, your never-ending support and encouragement. Kathryn

Contents

About the Editors

Susan R. Furr is a professor in the Department of Counseling at the University of North Carolina at Charlotte and a licensed psychologist. With over 20 years of full-time practice as a counselor and 25 years of experience as a counselor educator, she has both direct experience in working with grief issues and teaching experience in the area of grief and loss counseling. In addition, she has conducted research in the area of grief as it relates to issues of substance abuse. Her clinical experiences include working as a school counselor and as a counselor in the university counseling center. She presents frequently in the community on using cognitive behavioral therapy in clinical practice. She has published in the *Journal of Addictions and Offender Counseling* (*JAOC*) on grief issues with clients in recovery for substance abuse. She has served as the editor of the International Association of Addictions and Offender Counselors (IAAOC) newsletter for many years and is a member of the editorial board of *JAOC*. She is currently writing in the area of using rituals to facilitate the grieving process with a special focus on disenfranchised grief.

Kathryn Hunsucker received pastoral care specialist training from Presbyterian Hospital in Charlotte in 1996 and a master of arts in community/agency counseling from UNC Charlotte in 2000. She completed certification in clinical military counseling in 2017 from East Carolina University. She has a wide variety of experience working in outpatient treatment programs, hospitals, disaster services, and state/local government with children, youth, families, adults, and geriatrics with mental health, substance abuse, and developmental disabilities. She presents regularly at the North Carolina Counseling Association Conference and the American Counseling Association Conference. She is a national certified counselor, licensed clinical mental health counselor, licensed clinical mental health counselor supervisor, licensed clinical addictions specialist, approved clinical supervisor, and a certified clinical supervisor. In her current position, she conducts comprehensive clinical assessments and treatment focused on substance use disorders and mental health services.

About the Contributors

Lyndon P. Abrams, PhD, is an associate professor in the Department of Counseling at the University of North Carolina at Charlotte. He earned his PhD in counseling from Texas A&M Commerce in 2001 and has 20 years of experience as a counselor educator. He has served as the director of the doctoral program in counselor education and supervision and received the Bonnie E. Cone Early-Career Professorship in Teaching for his achievements as an instructor. His research interest areas have focused on social justice and multicultural issues with a focus on racial identity development, diversity in math and science careers, multicultural education, and social desirability.

Emily A. Barton, PhD, is an assistant professor of behavioral neuroscience at St. Edward's University in Austin, Texas. Her research focuses on the impact of alcohol use on the brain and cognitive functioning and the factors that lead to different patterns of drinking. She teaches courses in behavioral neuroscience and psychology. Her research interests include alcohol, exercise, glia, neuroimmune function, and behavior with a focus on the interplay between hormones, cognition, and patterns of alcohol drinking.

Kathleen Brown-Rice, PhD, is Associate Dean of Graduate Studies for the College of Education and Associate Professor of Counselor Education at Sam Houston State University. She is a licensed professional counselor (NC, TX); licensed clinical mental health counselor (SD); licensed clinical addiction specialist (NC); national certified counselor; and approved clinical supervisor. She has worked as a professional counselor in various clinical settings assisting clients with mental health, trauma, and substance abuse issues. Her scholarly research activity focuses on counselor supervision and training with an emphasis in ethical considerations, the implications of historical/generational trauma, and the impact of substance abuse on individuals, families, and the community.

Christine Chasek, PhD, LIMHP, LADC is an Associate Professor and Chair of the Counseling Department at the University of Nebraska Omaha and Workforce Director of the Behavioral Healthcare Center of Nebraska-University of Nebraska Medical Center. She is a practicing mental health and addictions counselor with experience in behavioral health care administration most currently focusing on behavioral healthcare in rural Nebraska. Her research interests include mental health and addiction counseling, counselor preparation, rural behavioral health, and clinical outcomes. Dr. Chasek also serves as the Chairman of the Nebraska Alcohol and Drug Licensing Board, Past President of the International Association of Alcohol and Drug Counselors, and a National Farm Medicine Research Fellow.

Michelle Colon, LPC, is a licensed professional counselor, counselor educator, and doctoral candidate at Regent University. She currently works in university counseling and teaches graduate courses in counseling at Regent. Her current research interests include addiction, collective self-esteem, counselor well-being, counselor burnout, and Latinx counselors in the field.

Stephanie Dorais, PhD, LPC, NCC, is a licensed professional counselor and counselor educator. She currently works in private practice and teaches graduate courses in counseling at New York University. Her research interests include contemplative science, trauma, and addiction recovery.

Sejal Foxx, PhD, is a professor and Chair of the Counseling Department at UNC Charlotte. She is also Director of the Urban School Counseling Collaborative. She has experience as an elementary and high school counselor. She is co-author of *School Counseling in the 21st Century* (6th ed.). In 2015, she received the Counselor Educator of the Year Award from the North Carolina School Counselors Association. She teaches both doctoral and master's level courses, and her special areas of interest are school counseling, multicultural issues and social justice, urban education, creating equity and access to college, and career readiness.

Gillian R. Galdy is a master's student in the Department of Counseling and Educational Development at UNC Greensboro, where she concentrates in couple and family counseling. Her areas of research and clinical interest include consent-based and gender-affirming sex education, best practices for supporting trans children and their families, domestic violence and sexual assault prevention, and social justice and intersectional feminist approaches to counseling.

Hannah Glenn, MA, is a licensed clinical mental health counselor, specializes in addiction, and works with children whose parent(s) live with a substance use disorder. She currently practices at Charlotte Counseling and Wellness and NorthStar Clinical Services, both located in Charlotte. Her area of research is parents' substance abuse and its impact on their children. She is a dedicated to helping others and serves on numerous charity boards in the Charlotte area.

Daniel Gutierrez, PhD, LPC, CSAC, is an associate professor of counselor education at the College of William and Mary. He is also a licensed professional counselor and a certified substance abuse counselor working in private practice. His research agenda focuses on addiction recovery, evidence-based practices with underserved and marginalized populations, and spirituality in counseling.

Henry L. Harris, PhD, is a professor in the Department of Counseling at UNC Charlotte. He is a former school counselor and Air Force veteran with 25 years of teaching and administrative experience as a counselor educator.

Leigh Falls Holman, PhD, has been a licensed professional counselor supervisor who has worked and conducted research with trauma, addictions, and offender populations for 25 years. She has served on the board of the International Association of Addiction and Offender Counseling (IAAOC) and the American Counseling Association (ACA). She is a department chair at the Dallas campus of the Chicago School of Professional Psychology. She has published a book on forensic mental health counseling, over 20 peer-reviewed research articles and book chapters, and has presented nationally and internationally on these topics.

Tahsin Ilhan, PhD, is a professor in the Department Psychology at Ankara Medipol University. His primary interest concerns supervision, individual, couple and family counseling, well-being, post-traumatic growth, and addiction. He regularly conducts counseling and training workshops in Turkey and Azerbaijan.

Vanessa Iverson, MA, is Behavioral Health Director at Wagner Indian Health Services in Wagner, SD. She is a licensed professional counselor (SD) and an approved clinical licensed professional counselor supervisor (SD). She has worked as a professional counselor in school settings, private practice, and now actively in the health care field. She prioritizes fostering a compassionate and safe relationship with her clients. Among her areas of expertise are anxiety, depression, trauma, boundary setting, and adjustments to life. Modalities used in treatment may include psychodynamic treatment approaches, internal family systems, and mindfulness-based interventions. Her approach focuses on how past experiences influence current behaviors and patterns. She has a passion for equal rights, social justice, multicultural education, and research.

Derrick Johnson, MA, is a PhD candidate at UNC Charlotte. His research area is disenfranchised grief experienced by support persons of those living with addiction, and he has published articles on grief and substance abuse in the *Journal of Addictions and Offender Counseling* (*JAOC*) and *Counseling Today*. He is Executive and Clinical Director of NorthStar Clinical Services in Charlotte and is a licensed clinical mental health counselor and licensed clinical addiction specialist. He also maintains a private practice where he works with issues surrounding addiction, grief and loss, LGBTQ issues, and trauma. He has been an instructor in the counseling department of the

Cato College of Education at UNC Charlotte and has spoken at numerous counseling and state mental health conferences.

Connie T. Jones, PhD, LCMHCA, LCAS, is a tenure-track assistant professor of Counseling and Educational Development at UNC Greensboro. She is a past president of the ACA's division of the IAAOC. Her background is in addiction and clinical mental health counseling. Her primary focus of scholarship concerns addictions, broaching, and social justice.

Pamela S. Lassiter, PhD, is a professor in the Department of Counseling at UNC Charlotte, where she served as program director for addiction counseling and graduate certificate in addiction counseling. She has served as editor of the *JAOC* and is a past president of IAAOC. Her specialty areas include sexual minority parenting, multicultural supervision, substance abuse counselor training, women's issues, and historical narratives in counseling.

Krupali Michaels, MEd, LPC, LPCC, is a counselor education doctoral student at Oregon State University. She received her master's degree in counseling from Malone University. She is a licensed professional (clinical) counselor (OH, OR).

Regina R. Moro, PhD, is an associate professor of counselor education at St. Bonaventure University. She is a licensed professional counselor (ID), licensed clinical addiction specialist (NC), and a licensed mental health counselor (FL). She is also a national certified counselor and a board-certified telemental health provider. Her clinical passion involves work with crisis and trauma, including a focus on addiction with individuals and families. She has experience working in community mental health, integrated care settings, and private practice. She is an active member of the ACA, the Association of Counselor Education and Supervision, and the IAAOC.

John C. Nance, PhD, LCMHC-S, NCC, ACS, is currently an assistant clinical professor in the counseling program at UNC Charlotte. He practices counseling in private practice, primarily working with adult survivors of early childhood trauma and torture. His background includes work as a pastor within the Christian faith and program coordination for chaplain and counseling internship training within a large hospital setting.

Christie Nelson, PhD, is a licensed clinical mental health counselor supervisor and a clinician at Novant Health in Winston-Salem, NC. She is also an assistant professor at Bradley University's online counseling program. Her areas of interest include spirituality, meditation, and contemplative pedagogy. She is a member of the ACA; the Association for Spiritual, Ethical, and Religious Values in Counseling; and the Association for Contemplative Mind in Higher Education. She has taken on the role of secretary for the 2021–2022 term of the North Carolina Counseling Association.

Kok-Mun Ng, PhD, LPC, LCMHC, ACS, NCC, is a professor of counselor education at Oregon State University. He is a Malaysian by birth who loves to engage with clients and students in growth-promoting encounters. His research interests include multicultural and cross-cultural counseling issues, internationalization of professional counseling, supervision, and postmodern counseling approaches.

Yun Shi, MA, MS, LMFT, is a counselor education doctoral student at Oregon State University. She received her master's degree in counseling from San Francisco State University. She is a licensed marriage and family therapist (CA, OR).

Michael S. Spivey, MA, LCMHC, NCC, works as a mental health clinician at Lenoir-Rhyne University's Student Support and Wellness Center. His areas of special interest include college, career, bereavement, and LGBTQIA+ counseling as well as research in the LGBTQIA+ arena. He holds a master of arts degree from UNC Charlotte in counseling and a master of arts degree from the George Washington University in education and human resource development.

Mark S. Woodford, PhD, is a professor in the Department of Counselor Education at the College of New Jersey. He is a licensed professional counselor, a master addiction counselor, and a national certified counselor who has worked in community-, family-, and school-based prevention and early intervention programs, as well as in a residential addiction treatment facility. In addition to his duties as chair, he teaches courses in treating addiction and co-occurring disorders and counseling boys and men, and he provides clinical supervision for graduate students in counselor education. His research interests are in the field of addiction counseling with a specific emphasis on the interplay of gender issues in substance abuse and addiction treatment. He is the author of *Men, Addiction, and Intimacy: Strengthening Recovery by Fostering the Emotional Development of Boys and Men* (Routledge, 2012).

Preface

We were approached about writing this book after presenting a Learning Institute at the American Counseling Association conference. We have been working on this concept for many years and believe grief and its connection to addictions is often overlooked in the field. At first, we wondered if we would have enough material for a book but also realized how much more we wanted to present but did not have the space at the conference to cover all of our topics in depth. Therefore, chapters 1–4 cover the foundational material that related grief counseling to addictions, which was the main focus of our presentation. To add to this foundational material, we were fortunate to find a young researcher in neuroscience, whose research focus is the effects of alcohol on the brain, to provide an expanded understanding of the connections between grief and substance use.

Because our program at UNC Charlotte is built around a multicultural core, we were excited about devoting chapters 5–19 to the dynamics that occur with substance use in different populations. We believe it is important for each of the topics to be presented by professionals who have a personal understanding of the values and meaning-making life experiences of each of the populations presented in these chapters. Although we had hoped to include additional chapters on multicultural groups in this section of the book, we were not always able to find someone who could address the issues from a culturally sensitive and knowledgeable perspective. We apologize if we did not address a cultural perspective that is important to you.

Finally, we both have years of providing direct services to clients, and we highly value ideas about how to directly work with clients. In chapters 20 and 21, we have shared a few approaches you may be able to use to engage clients in working on their grief issues as they arise in addictions counseling. Our hope is that this book will alert you to the importance of addressing grief and loss issues with those in recovery from substance use and that you will find new options that excite you about helping clients with their recovery journey.

Acknowledgments

Our collaboration began while at UNC Charlotte as student and professor. Kathryn designed a structured group on grief and substance abuse for Susan's group course. Susan also taught a course in grief counseling. After Kathryn's graduation, we joined efforts in developing a Learning Institute for the American Counseling Association's (ACA) annual conference that joined the topics of addiction counseling and grief. Over the years, we refined this presentation, which was the foundation for this book.

First, we want to express our appreciation to Dr. Sejal Foxx, chair of the Department of Counseling, and UNC Charlotte, which provided release time for developing this concept. UNC Charlotte has been a fertile ground for developing addiction counselors, beginning with Dr. Jane Carroll, who fostered the development of our addiction counseling program. Dr. Pam S. Lassiter continued to expand our program and our summer training institute, the Dr. Jonnie H. McLeod Institute. She is a frequent mentor for students who want to practice in the addictions field and inspires those who want to teach future addiction counselors. Dr. Jack Culbreth, as chair of the Board of the Council for Accreditation of Counseling and Related Educational Programs (CACREP), initiated the addition of addiction counseling as a specialty area, and Dr. Lassiter led the efforts for our program to become one of the first three programs in the country accredited by CACREP. Dr. Laura Veach brought a focus on Screening, Brief Intervention and Referral to Treatment (SBIRT) in the hospital setting. All of these wonderful people have been our guides. Other inspiration for our work has come from Dr. Geri Miller at Appalachian State University.

We have both been nurtured by our affiliation with the International Association for Addictions and Offender Counseling (IAAOC), a division of ACA. IAAOC provides cutting-edge research and professional development opportunities for those in the addictions and correction fields. Many of our contributors have been leaders in this outstanding organization. We encourage any counselor who works in the field of addiction counseling to seek out this organization.

Our knowledge has been enriched by our clients, colleagues, students, supervisees, and conference participants over the years. They have provided valuable insights into the impact of grief on addiction and recovery. We are grateful for their support and encouragement to pursue these ideas.

Finally, this book exists because of the generosity of the contributing authors. Each author has a strong connection to the content of their chapter and infuses the spirit of their commitment to the topic. Our goal has been to addressed a wide range of cultural perspectives with the hope of providing a deeper understanding of the intersection of culture, grief, and addiction. Some authors faced a new challenge of adding a grief perspective to their knowledge of substance abuse counseling. Others added the component of addiction to cultural knowledge. Each chapter adds a new and insightful understanding on blending the topics of grief and addictions. Bringing in the perspective of brain and neural processes, this book addresses the complex relationship between attachment formation, addiction, and grief by highlighting the shared neurological underpinnings that often are not addressed in treatment approaches. It is our hope that these chapters extend the reader's awareness of the importance of addressing grief issues related to recovery from addiction.

1 Is Addiction a Loss to Grieve?

Susan R. Furr

Unraveling the complexities of substance abuse is an ongoing exploration into the biopsychosocial model of addiction. This model moved the field of addictions from a biomedical model to an approach that examines the myriad factors that contribute to addiction. Because scientific findings have not established a single factor that explains why substance use leads to addiction for some individuals but not others, the field of recovery has moved to addressing multiple factors in helping overcome addiction (Skewes & Gonzalez, 2013). Much of the history of treatment for addictions has been built around the biological factors, which have been shown to be potent contributors to substance misuse. As a consequence of the biomedical model taking such a powerful role, treatment programs have focused on the biological factors connected to addiction, which is an approach necessary for treatment to be effective but one that does not capture all of the contributing elements. But addressing these biological factors alone is not enough to help those with substance use disorders (SUD) maintain abstinence. Thus, the movement to the biopsychosocial model was developed to acknowledge the importance of the biological/genetic, psychological, and sociocultural factors that research has shown to be connected to addiction (Skewes & Gonzalez, 2013). Moving treatment away from a singular view based on the biological factors of addiction created room to examine the losses that have occurred throughout the lives of those with SUDs. When a broad view of loss and grief is considered, where death is not the only loss to be mourned, clinicians can begin to recognize the wide range of losses that occurred in clients' lives. Throughout the process of becoming addicted and the journey through recovery, grief-related issues will emerge and will need to be recognized and processed as part of a comprehensive treatment strategy. Although grief counseling is just one component of treatment, research indicates grief also is related to trauma, which has been shown to be a contributor to substance use. In the seminal study on adverse childhood experiences (ACEs), researchers found a strong relationship with early alcohol use and the number of ACE events that a child experienced (Dube et al., 2006), and early use is associated with alcohol dependence later in life (Grant et al., 2001).

One theme that consistently emerges during treatment is centered on the number of losses experienced by clients. In fact, researchers have discovered

DOI: 10.4324/9781003106906-1

that the number of recent substance-related losses was related to the client's readiness to change when entering treatment. Those clients who recognized more losses demonstrated a higher readiness to change (Blume & Marlatt, 2000). Therefore, it is incumbent for clinicians to help clients recognize losses as a way of facilitating the change process. Keeping a careful balance between helping clients recognize losses without pushing them to experience the grief of each loss immediately entails great counselor sensitivity to each client's ability to cope with painful emotions while trying to maintain abstinence. An interactive process of building coping resources and then using these strengths to deal with small portions of the losses may emerge in which the counselor helps the client set limits and learn ways to take a break from grieving.

One of the early advocates for connecting addictions and mourning stated, "in order to successfully give up the drug, the addict must resolve his grief by completing the stages of mourning in the process of group therapy" (Skolnick, 1979, p. 281). Goldberg (1985) acknowledged the most appropriate focus initially was the loss related to giving up the substance itself, and only when sobriety was achieved could the deeper grief work be engaged. When other losses come up initially, these losses need to be acknowledged, but the clinician needs to use professional judgment in deciding how much to get the client to open up around the losses. A determination needs to be made around how much anxiety the client can manage. At least by acknowledging the losses, clients will be validated about the challenges created by their life experiences. In this way, clients will know the clinician understands the pain they have experienced and that their losses are an important part of what led to their addiction.

As acceptance of the biopsychosocial model has grown, emphasis has been placed on addressing a broader range of issues surrounding addiction. One factor that needs further attention is the role of loss as it relates to the unresolved grief that preceded substance use as well as losses that accompanied the behaviors surrounding addiction. Kinderman (2005) even proposed that the biological-psychological-social components did not occur in an equally divided manner; there were times when the psychological needed to be the primary focus. For this reason, clinicians who work with those experiencing SUD may need to incorporate grief counseling as part of their treatment protocol.

Integrating Grief and Loss Into Substance Abuse Treatment

Losses related to SUD can be divided into three phases: (a) losses upon entering treatment, (b) losses occurring while using, and (c) losses prior to using. This sequence has been supported by the work of Goldberg (1985), Beechem et al. (1996), and Furr et al. (2015). Losses are intertwined with substance use whether serving as a trigger to use substances as a coping mechanism or the substance use itself creating losses. One of the realities those with an SUD encounter is facing the damages caused by their addiction. Even the process of entering treatment and recovery can stimulate new losses to be addressed.

Not only do clients have to give up one of their primary coping strategies, but they also have to give up "people, places, and things" associated with their substance use. As much as a person may want to regain control of life, recovery means a loss of a former lifestyle that provided meaning for that person. For many, relapse will occur, where reentering treatment now has an added loss of having relapsed. As clients present in early treatment, the focus will be on the losses incurred just to be in treatment. Once the reality of entering treatment is addressed, a recounting of the losses precipitated by the addiction will emerge. Losses while using may include relationships, jobs, money, self-esteem, safety, status, goals/dreams, health, and mental abilities. Addressing these losses needs to be accompanied by strength building and developing coping resources. As treatment continues, deeper losses may emerge related to earlier life traumas. These challenges may not be experienced by all clients but can include abuse, relationships, deaths, and life opportunities.

As indicated by this three-level model, the counselor may only see the tip of the iceberg when the client first enters treatment. However, other issues will be lurking beneath the client's initial presentation of problems. The counselor's role will be to help the client manage issues as each emerges through helping the client "bookmark" issues they are not yet ready to address and then building the skills and strength necessary for each step of recovery. The following review highlights some of the losses incurred at each point and serves to illustrate what some of the losses are like. Developing a broad perspective on losses that occur throughout addiction and recovery will provide a new way to conceptualize the needs of each client.

Losses Associated With Entering Treatment

Once clients make the decision to enter treatment, they may experience a mixture of feelings. On one hand, a courageous choice that has taken much contemplation has occurred and may be accompanied by some hope of a better future. But given how often relapse occurs, there also may be some doubt about how successful they may be this time around. What often is unexpected is the sense of loss encountered over giving up both the substance and the associated relationships. Some may have been coerced into treatment by family, friends, or work and are still in denial about the seriousness of their substance use problem. This denial is often accompanied by anger over the loss of freedom to make their own choices. In her book *Necessary Losses*, Judith Viorst (1987) explored how loss is an important catalyst for growth, yet even desirable losses need to be grieved. Perhaps this is the reason why grief is such an integral component of the recovery process. To move forward, one must leave a part of one's self behind. This period of transition involves leaving the person one has become through addiction and moving to the person one wants to be. As positive as this sounds, it is not an easy journey for those addicted to substances. An open discussion of these losses may facilitate this process.

People, Places, and Things

In our own research, we found that over 75% of the participants identified substance use as a loss they encountered when entering treatment, with 62% citing loss of being able to escape from feelings through using (Furr et al., 2015). At least 50% identified loss of friendship with fellow users (57.6%), loss of way of life (50%), and loss of places where once used (50.8%). This time can be confusing for families and supportive friends who have anticipated the benefits of recovery for the person entering treatment. They may question why the person is reluctant to give up the substance when using has been such a destructive force. Chambers and Wallingford (2017) stated, "people not only like to do drugs and alcohol, but they like to do it together" (p. 455), which creates a social network. To give up the substance also means giving up these relationships, which can be another source of grief and loss. Families can be puzzled by the desire to keep these friendships that are often related to unhealthy and even illegal behaviors. Even the person with the SUD may not fully comprehend why these attachments are so strong.

Loss of Substance

For the person in treatment, giving up the substance is parallel to giving up a love affair. Chambers and Wallingford (2017) posited similar brain mechanisms are involved with addiction and attachment, resulting in a "love affair" with the drug. Goldberg (1985) also recognized the loss of alcohol was significant for those entering treatment, and exploration of this loss needed to become part of the grief work. Throughout this process, anxiety about being without the substance can be explored as part of the grieving. One treatment technique often utilized is writing a good-bye letter to one's substance of choice, which is described in Chapter 20. Through this experience, clients can recognize the meaning of the grief associated with losing their substance of choice.

Relapse as a Form of Loss

Relapse appears to be a common characteristic of SUDs with many theories developed to explain why relapse occurs (Brandon et al., 2007). While addiction might better be conceptualized as a chronic relapsing disorder that "demands ongoing monitoring and treatment adjustments, when necessary" (Brandon et al., 2007, p. 269), the individual may experience relapse as another loss caused by substance abuse. Research has provided a strong rationale for assisting clients in treatment for SUDs to develop the ability to recognize feelings associated with losses and the skills needed to tolerate the pain associated with grieving as part of the recovery process (Anand et al., 2017). Because the term *relapse* carries such negative connotations, reframing returning to treatment as a *"reoccurrence of use"* that can trigger a sense of loss may reduce the sense of stigma (Ashford et al., 2018, p. 132).

Losses While Abusing Substances

The costs associated with having an SUD are high, whether financial, health, emotional, or social. From a financial perspective, the estimated costs of problematic drinking in the United States were $223.5 billion due to lost productivity (72.2%), health care costs (11.0%), criminal justice costs (9.4%), and other effects such as property damage and accidents (7.5%; Bouchery et al., 2011). However, these financial costs do not show the full picture of the costs related to how the individual with an addiction experiences these losses.

HEALTH LOSSES

Health care costs increase for those with an SUD. Compared to patients without a mental health or substance abuse problem, those with either a substance abuse problem or co-occurring problems had the highest use of all types of medical services, with the co-occurring group having the highest needs (Graham et al., 2017). There were more health-related problems in general for this group as well as more intentional and unintentional injuries. What this means for the individual is that substance use has a devastating effect on one's health. When entering a recovery program, the motivation to change often comes from encountering losses related to substance use. One study of a residential treatment program indicated that 42.2% of clients who abused alcohol encountered accidental injury, 25.4% experienced physical violence, and 23.5% had an overdose (Macdonald et al., 2014). The awareness that substance misuse has created problems may come from a brief intervention at a hospital, where staff may confront patients with the consequences of using. Whether the crisis was a car accident, violent act, or overdose, the reality of physical harm or even narrowly escaping death may create the "teachable moment" that begins the journey toward recovery (Graham et al., 2019).

SOCIAL

Much of substance use takes place in social settings where it is viewed as a positive behavior. But problematic substance use often creates a stigma that damages important social relationships and leads to social exclusion and marginalization from the social group (Room, 2005). A substance that once was part of the social fabric soon becomes a demarcation between acceptable and unacceptable behavior. Although professionals in the field may view addiction as a disease, society may judge the behaviors of the addicted person from a moral perspective and find them to be unacceptable. Of 18 behaviors identified as carrying social disapproval or stigma, alcoholism and drug addiction were ranked near the top in terms of stigma (Room, 2005).

Perhaps the relationship most damaged by addiction is marriage. Marriage can be a protective factor in substance use, yet alcohol dependence has a strong association with early separation (Waldron et al., 2011). In one national survey, almost 11% of men and women cited substance use as the primary reason for divorce (Amato & Previti, 2003), while another study found 34.6% of participants stated substance abuse was a major contributing factor to the divorce (Scott et al., 2013).

EXTERNAL LOSSES

Those who develop an addiction problem may encounter many losses over time related to roles that they previously fulfilled. One loss, which also may trigger other losses, is the loss of a job due to substance use, which can be the catalyst for other losses such as health care, financial problems, and reduced social support (Zemore et al., 2017). These authors found job loss was significantly associated with binge drinking and alcohol dependence. In a longitudinal study, alcohol, tobacco, and cannabis use were independently associated with job loss, and rates of unemployment increased with increased use of a substance (Airagnes et al., 2019).

Those in treatment for addiction have identified a number of losses as occurring while using, including loss of material possessions (66.2%), financial problems (76.5%), and revocation of driver's license (54.4%; Furr et al., 2015). These visible losses often are intertwined, with one loss creating or impacting another. Loss of a driver's license may affect the ability to get to work, and loss of a job can force a change in living arrangements, even leading to homelessness. Clients may minimize these non-death losses in terms of needing to grieve, but such losses need to be acknowledged as a source of grief.

INTERNAL LOSSES

Problematic substance use can create a direct causal pathway with an SUD leading to increased symptoms of the internalizing disorders of depression and anxiety. Using longitudinal data, Fergusson et al. (2013) found a reciprocal path in which an increase in anxiety disorder symptoms led to increased symptoms of alcohol abuse/dependence, thus creating an ongoing cycle. Knowing there is an interaction between substance use and anxiety or depression, the importance of addressing these disorders in treatment needs to be recognized. Both of these disorders respond well to a variety of treatments, with cognitive behavioral therapy demonstrating effective treatment. Brain research has also demonstrated that the logical center of the brain (prefrontal cortex) cannot be fully engaged until regions involved with emotional processing, such as the amygdala and insula, are calmed. The amygdala grows calmer in the presence of a trusted person, and through this relationship, implicit memories of past traumas can be awakened and healed (Badenoch, 2018). Because of the emotional impact of traumatic events, the counselor needs to create a safe space for grieving the pain and sorrow associated with the losses before engaging in cognitive treatment.

Internalized Stigma and Self-Esteem

Goldberg (1985), one of the early adopters of addressing grief in recovery, identified loss of self-esteem, self-respect, and self-confidence as losses associated with alcoholism. While alcohol and even some illicit drug use can be a component of positive social interactions, there is often a tipping point where excessive use is criticized and results in stigmatization of those who have an SUD. Often society has attempted to control behavior through stigmatization (Schomerus et al., 2011), but shame generated by this stigma may have the opposite effect and lead to increased substance use. Treatment programs that induce shame are not recommended and instead need to focus on interventions to reduce shame (Wiechelt, 2007). Addicted individuals experience more social rejection and negative emotions than found for other mental health disorders and encounter a greater likelihood of being discriminated against (Schomerus et al., 2011). Even health care professionals have been found to hold negative attitudes toward patients who exhibit an SUD (van Boekel et al., 2014). Perceived stigma can evolve into internalized stigma in which the individual begins to apply the stigma to self, creating feelings of worthlessness. Internalized stigma has been found to be associated with greater substance use problems (Kulesza et al., 2017), and Schomerus et al. (2010) demonstrated stigma is not an effective strategy to promote abstinence.

Cognitive Losses

One of the primary losses during times of active substance use is the loss of cognitive functioning, with 64.7% citing memory problems and 73.5% expressing concern about the loss of ability to think clearly and logically (Furr et al., 2015). Extensive research has addressed the issue of cognitive impairment in those entering treatment for addiction (Mulhauser et al., 2018; Ramey & Regier, 2018; Sampedro-Piquero et al., 2019). One general finding is someone with an SUD has altered cognitive functioning in the executive domains of functioning, including working memory, decision-making, and attention (Ramey & Regier, 2018; Sampedro-Piquero et al., 2019). In a study of 28 clients entering treatment, Mulhauser et al. (2018) found that 93% met diagnostic criteria for a mild or major neurocognitive disorder after completing acute detoxification, with 71% still impaired in at least one of five domains after completing 10 days of treatment; executive functioning appeared to remain impaired during this short-term treatment.

When cognitive processes are affected, treatment efficacy suffers because many of the psychosocial treatments rely on basic executive and memory abilities (Mulhauser et al., 2018). In a review of the literature, Sampedro-Piquero et al. (2019) found cognitive impairment is one of the most consistent factors for dropping out of treatment and has been identified as a predictor of relapse. Clients recognize memory problems and impaired thinking ability as being losses that occurred during times of using and may worry about whether they will be able to recapture these abilities. Research supports that many of these cognitive abilities can be restored with continued abstinence. While cognitive impairment associated with substance use may remain during short-term and intermediate-term abstinence, Schulte et al. (2014) found these abilities often return with sustained abstinence. This type of information may be encouraging to clients who fear never regaining cognitive abilities.

One area of challenge for many clients is the capacity to deal with emotions triggered by entering treatment. Frequently there is a lack of ability to identify or label the emotions experienced. Consequently, clients may not have words to express the pain of their losses and may have a reduced awareness of the learned emotional warning signals from the body, which can lead to risky decision-making (Verdejo-García et al., 2007). Van der Kolk (2015) stated, "the only way we can begin to change the way we feel is by becoming aware of our inner experience and learning to befriend what is going on inside ourselves" (p. 206). Ramey and Regier (2018) have identified meditation as having promise to improve awareness of internal states and the ability to label emotions. Such a process could assist clients in addressing the feelings they have often blocked through using substances. Avoidance of grieving may be related to lack of skills in recognizing the feelings associated with loss.

Losses Prior to Addiction

No one begins life wanting to become an addict. With the exception of children born to a mother in active substance use, there is a period of life when substances are not part of daily living. Throughout childhood and spanning into adulthood, there are numerous losses that occur and need to be grieved. Not everyone encounters these losses, and of those who do face a significant life loss, there may have been healthy coping mechanisms. For those who take the pathway of substance use to deal with life's challenges, many will develop problematic issues with substance use. Clinicians need to be aware of losses related to clients' initial substance use and how grieving these losses may be necessary for healthy recovery.

Adverse Childhood Experiences

There is increasing recognition of the impact of ACEs on adult behavior. While causation cannot be attributed to these experiences, there are strong indications that those who experience traumatic events are more likely to encounter negative health outcomes. Simpson and Miller (2002) conducted an extensive review of the empirical research to examine whether factors of childhood sexual and/or physical abuse could be "implicated in the genesis, maintenance, and recurrence" of substance use problems (p. 28) and believed these factors may be important in the development of substance use issues for women. Fuller-Thomson et al. (2016) found three types of ACEs (witnessing domestic violence, physical abuse, and sexual abuse) before age 16 were independently and significantly associated with alcohol dependence. Raghavan and Kingston (2006) discovered childhood sexual abuse for females was significantly correlated with younger age of first use of substances than for those who were not sexually abused. These authors recommended routine screening for post-traumatic stress disorder (PTSD) for women entering substance abuse treatment programs. In the most extensive study of ACEs in California, an increased likelihood of early adolescent drinking was associated with each category of ACEs, with those who experienced sexual abuse being three times more likely to begin alcohol use during mid-adolescence than those who did not experience sexual abuse. These researchers found that multiple early stressors and traumatic events in childhood were strong predictors of early drinking for females and males (Dube et al., 2006). Some gender differences have been detected in sexual assault, which was a common predictor for drug and alcohol abuse for young women, and physical assault and PTSD, which were common predictors for drug and alcohol abuse among young men (Danielson et al., 2009).

Homelessness

While much of the focus of early life losses has been related to childhood trauma, other losses may also be contributors to substance use. One issue identified as a loss prior to developing an SUD is homelessness. In our study, 28.4% of our participants identified homelessness as an issue prior to abusing substances (Furr et al., 2015). In the general population, about 7.4% of adults have been homeless at some time during their lives (Link et al., 1994), thus indicating homelessness prior to addictive behavior may be a factor in subsequent substance abuse. However, comprehending the relationship between homelessness and later substance use can be complex. Many adolescents who are homeless become so because of running away from situations where they have been victimized (Tyler et al., 2013). The decision to run away often is fraught with traumas that occurred in the home and can lead to other traumas, such as being coerced into the sex trade. Homelessness is particularly prevalent among the LGBT population, with as much as 48% of the population becoming homeless through either running away or being evicted (Rosario et al., 2012). These researchers found substance use for their population of homeless youth occurred simultaneously with or after their initial episode of homelessness, making substance use a consequence of homelessness.

Death of Significant Person

Other losses early in life can be contributors to substance use because of disruption to the development of healthy coping skills (Høeg et al., 2017). Death of a parent prior to age 17 was found to be associated with alcohol dependence in a sample of male twins ($n = 584$), and parental separation, particularly maternal separation, was a risk factor for alcohol dependence (Otowa et al., 2014). When examining parental loss prior to age 30, those who were bereaved scored significantly higher for substance use than non-bereaved individuals, with those who lost both parents and those whose parent died when they were between the ages of 6 and 18 being most vulnerable to substance use as adults (Høeg et al., 2017).

Unexpected death at any age can precede an SUD. Keyes et al. (2014) found an increased incidence of alcohol use disorders following the unexpected death of a loved one for all age groups but particularly for those over 45 years of age. These researchers also found that as the number of unexpected deaths increased, alcohol use disorders also increased. Youth who experience parental death, especially through suicide, were found to demonstrate significantly higher levels of alcohol or substance use than those from non-bereaved families; those who experienced a parent's death by suicide showed higher rates 21 months after the death (Brent et al., 2009). It is important to note that unexpected and traumatic deaths may be associated with many other life disruptions that may include the impact on one's support system, loss of financial resources, or change in living arrangements. This combination of losses may create a sense of hopelessness about how to face the future without this significant person and the emotional and physical resources provided by this person.

Loss of Children

When we think of loss of a child, our first thought is often the death of a child and the intense grief that accompanies such a loss. Often parents cannot make sense of this type of loss (Bogensperger & Lueger-Schuster, 2014). When an infant dies, parents may engage in self-blame, which can be a common aspect of grief (Garstang et al., 2016). Emergence of a substance abuse problem among men was just one of many negative changes that occurred in the relationship of couples who experienced an infant's or child's death, with men more likely to engage in increased alcohol consumption than women (Jones et al., 2019). Harper et al. (2014) found substance use was significantly associated with depression following the loss of a child.

However, other circumstances can lead to a separation from children through custody issues or circumstances that lead to a child being placed in foster care. While substance use can be a factor in a child being taken from the home, it can also be a consequence of having a child removed from the home. Wall-Wieler et al. (2017) found the percentage of SUDs in mothers almost doubled in the two years after a child was taken into care, creating a condition that may prevent reunification with children. Being exposed to intimate partner violence (IPV) can lead to involvement with child protective services because this violence is considered a form of child mistreatment. Nixon et al. (2013) found prescription drugs and alcohol were used by some mothers to deal with the pain of losing their children through involvement with child protective services. These mothers expressed a strong experience of grief over losing their children that included profound sadness and depression.

End of Relationship

Divorce, separation, and the end of an intimate relationship can be devastating to the individuals who are involved as well as to children and family members. All one needs to do is to check out the number of country songs about alcohol and heartbreak to see the connection substance use has to losing a significant person in one's life. A longitudinal study found those participants with an alcohol abuse/dependence issue were 1.66 times more likely to have a relationship end, even when confounding variables were controlled, with no gender differences found (Boden et al., 2013).

Parental divorce has the largest impact of any family stressor on subsequent increases in drinking behavior among adolescents (Fletcher & Sindelar, 2012). Among young adults, ending a romantic relationship has been associated with increases in heavy drinking and marijuana use. However, marriage has often been viewed as a protective factor in terms of alcohol use (Scott et al., 2010). Using data from a large international population, these authors found that marriage was a protective factor in alcohol use for both men and women, with women experiencing a significantly strong protective pattern.

Unemployment

Job loss can be a trigger for substance use, whether the unemployment was due to a major economic downturn or personal factors. Many of the studies of the past 10 years have related to the economic crisis that began in 2008, but any type of unemployment can create similar distress. Some will cope through using substances, and our culture often encourages drinking as a means of dealing with loss. For example, a bar in a large city reportedly gave a free drink for each job rejection letter brought in and posted on their wall. We often do not think of job loss as a loss to be grieved, yet this type of loss carries an emotional burden.

In a review of research on the impact of the 2008 economic recession in the United States, there were higher rates of heavy alcohol and illicit drug use as well as alcohol use disorders and illicit drug disorders in those who were unemployed (Compton et al., 2014). de Goeij et al. (2015) found comparable results where psychological distress resulting from unemployment was related to increased drinking problems in some populations, but also tighter budgets reduced money spent on alcohol in other populations. Drinking as a means to relieve distress was observed mainly in men. These results can only provide the association of substance use with unemployment, so more research is needed in terms of the how job loss may precede substance use; however, substance misuse is an important issue to examine among the unemployed. The loss of one's job may be a catalyst to using alcohol or drugs as a coping mechanism that can later become a problem in itself.

These are just a few of the losses experienced in life prior to substance abuse. Using substances to cope with earlier life experiences may create unhealthy coping patterns and contribute to addiction becoming its own problem. The losses only mount during the time of active addiction. By the time a person enters treatment, unacknowledged or unaddressed grief often lurks in the background of learning to manage the biological aspects of the addiction. However, the recovery process can be facilitated by a compassionate approach that allows for exploration of losses and provides space for grieving. This process needs to be mindful of the individual's internal coping mechanisms to handle the powerful emotions that accompany loss and trauma. The grief process during addiction treatment will be a constant interplay of the emerging of losses and the building of strengths to face and mourn those losses.

Suggestions for Counselors

- Listen for losses as clients tell their stories. Most people first think of death as the primary loss to be grieved. Even though loss of a marriage, relationships, home, or finances may be labeled as losses, society has not recognized a need to grieve these losses and often dismisses them as "things that just happen." Acknowledging these losses gives credence to what clients have experienced.
- Pay attention to disenfranchised losses. These are the losses dismissed by others as lacking value or meaning. For example, family and friends may not comprehend that giving up one's substance creates a sense of loss or that separating from friends who use creates a vacuum in relationships. Bring up these losses in group sessions so there can be discussion about what it means to face the losses of people, places, and things as clients enter treatment. Giving up a way of life, no matter how dysfunctional, can create loss.
- Be careful not to move into deeper losses too quickly. Many clients have significant traumas and may not yet have the necessary coping skills. While it is important to understand the impact these losses have had on the substance use, the client may not be ready to experience the pain of the loss. Teaching skills to contain emotions when feelings become overwhelming and being careful not to probe more deeply until the client has the strength to encounter the loss are essential to maintaining progress.
- Because internalized stigma is related to poorer treatment outcomes (Kulesza et al., 2017), consider approaches to help clients challenge the negative beliefs they have developed about themselves. Approaching this from the grief and loss perspective may help clients recognize how they have let the views of others influence how they view themselves. Support can be crucial to counteract the impact of stigma.

References

Airagnes, G., Lemogne, C., Meneton, P., Plessz, M., Goldberg, M., Hoertel, N., . . . Zins, M. (2019). Alcohol, tobacco and cannabis use are associated with job loss at follow-up: Findings from the CONSTANCES cohort. *PLoS One, 14*(9), e0222361. https://doi.org/10.1371/journal.pone.0222361

Amato, P., & Previti, D. (2003). People's reasons for divorcing: Gender, social class, the life course, and adjustment. *Journal of Family Issues, 24*(5), 602–626. https://doi.org/10.1177/0192513X03024005002

Anand, D., Chen, Y., Lindquist, K., & Daughters, S. (2017). Emotion differentiation predicts likelihood of initial lapse following substance use treatment. *Drug and Alcohol Dependence, 180*, 439–444. https://doi.org/10.1016/j.drugalcdep.2017.09.007

Ashford, R., Brown, A., & Curtis, B. (2018). Substance use, recovery, and linguistics: The impact of word choice on explicit and implicit bias. *Drug and Alcohol Dependence, 189*. http://search.proquest.com/docview/2100878951/

Badenoch, B. (2018). *The heart of trauma: Healing the embodied brain in the context of relationships*. W. W. Norton & Company.

Beechem, M., Prewitt, J., & Scholar, J. (1996). Loss-grief addiction model. *Journal of Drug Education, 26*(2), 183–198. https://doi.org/10.2190/0GXH-9Q2Y-9NUG-UQ24

Blume, A., & Marlatt, G. (2000). Recent important substance-related losses predict readiness to change scores among people with co-occurring psychiatric disorders. *Addictive Behaviors, 25*(3), 461–464. https://doi.org/10.1016/S0306-4603(98)00133-6

Boden, J., Fergusson, D., & Horwood, L. (2013). Alcohol misuse and relationship breakdown: Findings from a longitudinal birth cohort. *Drug and Alcohol Dependence, 133*(1), 115–120. https://doi.org/10.1016/j.drugalcdep.2013.05.023

Bogensperger, J., & Lueger-Schuster, B. (2014). Losing a child: Finding meaning in bereavement. *European Journal of Psychotraumatology, 5*(1), Article 22910. https://doi.org/10.3402/ejpt.v5.22910

Bouchery, E., Harwood, H., Sacks, J., Simon, C., & Brewer, R. (2011). Economic costs of excessive alcohol consumption in the U.S., 2006. *American Journal of Preventive Medicine, 41*(5), 516–524. https://doi.org/10.1016/j.amepre.2011.06.045

Brandon, T., Vidrine, J., & Litvin, E. (2007). Relapse and relapse prevention. *Annual Review of Clinical Psychology, 3*(1), 257–284. https://doi.org/10.1146/annurev.clinpsy.3.022806.091455

Brent, D., Melhem, N., Donohoe, M., & Walker, M. (2009). The incidence and course of depression in bereaved youth 21 months after the loss of a parent to suicide, accident, or sudden natural death. *American Journal of Psychiatry, 166*(7), 786–794. https://doi.org/10.1176/appi.ajp.2009.08081244

Chambers, R., & Wallingford, S. (2017). On mourning and recovery: Integrating stages of grief and change toward a neuroscience-based model of attachment adaptation in addiction treatment. *Psychodynamic Psychiatry, 45*(4), 451–473. https://doi.org/10.1521/pdps.2017.45.4.451

Compton, W., Gfroerer, J., Conway, K., & Finger, M. (2014). Unemployment and substance outcomes in the United States 2002–2010. *Drug and Alcohol Dependence, 142*, 350–353. https://doi.org/10.1016/j.drugalcdep.2014.06.012

Danielson, C., Amstadter, A., Dangelmaier, R., Resnick, H., Saunders, B., & Kilpatrick, D. (2009). Trauma-related risk factors for substance abuse among male versus female young adults. *Addictive Behaviors, 34*(4), 395–399. https://doi.org/10.1016/j.addbeh.2008.11.009

de Goeij, M. C., Suhrcke, M., Toffolutti, V., van de Mheen, D., Schoenmakers, T. M., & Kunst, A. E. (2013). How economic crises affect alcohol consumption and alcohol-related health problems: A realist systematic review. *Social Science & Medicine, 131*, 131–146. https://doi.org/10.1016/j.socscimed.2015.02.025

Dube, S., Miller, J., Brown, D., Giles, W., Felitti, V., Dong, M., & Anda, R. (2006). Adverse childhood experiences and the association with every using alcohol and initiating alcohol use during adolescence. *Journal of Adolescent Health, 38*(4), 444. e1–444.e10. https://doi.org/10.1016/j.jadohealth.2005.06.006

Fergusson, D., Boden, J., & Horwood, L. (2013). Alcohol misuse and psychosocial outcomes in young adulthood: Results from a longitudinal birth cohort studied to age 30. *Drug and Alcohol Dependence, 133*(2), 513–519. https://doi.org/10.1016/j. drugalcdep.2013.07.015

Fletcher, J. M., & Sindelar, J. L. (2012). The effects of family stressors on substance use initiation in adolescence. *Review of Economics of the Household, 10*(1), 99–114. https://doi.org/10.1007/s11150-010-9116-z

Fuller-Thomson, E., Roane, J., & Brennenstuhl, S. (2016). Three types of adverse childhood experiences, and alcohol and drug dependence among adults: An investigation using population-based data. *Substance Use & Misuse, 51*(11), 1451–1461. https:// doi.org/10.1080/10826084.2016.1181089

Furr, S., Johnson, W., & Goodall, C. (2015). Grief and recovery: The prevalence of grief and loss in substance abuse treatment. *Journal of Addictions & Offender Counseling, 36*(1), 43–56. https://doi.org/10.1002/j.2161-1874.2015.00034.x

Garstang, J., Griffiths, F., & Sidebotham, P. (2016). Parental understanding and self-blame following sudden infant death: A mixed-methods study of bereaved parents' and professionals' experiences. *BMJ Open, 6*(5), e011323. https://doi.org/10.1136/ bmjopen-2016-011323

Goldberg, M. (1985). Loss and grief: Major dynamics in the treatment of alcoholism. *Alcoholism Treatment Quarterly, 2*(1), 37–46. https://doi.org/10.1300/ J020V02N01_04

Graham, H., Copello, A., Griffith, E., Clarke, L., Walsh, K., Baker, A., & Birchwood, M. (2019). Mental health hospital admissions: A teachable moment and window of opportunity to promote change in drug and alcohol misuse. *International Journal of Mental Health and Addiction, 17*(1), 22–40. https://doi.org/10.1007/ s11469-017-9861-9

Graham, K., Cheng, J., Bernards, S., Wells, S., Rehm, J., & Kurdyak, P. (2017). How much do mental health and substance use/addiction affect use of general medical services? Extent of use, reason for use, and associated costs. *Canadian Journal of Psychiatry, 62*(1), 48–56. https://doi.org/10.1177/0706743716664884

Grant, B., Stinson, F., & Harford, T. (2001). Age of onset of alcohol use and DSM-IV alcohol abuse and dependence: A 12-year follow-up. *Journal of Substance Abuse, 13*, 493–504.

Harper, M., O'Connor, R., & O'Carroll, R. (2014). Factors associated with grief and depression following the loss of a child: A multivariate analysis. *Psychology, Health & Medicine, 19*(3), 247–252. https://doi.org/10.1080/13548506.2013. 811274

Høeg, B., Appel, C., Von Heymann-Horan, A., Frederiksen, K., Johansen, C., Bøge, P., . . . Bidstrup, P. (2017). Maladaptive coping in adults who have experienced early parental loss and grief counseling. *Journal of Health Psychology, 22*(14), 1851–1861. https://doi.org/10.1177/1359105316638550

Jones, K., Robb, M., Murphy, S., & Davies, A. (2019). New understandings of fathers' experiences of grief and loss following stillbirth and neonatal death: A scoping review. *Midwifery, 79*, 102531. https://doi.org/10.1016/j.midw.2019.102531

Keyes, K., Pratt, C., Galea, S., McLaughlin, K., Koenen, K., & Shear, M. (2014). The burden of loss: Unexpected death of a loved one and psychiatric disorders across the life course in a national study (Report) (Author abstract). *American Journal of Psychiatry*, *171*(8).

Kinderman, P. (2005). A psychological model of mental disorder. *Harvard Review of Psychiatry*, *13*(4), 206–217. https://doi.org/10.1080/10673220500243349

Kulesza, M., Watkins, K., Ober, A., Osilla, K., & Ewing, B. (2017). Internalized stigma as an independent risk factor for substance use problems among primary care patients: Rationale and preliminary support. *Drug and Alcohol Dependence*, *180*, 52–55. https://doi.org/10.1016/j.drugalcdep.2017.08.002

Link, B., Susser, E., Stueve, A., Phelan, J., Moore, R., & Struening, E. (1994). Lifetime and five-year prevalence of homelessness in the United States. *American Journal of Public Health*, *84*(12), 1907–19012. https://doi.org/10.2105/AJPH.84.12.1907

Macdonald, S., Pakula, B., Martin, G., Wells, S., Borges, G., Roth, E., . . . Callaghan, R. (2014). Health profiles of clients in substance abuse treatment: A comparison of clients dependent on alcohol or cocaine with those concurrently dependent. *Substance Use & Misuse*, *49*(14), 1899–1907. https://doi.org/10.3109/10826084.2014.935791

Mulhauser, K., Weinstock, J., Ruppert, P., & Benware, J. (2018). Changes in neuropsychological status during the initial phase of abstinence in alcohol use disorder: Neurocognitive impairment and implications for clinical care. *Substance Use & Misuse*, *53*(6), 881–890. https://doi.org/10.1080/10826084.2017.1408328

Nixon, K., Radtke, H., & Tutty, L. (2013). "Every day it takes a piece of you away": Experiences of grief and loss among abused mothers involved with child protective services. *Journal of Public Child Welfare*, *7*(2), 172–193. https://doi.org/10.1080/15548732.2012.715268

Otowa, T., York, T., Gardner, C., Kendler, K., & Hettema, J. (2014). The impact of childhood parental loss on risk for mood, anxiety and substance use disorders in a population-based sample of male twins. *Psychiatry Research*, *220*(1–2), 404–409. https://doi.org/10.1016/j.psychres.2014.07.053

Raghavan, C., & Kingston, S. (2006). Child sexual abuse and posttraumatic stress disorder: The role of age at first use of substances and lifetime traumatic events. *Journal of Traumatic Stress*, *19*(2), 269–278. https://doi.org/10.1002/jts.20117

Ramey, T., & Regier, P. (2018). Cognitive impairment in substance use disorders. *CNS Spectrums*, *24*(1), 1–12. https://doi.org/10.1017/S1092852918001426

Room, R. (2005). Stigma, social inequality and alcohol and drug use. *Drug and Alcohol Review*, *24*(2), 143–155. https://doi.org/10.1080/09595230500102434

Rosario, M., Schrimshaw, E., & Hunter, J. (2012). Homelessness among lesbian, gay, and bisexual youth: Implications for subsequent internalizing and externalizing symptoms. *Journal of Youth and Adolescence*, *41*(5), 544–560. https://doi.org/10.1007/s10964-011-9681-3

Sampedro-Piquero, P., Ladrón de Guevara-Miranda, D., Pavón, F., Serrano, A., Suárez, J., Rodríguez de Fonseca, F., . . . Castilla-Ortega, E. (2019). Neuroplastic and cognitive impairment in substance use disorders: A therapeutic potential of cognitive stimulation. *Neuroscience and Biobehavioral Reviews*, *106*, 23–48. https://doi.org/10.1016/j.neubiorev.2018.11.015

Schomerus, G., Corrigan, P., Klauer, T., Kuwert, P., Freyberger, H., & Lucht, M. (2010). Self-stigma in alcohol dependence: Consequences for drinking-refusal self-efficacy. *Drug and Alcohol Dependence*, *114*(1), 12–17. https://doi.org/10.1016/j.drugalcdep.2010.08.013

Schomerus, G., Lucht, M., Holzinger, A., Matschinger, H., Carta, M., & Angermeyer, M. (2011). The stigma of alcohol dependence compared with other mental disorders: A review of population studies. *Alcohol and Alcoholism (Oxford, Oxfordshire)*, *46*(2), 105–112. https://doi.org/10.1093/alcalc/agq089

Schulte, M., Cousijn, J., Den Uyl, T., Goudriaan, A., van Den Brink, W., Veltman, D., . . . Wiers, R. (2014). Recovery of neurocognitive functions following sustained abstinence after substance dependence and implications for treatment. *Clinical Psychology Review*, *34*(7), 531–550. https://doi.org/10.1016/j.cpr.2014.08.002

Scott, K. M., Wells, J. E., Angermeyer, M., Brugha, T. S., Bromet, E., Demyttenaere, K., . . . Kessler, R. C. (2010). Gender and the relationship between marital status and first onset of mood, anxiety and substance use disorders. *Psychological Medicine*, *40*(9), 1495–505. https://doi.org/10.1017/S0033291709991942

Scott, S., Rhoades, G., Stanley, S., Allen, E., & Markman, H. (2013). Reasons for divorce and recollections of premarital intervention: Implications for improving relationship education. *Couple & Family Psychology*, *2*(2), 131–145. https://doi.org/10.1037/a0032025

Simpson, T., & Miller, W. (2002). Concomitance between childhood sexual and physical abuse and substance use problems: A review. *Clinical Psychology Review*, *22*(1), 27–77. https://doi.org/10.1016/S0272-7358(00)00088-X

Skewes, M. C., & Gonzalez, V. M. (2013). The biopsychosocial model of addiction. In P. M. Miller (Ed.), *Principles of addiction* (pp. 61–70). Academic Press.

Skolnick, V. (1979). The addictions as pathological mourning: An attempt at restitution of early losses. *American Journal of Psychotherapy*, *33*(2), 281–290. https://doi.org/10.1176/appi.psychotherapy.1979.33.2.281

Tyler, K., Gervais, S., & Davidson, M. (2013). The relationship between victimization and substance use among homeless and runaway female adolescents. *Journal of Interpersonal Violence*, *28*(3), 474–493. https://doi.org/10.1177/0886260512455517

van Boekel, L., Brouwers, E., van Weeghel, J., & Garretsen, H. (2014). Healthcare professionals' regard towards working with patients with substance use disorders: Comparison of primary care, general psychiatry and specialist addiction services. *Drug and Alcohol Dependence*, *134*(1), 92–98. https://doi.org/10.1016/j.drugalcdep.2013.09.012

Van der Kolk, B. (2015). *The body keeps the score: Brain, mind, and body in the healing of trauma*. Penguin Books.

Verdejo-García, A., Rivas-Pérez, C., Vilar-López, R., & Pérez-García, M. (2007). Strategic self-regulation, decision-making and emotion processing in poly-substance abusers in their first year of abstinence. *Drug and Alcohol Dependence*, *86*(2–3), 139–146. https://doi.org/10.1016/j.drugalcdep.2006.05.024

Viorst, J. (1987). *Necessary losses*. Ballantine Books.

Waldron, M., Heath, A., Lynskey, M., Bucholz, K., Madden, P., & Martin, N. (2011). Alcoholic marriage: Later start, sooner end. *Alcoholism, Clinical and Experimental Research*, *35*(4), 632–642. https://doi.org/10.1111/j.1530-0277.2010.01381.x

Wall-Wieler, E., Roos, L., Bolton, J., Brownell, M., Nickel, N., & Chateau, D. (2017). Maternal health and social outcomes after having a child taken into care: Population-based longitudinal cohort study using linkable administrative data. *Journal of Epidemiology and Community Health*, *71*(12), 1145–1151. https://doi.org/10.1136/jech-2017-209542

Wiechelt, S. (2007). The specter of shame in substance misuse. *Substance Use and Misuse, 42*, 399–409. https://doi.org/10.1080/10826080601142196

Zemore, S., Mulia, N., Williams, E. D., & Gilbert, Pl. (2017). Job loss and alcohol dependence among Blacks and Whites in a national, longitudinal survey. *Journal of Ethnicity in Substance Abuse, 16*(3), 314–327. https://doi.org/10.1080/15332640.2016.1209144

2 A Primer on Grief Theories and Their Application to Substance Use Recovery

Susan R. Furr

Grief theories take many forms, whether the focus is on stages, phases, tasks, or models of oscillation. There are even those who advocate moving away from theories to focus on the unique needs of each individual (Corr, 2019; Humphrey, 2009). When theories are applied in a rigid way that tries to make the client fit the theory, there may be a good reason to step away from the theories. A good theory just provides a tool for making sense of the client's experience and should not be used as a weapon to force the client in a particular direction. The theory opens up possibilities for explaining the client's journey and potential directions for moving forward with the client's issues. A theory should not become a barrier between the counselor and the client (Corr, 2019) but should create a path that gives insight to client experiences. When a theory does not provide helpful insight or even becomes a hindrance to client progress, we need to move beyond what the theory has to offer and listen to what our clients have to say. "All models are useful insofar as the model assists the therapist or offers insight to the client" (Doka & Martin, 2010, p. 164). After examining a number of theories related to grief and loss, some commonalities of grief theories emerge. First, grief theories acknowledge the disruption that loss creates for those experiencing loss. Loss can be hard to comprehend and may create a sense of disbelief. The human psyche often cannot comprehend that this loss has actually occurred and protects itself by denying the full impact of the loss. If we had to fully embrace the meaning of a loss when it is first faced, the emotional impact could be too much to bear. A second aspect of grieving is working through all of the emotions triggered by the loss. As the loss becomes more real and the denial dissipates, the range of emotions that emerges can be quite surprising to the grieving individual. Sadness is expected, but other emotions such as anger and fear can catch the person by surprise. There can be an extended period where emotions dominate daily life and come unexpectedly in ways that disrupt the ability to complete everyday tasks. As one begins facing the loss and accepting these new feelings, most theories move to a space of learning to live with the fact that life has changed in some sort of permanent way. New adjustments have to be made and perhaps new skills developed. Finally, the "new normal" emerges, where the loss becomes part of how one views everyday life. We never get over the loss but learn to

DOI: 10.4324/9781003106906-2

integrate it in how we see the world. These components may not necessarily occur in some neat, linear fashion but can occur simultaneously or fluctuate back and forth. Because of similarities found by different theorists, the theoretical models have acquired validity. All of the models were formulated from observing those who experienced losses and were grieving those losses. These theories draw from the human experience and merely organize these observations into models that help explain the possible experiences those grieving may share. For the clinician, finding a "road map" that assists the client in normalizing the loss experience is one of the values of employing a theoretical perspective. However, we need to be cautious with clients trying to adhere to what they believe are the steps they should follow given the human tendency to seek patterns to organize life experiences in a way that makes change seem predictable and thus puts them in control (Holland & Neimeyer, 2010).

However, one of the difficulties of applying many of the theories is they were built around the concept of the loss being associated with the death. Although there has been some acknowledgment that other losses result in feelings of grief, the language of the theories is primarily death oriented. The purpose of this chapter is to examine the major grief theories in terms of the grief encountered through all of the phases of substance use and recovery. Learning about the different theories will provide a number of perspectives to use with clients in recovery. Applying grief theories to recovery will take the client to a deeper level of understanding to address hidden feelings that hold them back from maintaining their recovery. Grief that is not addressed has a way of reemerging and feeding relapse.

Disenfranchised Grief

An important aspect of grief that needs to be noted is *disenfranchised grief*, or those losses that are not acknowledged by others or society in general because of social stigma (Mortell, 2015). Doka (2002) identified *loss not acknowledged* as one aspect of disenfranchised grief. It is particularly important for addiction counselors to keep this concept in mind because of how others view those who abuse substances. Losses accrued while abusing substances may be viewed as a just reward for those who are addicted. The person who experiences addiction may feel shame and even engage in self-disenfranchisement, believing they deserve the losses and have no right to grieve. Thus, they may silence themselves and not discuss their losses. From another perspective, the idea of needing to grieve the loss of the addictive substance may seem foreign to clients, yet leaving the substance behind can be a powerful source of grief. Nevertheless, receiving empathy for loss is part of making meaning of one's losses. Although Mortell (2015) did not consider addiction in her discussion of disenfranchised grief, her suggestions about how to support clients can easily be applied. She highlighted the importance of providing empathy through actively listening to the loss experience. Because these types of losses do not have any type of rituals, counselors can help the client to create meaningful rituals for saying good-bye to the substance and other attachments related to using. Finally, she suggested the use of support groups to provide validation for the meaning of the loss, an option readily available for most clients in treatment for substance use.

In this chapter, several grief theories are adapted to address losses related to substance use. Although Kübler-Ross (1969) is perhaps the most well known of the grief theorists, she only studied those who were dying. For this reason, her work is not included in this section.

Therese Rando: The Six Rs

Rather than conceive of the grief process as stages, Rando (1993) created the concept of reactions to examine how individuals experience grieving, with the concept that individuals move back and forth among the reactions. She established three phases with different processes or reactions accompanying each phase. Phase 1 is the *Avoidance Phase*, which is characterized first by shock when confronted by a loss and is followed by denial, which allows the reality of the loss to be absorbed a little at a time. Avoidance may show up in two major ways for those in recovery. For people who have abused substances, there may be many instances throughout their lives where they have avoided dealing with losses, so they have never grieved them. As described in Chapter 1, losses occur throughout life for those who are addicted, with substance use related to avoiding the pain of the losses. The second type of avoidance occurs when facing the fact that one is addicted. No matter how many people have confronted them, there is a good chance they have experienced shock and denial of their substance use problem. Those who are more outgoing may have verbal outbursts when confronted, while the more introverted may withdraw. Coming to the reality that one's substance use has created such losses can be hard to admit. Even more difficult may be facing the losses that accompany giving up the substance. The process that Rando associates with this phase is *recognizing the loss*. Initially the recognition of loss may be on a level of intellectualized acceptance but will need to move to a recognition of the emotional impact of the loss. Part of this initial understanding will be to examine the lasting impact of the loss of one's substance, but there will also be a need to recognize the deeper significance of the long-term changes on one's life.

Phase 2 is the *Confrontation Phase*, where grief is felt most intensely and extremes of emotions are experienced. While some have the ability to express emotions readily, others may not be able to recognize what they are feeling or may not know appropriate ways to express emotions and could benefit from psychoeducation in this area. Others have been conditioned to avoid expressing feelings and need to examine and revise internalized prohibitions around emotional expression. During this phase, individuals may encounter anxiety or panic over the unknown and may fear they will not be able to recover from their substance abuse. They may be frightened they cannot make it alone so can benefit from being in a supportive community. Two emotions that might create problems because of societal attitudes are anger and guilt. Clinicians need to reassure them these emotions are to be expected and can be worked through. Anger is a natural consequence of being deprived of something desired, and there is a risk of displacing anger onto other people. Those grieving their loss of substance use may become bitter, easily hurt, and have exaggerated sensitivity to real or imagined slights. They may even feel envy for those not going through the same losses associated with giving up the substance. Clinicians may be the recipient of some of the anger and need to understand the source of the anger while also setting appropriate and clear boundaries. In child-centered play therapy, there are only three rules in the play room: you cannot hurt self, you cannot hurt others, and you cannot destroy property. These rules may apply well for clients in the confrontation phase.

Three processes occur in the confrontation phase. First is *reacting to the separation*, which for those in recovery means reacting emotionally to all the losses that occur upon entering treatment and separating from the substance as well as the people, places, and things associated with using. Recognizing life will not be the same without these relationships may lead to strong feelings of sadness and even anger over giving up this part of life. Important in this process is learning to identify feelings and ways to express them appropriately. Secondary losses may emerge as past actions are recalled and the impact is examined. For example, loss of job due to drinking may lead to loss of financial security or loss of home. A second aspect of this phase is *recollecting and reexperiencing the losses*. As clients review memories of their primary loss of substance use, they may recall happy times that occurred while using that will not occur again as part of their commitment to abstinence. Before substance use became problematic, pleasant experiences in life may have been associated with having a drink or getting high. Knowing these experiences will not occur the same way again may lead to sadness that needs to be acknowledged and processed. A final aspect of this phase is *relinquishing old attachments*, which refers to putting losses behind them by realizing and accepting their world has truly changed. Clients will need to accept there is no turning back to their former life without risking a return to addiction.

Phase 3 in Rando's model is the *Reestablishment Phase*, characterized by a decline in the feelings of grief. This phase is the beginning of the clients' social and emotional reentry into the everyday world, where they are learning to live with their loss of substance use. For this phase to be successful, clients need to reinvest emotional energy into new persons, things, and ideas. Building a network with those in recovery through group meetings, establishing friendships with nonusers, and forming new ideas about the type of life one wants to live are part of this process. However, this process is not all-or-nothing, so there may be movement in and out of this phase. For this reason, some type of continuous aftercare program is needed to support the changes the person has made. Clinicians also need to be sensitive to any guilt clients may experience for making progress while other friends may not be so fortunate. There are two processes in this phase, with the first being *readjusting to move into a new world.* Leaving treatment to return to daily life is a crucial move that if not handled well can lead to relapse. Remembering one's old world and the reasons for not going back can be an essential component of maintaining change. Continued support may be needed to learn skills to adapt to this new world. As the person in recovery reenters a family system, assistance with communication skills for the family may be helpful. Family and friends need to understand the challenges of recovery and ways they can be supportive while also holding the person accountable for recovery efforts. The final aspect of this model is *reinvesting emotional energy* in one's new life. Forming new relationships and commitments is part of this process. Those in recovery need to accept the changes that have occurred through losing the substance and move past them. Some of this reinvestment may include involvement in the recovery community, which will understand that losing one's substance is a loss that will need to be grieved.

J. William Worden: Tasks of Mourning

As a way of departing from the concept of stages or phases, which implies that grieving individuals move through a specific order of steps, Worden (1982) introduced the concept of *tasks of mourning*. Since his original work, he has evolved his model and redefined the description of the tasks. Even though his model was based on grieving a death, we have found the wording of his tasks in the third edition of his book (Worden, 2002) most related to the grieving that occurs for those in recovery for substance use. These tasks are (a) to accept the reality of the loss, (b) to work through the pain of grief, (c) to adjust to an environment in which the deceased is missing, and (d) to emotionally relocate the deceased and move on with life. He promoted the concept that the grieving person needed to complete the four tasks for mourning to be accomplished. The term *mourning* is used to define the process one goes through to adapt to the loss, while *grief* refers to the personal experience of the loss.

Worden (2018) has favored the concept of tasks because the grieving person can be actively engaged in the mourning process rather than being just a passive observer. Stage theories imply that individuals go through the stages passively, hoping they feel differently at some type of ending of their grief. By engaging in action, individuals have hope they can do something to get through the loss. While taking action may seem overwhelming initially to someone devastated with pain of grief, action can provide some sense of control and reduce the sense of helplessness experienced by those grieving. Worden emphasized that the tasks do not have to be addressed in a particular order, although there is some suggestion the first task of accepting the reality of the loss has to occur to some degree in order to work on the other tasks. Tasks can be worked on simultaneously and be revisited to work through again over time. Being able to identify tasks that need to be tackled can help provide direction for facing one's grief in a way that moves beyond emotional expression and gives hope to the mourner. Rather than the idea of getting over grief, the focus is on adapting to grief in a way that allows for living a full life in the present while honoring the loss of the past, which he termed as grief work.

Below is our adaptation of Worden's Four Tasks of Mourning to the recovery process. This framework is helpful for those who have not considered giving up their addiction as a loss to be grieved. Clients need to acknowledge and process that the use of one's drug of choice has had a defining role in one's life and to leave this behind creates a hole that may be filled with sorrow. As clients move through the treatment program, other life losses as described in Chapter 1 will begin to emerge. It is almost as if the time of active addiction can be defined as *living a loss* in which all that one has valued and has been is gone. The journey to recovery means redefining and rebuilding who one is. Clients may go through a cycle where the first layer of losses are those incurred by entering treatment, followed by recognizing and reconciling with the losses that happened while in active addiction. Throughout the process, pre-addiction losses will emerge that may be the epicenter of the addiction. The Tasks of Mourning may recycle through each of these levels.

Task I: To Accept the Reality of the Loss

Coming to grips with a loss takes time, and denial is a natural part of the loss response. For the person who abuses substances, there often is much avoidance behavior and denial before entering treatment. Anyone who works in the field knows how frequently people state that they do not have a substance use problem and can quit at any time. Eventually, that level of denial cannot be sustained in light of all of evidence of their continual failures to manage everyday life. Once entering treatment, a new level of loss is faced in having to give up the substance. Not only does the substance represent a lifestyle, but it is also a means of coping with life, maintaining social relationships, and a way of defining self. This is the first reality that has to be confronted. While clients may be aware of this loss on an intellectual level, it may take time for them to reach this awareness on an emotional level. Complicating this process is the physiological aspects of withdrawing from drugs or alcohol. Even after going through a detoxification process before entering treatment, the first 10 days of treatment will still be plagued by anxiety, low mood, and disturbed sleep. Dealing with these physical symptoms takes precedence in treatment before emotional work can begin. Many entering treatment believe they can go back to controlled use of their substance so may not be accepting the reality of their loss. Although some clinicians advocate for controlled use as a treatment outcome, the seriousness of those with severe physical dependency may require abstinence (Musalek, 2013), thus creating a loss to be grieved.

One part of moving through this task is addressing the denial of the facts of the loss. In order to grieve a loss, the first step is to accept the fact that the loss occurred. Frequently those dealing with addiction have blocked their memories of destructive behaviors or have minimized the impact of those behaviors on others as well as themselves. It is not unusual for people to engage in "selective forgetting" and not recall the negative aspects of using. This is an area where group treatment is effective. Clients who are further along in their treatment can easily spot the denial and confront newcomers on the games they are playing. Once clients recognize the facts of what has happened in their lives, they can begin to get to the meaning of their use of substances and the significance of giving up use. Another way to avoid dealing with the loss is to deny the meaning of the loss, which can be the more difficult aspect of denial to confront. This type of denial creates the illusion that the loss was not very significant. Clients may report that the loss of a drinking companion was not important, although this individual may have been a constant presence for years. Not being able to go to a favorite bar might just be dismissed as not a big deal, even though this was primary source of social connection. Both the facts of the loss and the meaning of the loss need to be recognized for clients to address Task I.

Questions for the Clinician to Consider

- What losses will a person entering treatment for substance use encounter?
- Once a person stops using, what losses might be discovered?
- How does accepting the loss of the substance lead to recognizing other losses?

Task II: To Work Through the Pain of Grief

Not only does grief create emotional pain, there also is physical and behavioral pain. People dealing with significant losses often suffer from physical symptoms including fatigue, aches and pains, tightness in chest and shortness of breath, headaches, forgetfulness, inability to focus, and appetite issues. Behavioral issues may manifest in the form of aberrant behavior, such as impulsive and aggressive behaviors. Society may not give permission to experience grief related to substance abuse, so clients are not permitted to express these intense emotions, and emotions may be redirected in ways that are harmful to the individual and others. However, losses related to entering treatment need to be acknowledged, and the client needs to work through the pain. Avoiding or suppressing the pain prolongs the period of mourning. While most grief is easier to work through at the time of the loss, the clinician needs to be aware of how much exploration of painful emotions the client can tolerate while also working on abstinence. Perhaps the most pressing loss that often is forbidden to discuss outside of treatment is the loss of the substance and the accompanying people and places. This type of discussion can validate client feelings that people outside of treatment would deny. Keep in mind clients entering treatment may lack the coping skills needed to manage powerful emotions so psychoeducation may be necessary such as how to identify and cope with these unexpected feelings of loss. As clients progress through treatment, they will be confronting both the destructive behaviors and actions they committed while using and losses they may have experienced early in life. Putting these events in the context of loss may provide the permission they need to process these feelings and learn that they can face feelings, knowing that in time, the intensity will lessen. This is not a time for clients to feel sorry for themselves or use the role of victim as an excuse for past behaviors. It is a time where empathy and compassion from the clinician for the pain the client is experiencing can lead to the client regaining a sense of self-worth, which then can support staying in treatment.

Questions for the Clinician to Consider

- How has the person coped with pain in the past?
- What is the client's ability to tolerate emotional pain?
- What coping skills have they utilized?
- How healthy are these coping skills?
- What coping skills need to be developed?

Task III: To Adjust to an Environment Without Substance Use

Sometimes it is hard to know the meaning of something until it is no longer present. Like the lyrics of the old song, "you don't know what you've got (until you lose it)," life without substance use will reveal unanticipated losses. For the person who has abused substances, the role of the substance may not be obvious until it can no longer be a part of daily life. On one level, using a substance might have centered on socializing and friendships. Having a common place to go, around people who share a mutual lifestyle, makes social life easy, particularly for those who may have some anxiety in social situations. Individuals also may just like the mood and feelings created by the substance and feel at ease with others when using. For others, substance use might have evolved into a way of coping with life stressors and mental health issues. Some conditions such as depression, anxiety, and post-traumatic stress disorder (PTSD) create a higher risk of developing an addiction, leading individuals to use substances to cope with difficult situations. Learning to manage mental health issues such as anxiety and depression without the crutch of the substance will be a new challenge to learning to live substance free. Unlike dealing with death, where the loss is an absolute that cannot be reversed, the temptation to go back to old habits is always present. Helping clients develop coping skills in small steps can help them recognize success and build strengths for continued abstinence.

Part of this new challenge is readjusting one's sense of self. Identity will change once a client gives up substance use as a core part of self. Worden (2018) identified three areas of adjustment after a loss. The first is *external adjustments*, which in the case of the loss being a substance means identifying all of roles the substance played. This change may be related to the places and people who were part of the substance-abusing world. New skills may be needed in how to form new relationships and make choices about where to go and how to interact without using substances. The second area is *internal adjustments*, which refers to adjusting one's own sense of self. Self-esteem and self-efficacy probably suffered during the time of active addiction. Now the task is to develop a definition of self without substances. Learning to recognize personal strengths and understand one's own worth can be difficult after having engaged in negative behaviors but is an essential part of recovery. Self-efficacy, the degree to which individuals believe they have some control over what happens to them, needs to be encouraged and developed through taking positive actions. However, this can be a challenging process for someone who has felt a loss of all control. The importance of having positive models and receiving consistent encouragement will be a core part of treatment. The third area is *spiritual adjustments*, which refers to fundamental life values and beliefs about the world. The search for meaning in all of the losses that have occurred may raise questions about one's basic assumptions about the world. Perhaps the world has not been a safe place for them, or people have not been trustworthy throughout their lives. Hope for a better life may seem a foreign concept, yet hope is a necessary part of making these adjustments. New beliefs may need to be developed, as old ones are dropped as no longer being valid. Finding new meaning in life is key to regaining a sense of control in life. What can interrupt this exploration is failing to develop the skills needed to manage everyday life. Some even promote their own helplessness and seek relationships with those who will take care of them, while others might just withdraw and not face the changes they need to make. Both of these approaches may lead to relapse.

Questions for the Clinician to Consider

- Once the client stops using, what life changes does the person have to face?
- What confidence in self does the client need to build to face these changes?
- What skills are missing that are needed for readjustment?
- How will the client develop these skills?

Task IV: To Emotionally Relocate the Past Use and Move On With Life

Living a life of recovery does not erase the life lived while using. Part of recovery is learning to live with the past in a way where the past informs current living. Here, the clinician can assist the client in finding an appropriate space for the past related to substance abuse while not letting the past take away from living in the present. Stopping use is not enough; one needs to learn to live fully in everyday life. This process will involve investing energy in new aspects of life as well as reconstructing and reinvesting in previous aspects of one's life. People begin to rebuild careers or even return to school to develop a new career. New interest may include being part of a recovery network and building relationships with those who understand the ongoing nature of recovery. Helping families understand the importance of these new relationships may help ease the tension caused by devotion to recovery. One complication may be related on how to interact with those family and friends who are still using. The client may have to figure out how to build a world without the presence of those who can disrupt recovery and find ways to compensate for roles and skills that were performed by those still using. Ending relationships may cause some pain of separation and create feelings of loss that need to be acknowledged.

Although challenging, rebuilding damaged relationships with family and friends may be part of this task. Unfortunately, many treatment programs do not extend to work with family beyond a few family informational sessions. Yet maintaining recovery can be more successful with family support. The person in recovery can benefit from recognizing the losses the family has experienced and understand that rebuilding trust will take time and effort. This task is congruent with Steps 8 and 9 in AA, which will help clients see the importance of this task.

Questions for the Clinician to Consider

- How does the client say good-bye to the past?
- Where does the past fit into the client's present view of self?
- What actions facilitate "moving on"?
- What meaning does past use give to life in the present?

Stroebe and Schut: Dual Process Model

To avoid the limitations presented by linear stage, phase, and task models, Stroebe and Schut (1999, 2010) evolved the Dual Process Model, which builds on the strengths of previous models (Stroebe & Schut, 2016). These authors defined grief work as a "cognitive process of confronting a loss, of going over the events before and at the time of death, of focusing on memories, and working toward detachment from the deceased," which "requires an active, ongoing, effortful attempt to come to terms with loss" (Stroebe & Schut, 1999, p. 199). In a review of quantitative studies, Fiore (2019) concluded that interventions based on the Dual Process Model may be more effective than traditional grief therapy approaches.

Stroebe and Schut (1999, 2010) conceptualized grieving as a highly individualized movement or *oscillation* between two dimensions, which they identified as loss-oriented stressors and restoration-oriented stressors. *Loss-oriented stressors* are those associated with the loss experience itself with a focus on the relationship, life together, and the circumstances and events surrounding the death. This process can involve rumination and yearning for the deceased and a depth of emotional expression over the loss. As losses are confronted by those in treatment for substance use disorder (SUD), a similar grief process may emerge that may be repeated over time as more losses come to the forefront. The focus will be on the disrupted bonds with the object of the loss. As discussed in Chapter 1, the emotional impact of losing one's substance triggers a similar physiological response as the one experienced when losing a relationship. This grief may not have been recognized at the time the loss occurred, but once recognized, the negative affect will be the focus, and loss-oriented coping will dominate. At times, the person may avoid the stressors associated with the loss only to confront them at other times. This fluctuation in confrontation and avoidance is a normal process in loss adaptation, as there will be times when avoiding is a normal reaction. In this process, clients may experience an intrusion of grief and engage in grief work that involves addressing continuing bonds. The focus is on the emotional aspects of grieving.

Because this is not a phase model, there will be a waxing and waning of the two coping processes. The other process, *restoration-oriented stressors*, includes those stressors associated with the consequences of the loss. Many changes result from a primary loss such as identity changes, role changes, and the need to learn skills. Restoration does not refer to any particular outcome variable but is a focus on identifying those things that need to be dealt with and how a person can manage them. The primary work in this process is to attend to life changes, do new things, and avoid the more emotional aspects of grief. It is important to keep in mind that having to learn new roles, develop a new identity, and reorganize one's life can create their own anxiety, so it is not unusual for someone to want to avoid confronting all of these changes. Taking a break from grieving stressors may not necessarily be negative but can represent a healthy way of coping. For those in recovery, developing an identity that is not based on substance use is a developmental process that will involve grieving the loss of who one has been and developing a sense of who one can be.

Both of these processes involve a combination of confrontation and avoidance of stressors, which produces a dynamic back-and-forth process distinctly different from sequential models of grief. Clients may choose to take time off, be distracted, or attend to new things. As a clinician, it is important to acknowledge the benefits of denial or avoidance but also be attuned to extreme forms of denial. Totally avoiding emotional expression has been shown to have negative health effects (Stroebe & Schut, 1999). Healthy adjustment appears to be related to the oscillation process in dealing with these two aspects of coping with loss. Either extreme rumination or extreme denial may disrupt oscillation and thus derail the grieving process. For example, clients in recovery may have such a desire to engage in the activities (restoration-orientation) to rebuild damaged relationships that they neglect their own damaged emotions over the losses they experienced throughout life. While there are many positive benefits from building a new sense of self and making amends for past actions, healing the hurt underneath is needed to maintain this progress.

One benefit of the Dual Process Model is it addresses gender differences in a way not addressed by other models. Women appear to be more loss oriented, with a desire to feel and express their distress. Men appear to be restoration oriented, actively engaging with problem-solving and practical issues associated with loss (Stroebe & Schut, 2010). Clinicians can focus on the stressors that seem to best fit the client's style while also watching for lack of oscillation. However, some benefit has been found for teaching men and women dealing with grief to cope in the way the opposite sex usually adopts. This approach was found to lower distress for both groups (Schut et al., 1997). Because this model allows flexibility for emotional experiencing and action behaviors, it has the ability to be more culturally sensitive by not valuing one process over the other. The value of this model for those in treatment for SUD is the focus it provides for those who grieve using the restoration-oriented style and who may have difficulty expressing emotions. Although these clients may need assistance in learning to identify emotions they may be avoiding, they will also be valued for their different style of grieving.

Facilitative Questions

- When you are faced with a significant loss, how do you typically respond?
- How comfortable are you crying in front of others? Do you seek out others with whom you can share your grief?
- What actions have you taken that have helped you cope with your grief?
- How easy is it for you to put your feelings into words?

Neimeyer: Meaning Reconstruction

Taking a different approach, Neimeyer (2001) began to view grief therapy as a process of reconstructing one's world of meaning that has been challenged by a loss. This process involves identity reconstruction and can include taking on new roles, revisiting old priorities, and finding new meaning in a world that has changed because of the loss. In general, people have deep-seated beliefs through which they filter life events, which include believing that they are worthy and deserving of positive outcomes, have significant control over their lives, and view the world as a just and benevolent place (Neimeyer et al., 2010). When a significant loss occurs, these assumptions are challenged, and meaning is lost. The path of finding meaning is not an easy one, and some types of losses, such as tragic and accidental deaths, may not lead to finding meaning from the loss. Neimeyer's Meaning Reconstruction approach to grief therapy is considered a constructivist approach that is tailored to each individual's understanding of the world and what gives life meaning.

Neimeyer and Thompson (2014) found about one-third of those grieving experienced few of the intense feelings associated with the classic stage model, while 10%–15% struggled with prolonged, intense feelings associated with complicated grief. Although most cope effectively with loss and the distress it creates, as many as 40% experience prolonged distress in the form of neuroendocrine disturbance, anxiety or panic, and sleep disturbance (Neimeyer et al., 2002). Not only is loss through death a source of meaning disruption, but Neimeyer and Thompson viewed the process of meaning making as applicable to losses other than death such as loss of career, relationships, and goals as well as personal injury. Although having an SUD was not mentioned, there are many losses surrounding substance use that disrupt life meaning. Research has shown that meaning making is associated with more favorable outcomes in bereavement, and struggles for meaning have been linked to bereavement complications (Neimeyer, 2019). Some of these complications include separation distress, preoccupations with the loss that impairs social and work functioning for a year or longer, a struggle to accept reality, avoidance of triggers, feeling a lack of purpose, and a disruption of relationships. Neimeyer and Thompson conceptualized meaning making as a coping resource that facilitates the grief process. Corr (2019) stated that meaning reconstruction includes making sense out of the events associated with the loss, which can be a challenge for those in recovery. Many of their losses may be associated with personal decisions made and actions taken related to substance use. Finding meaning within one's existing meaning framework and constructing meaning in new ways will be an ongoing process as clients in recovery face the losses they have experienced while using. The focus on constructing new meaning may focus on making sense of the losses and finding some important life lessons that have emerged from these losses (Neimeyer et al., 2002).

It is a human tendency to organize one's life experience in a narrative form (Neimeyer et al., 2002), and when loss interrupts this story, meaning must not only be reconstructed, it must also be integrated into one's identity (Neimeyer, 2001). There is a need both to preserve a sense of who one has been prior to the loss and to integrate the new reality of who one must become because of the loss (Neimeyer et al., 2002). Because the best predictor of adapting to the loss is one's ability to make sense of the loss and find some important life lesson or existential benefit, those who are in recovery for SUD will need to use this experience to redefine who they want to become and what they want their life to mean. An inability to make sense of losses has been shown to strongly predict complicated grief, while meaning making has been associated with alleviation of grief symptoms (Neimeyer, 2019).

Feelings of distress triggered by loss initiate the process of meaning making. Loss shatters the life-guiding cognitive schema, which often results in questioning the worthiness of self. Loss also impacts basic trust in the world, and as discussed in Chapter 1, early life traumas and losses are prevalent among those who abuse substances. For these clients, the cognitive schema already contains negative messages about their personal worth and the safety of the world. When additional losses occur, it is not unusual for someone to want to create a buffer from this shock by denying and numbing one's self, perhaps even using substances as part of this avoidance. To adapt to the loss, clients need to cognitively reframe the negative experience as part of meaning-based coping (Gillies & Neimeyer, 2006).

Gillies and Neimeyer (2006) have identified three activities that facilitate the process of meaning making. These include *sense making, benefit finding*, and *identity change*. Central to the process of grieving is the ability to make sense of the loss, and the most difficult losses are those that fail to make sense. While these authors discussed untimely and tragic deaths, there are losses and traumatic experiences that do not make sense, such as children who experience physical or sexual abuse, which is a common experience among those who abuse substances. When a reason cannot be found for what happened, the person may blame self as the cause, which can result in a damaged self-worth. Even becoming addicted itself may not make sense to clients who may question why they have an SUD when others they know have not developed a problem. Benefit finding from the loss can help individuals adapt to the loss and is a means of building new meaning structures. However, this process will not be seen soon after the loss, may take months or years, and is by no means a certain outcome. On one side, the initial losses caused by substance use may not appear to be benefits, such as loss of relationships, physical health, or jobs. The benefits that may emerge are increased awareness of taking care of relationships and one's self and the motivation to do a better job of managing one's life. On the other side, the loss of one's substance may initially be difficult, but benefits become apparent over time as one's thinking and cognitive functions improve and family relationships are rebuilt. Gillies and Neimeyer reported that making sense of a loss is an effective coping means in early months, while benefit finding is a better ongoing means of coping. Some of the positive changes that can occur due to loss include a changed sense of self that incorporates becoming more resilient, developing a greater awareness of life's fragility, and increased capacity for empathy (Gillies & Neimeyer, 2006). In their review of the research, they found several emergent qualitative themes, one of which was the importance of personal responsibility and growth, a theme that would be valuable to explore for those in treatment for SUD. In the quantitative research, greater grief was found in those who harbored perceptions that the world was random and uncontrollable. The processes of sense making and benefit finding were not found to be correlated, suggesting they are independent processes. Finally, identity change focuses on evolving purpose and meaning in life as a result of the loss, which means reconstructing the self. When a client responds to loss in adaptive ways, the result is a changed sense of self. These changes can be recognized when someone takes on new roles, experiences spiritual growth, and is able to become closer emotionally to others. However, one realization that may surface is finding life is more painful and challenging than they had expected, and achieving goals may be more difficult than anticipated (Gillies & Neimeyer, 2006). This realization may be particularly potent for those in treatment for SUD, where the challenges of abstinence take much energy and devotion. While personal growth can create distress, "learning how to become someone who can carry the weight of his or her distress" (p. 53) can be a focus of addictions counseling.

Meaning making is viewed as an individualized grief therapy experience, with each client examining how loss has affected one's views of self, others, and the world. Each person is the author of a personal narrative that tries to make sense of the loss event. The grieving process involves reconstructing the narrative in ways that foster coping with the loss and moving forward with a new story that incorporates the meaning of the loss. The therapist's challenge is to create the conditions for exploring meaning without trying to impose meaning on the client. Many of the techniques employed will involve storytelling, writing, analogies, and even empty chair work. Given that those in treatment for SUD will need to build skills to cope with powerful emotions, pacing will be critical. Treatment may oscillate between building coping skills and probing for deeper meaning of the loss. This approach will be enhanced through the development of a strong therapeutic alliance with clients, in which clients experience support and profound listening from the therapist.

Facilitative Questions

- Losses upon entering treatment:

  - What has been the impact of entering treatment in terms of relinquishing former relationships and activities that defined your life?
  - How do you compare the person you are now to the person you were before substance use became problematic? What did you lose by using? What did you gain?
  - How do you envision yourself in the next year after giving up substance use?
  - What will make your life worth living in the future?

- Losses while using:

  - What was important in your life that changed because of using substances?
  - How was your sense of who you were and who you wanted to be affected by substance use?
  - What did you like about yourself while using substances? What did you not like about yourself?
  - How has substance use changed your life story?
  - What memories of your substance use bring pain, guilt, or sadness? Where do you need to seek forgiveness for these actions?
  - How do you deal with feelings caused by behaviors that hurt someone else? How do you forgive yourself?

- Losses prior to using:

- Was there a time in your life where you felt hopeful about the future? What happened to change that feeling?
- What were your hopes and dreams, and who supported you in seeking these?
- What losses occurred that changed your view of the future?
- When you look back on your earlier life losses, how much do you blame yourself for what happened? How much did others blame you?

Summary

Each of the theories presented contains perspectives that can be helpful to clients' understanding of their grief and loss experiences. By focusing on the needs of clients and ways to strengthen their coping resources, the clinician can choose an approach that fosters the client's ability to recognize the reality of the loss and the emotional, cognitive, and spiritual/existential balance needed to address their grief. Each theory offers a different perspective that can foster clients' understanding of how to navigate the turbulent waters of the grief journey. When grief is recognized as part of the recovery process for those who are addressing SUD, clients are able to make sense of the deeper impact substance use has had on their well-being, and they increase their ability to achieve resolution of unaddressed issues. Theory creates a pathway to rebuilding a sense of meaning that was shattered by loss.

References

Corr, C. (2019). The "five stages" in coping with dying and bereavement: Strengths, weaknesses and some alternatives. *Mortality, 24*(4), 405–417. https://doi.org/10.108 0/13576275.2018.1527826

Doka, K. (2002). Disenfranchised Grief. In Kenneth J. Doka (Ed.), *Living with grief: Loss in later life* (pp. 159–168). The Hospice Foundation of America.

Doka, K., & Martin, T. (2010). *Grieving beyond gender: Understanding the ways men and women mourn* (2nd ed.). Brunner-Routledge.

Fiore, J. (2019). A systematic review of the dual process model of coping with bereavement (1999–2016). *Omega,* 30222819893139. https://doi.org/10.1177/003022281 9893139

Gillies, J., & Neimeyer, R. (2006). Loss, grief, and the search for significance: Toward a model of meaning reconstruction in bereavement. *Journal of Constructivist Psychol ogy, 19*(1), 31–65. https://doi.org/10.1080/10720530500311182

Holland, J., & Neimeyer, R. (2010). An examination of stage theory of grief among individuals bereaved by natural and violent causes: A meaning-oriented contribution. *OMEGA—Journal of Death and Dying, 61*(2), 103–120. https://doi.org/10.2190/ OM.61.2.b

Humphrey, K. M. (2009). *Counseling strategies for loss and grief.* American Counseling Association.

Kübler-Ross, E. (1969). *On death and dying.* Macmillan.

Mortell, S. (2015). Assisting clients with disenfranchised grief: The role of a mental health nurse. *Journal of Psychosocial Nursing & Mental Health Services, 53*(4), 52–57. https://doi.org/10.3928/02793695-20150319-05

Musalek, M. (2013). Reduction of harmful consumption versus total abstinence in addiction treatment. *Neuropsychiatry, 3*(6), 635–644. https://doi.org/10.2217/npy.13.84

Neimeyer, R. (2001). Reauthoring life narratives: Grief therapy as meaning reconstruction. *Israel Journal of Psychiatry and Related Sciences, 38*(3–4), 171–183.

Neimeyer, R. (2019). Meaning reconstruction in bereavement: Development of a research program. *Death Studies, 43*(2), 79–91. https://doi.org/10.1080/07481187.2018.1456620

Neimeyer, R., Burke, L., Mackay, M., & van Dyke Stringer, J. (2010). Grief therapy and the reconstruction of meaning: From principles to practice. *Journal of Contemporary Psychotherapy, 40*(2), 73–83. https://doi.org/10.1007/s10879-009-9135-3

Neimeyer, R., Prigerson, H., & Davies, B. (2002). Mourning and meaning. *American Behavioral Scientist, 46*(2), 235–251. https://doi.org/10.1177/000276402236676

Neimeyer, R., & Thompson, B. E. (2014). Meaning making and the art of grief therapy. In B. E. Thompson & R. A. Neimeyer (Eds.), *Grief and the expressive arts: Practices for creating meaning* (pp. 3–13). Routledge.

Rando, T. (1993). *Treatment of complicated mourning*. Research Press.

Schut, H. A. W., Stroebe, M., de Keijser, J., & van den Bout, J. (1997). Intervention for the bereaved: Gender differences in the efficacy of grief counselling. *British Journal of Clinical Psychology, 36*, 63–72. https://doi.org/10.1111/j.2044-8260.1997.tb01231.x

Stroebe, M., & Schut, H. (1999). The dual process model of coping with bereavement: Rationale and description. *Death Studies, 23*(3), 197–224. https://doi.org/10.1080/074811899201046

Stroebe, M., & Schut, H. (2010). The dual process model of coping with bereavement: A decade on. *OMEGA—Journal of Death and Dying, 61*(4), 273–289. https://doi.org/10.2190/OM.61.4.b

Stroebe, M., & Schut, H. (2016). Overload: A missing link in the dual process model? *OMEGA-Journal of Death and Dying, 74*(1), 96–109. https://doi.org/10.1177/0030222816666540

Worden, J. W. (1982). *Grief counseling and grief therapy: A handbook for the mental health practitioner*. Springer.

Worden, J. W. (2002). *Grief counseling and grief therapy: A handbook for the mental health practitioner* (3rd ed.). Springer.

Worden, J. W. (2018). *Grief counseling and grief therapy: A handbook for the mental health practitioner* (5th ed.). Springer.

3 The Counselor's Own Grief

Susan R. Furr

Counseling is not just what therapists do; it becomes who they are. Often, students entering the field describe it as a calling they just could not ignore. Individuals enter the field for many reasons, but for a large number of clinicians, the motivation to help others arises from personal woundedness that began in childhood (Conchar & Repper, 2014). These authors found themes in the literature relating to the desire to self-heal as part of the motivation to become a therapist. Whatever the reason for entering the field, therapists need to be aware of personal experiences and challenges that can impact the therapeutic process.

Therapists, however, do not enter the therapy room as blank slates but bring their history of loss and trauma that can both help and hinder clients. The focus of this chapter is on how grief and loss affect those in the helping professions with particular emphasis on clinicians who also deal with their own recovery while assisting others in recovery. The role of the supervisor in assisting clinicians dealing with their own losses will be discussed as one of the primary coping strategies. The chapter concludes with a personal exploration exercise that can be helpful in identifying areas that may need more attention in the dealing with personal grief.

Therapist myths and concerns

One of the common myths therapists encounter is the idea of being immune to problems (Rudick, 2012). Because we have learned strategies to live mentally healthy lives and practice wellness, it is easy to forget that our control over life losses is limited. We can do all of the right things and still have bad things happen. When a local grief counselor lost her young adult son to an accident, the entire staff was in shock. One of the counselors realized they had learned to operate under the premise they "gave at the office" every day in helping families who had lost children so felt immune to the possibility it could happen to them. This response may appear irrational on the surface, but therapists often develop cognitive strategies that provide self-protection. By hearing so many traumatic stories on a regular basis, therapists can begin seeing the world as an unsafe and tragic place. To cope with exposure to all of these painful events,

DOI: 10.4324/9781003106906-3

it is not unusual for therapists to develop rationale for why this trauma would not happen to them. Our desires for self-protection may arise from the stigma of admitting our own vulnerabilities. Therapists are supposed to be strong and know how to cope, so when loss happens, it may become difficult to admit one is having difficulty. Lack of acknowledging that one is vulnerable to loss may trigger seeing self as a failure when loss occurs (Rudick, 2012). Therapists face one of their greatest challenges in figuring out how to balance knowing they are not immune to losses while also not becoming fearful of encountering the same losses as their clients. Choosing to work in the field of substance abuse means working with a population that has a high exposure to trauma, which can have secondary impact on the therapist. Being able to admit vulnerability is key to managing this stress.

While personal trauma may have initiated the desire to become a therapist, there may be an underlying expectation therapists should be strong, leading to not wanting to expose any imperfections (Conchar & Repper, 2014). After all, what would clients think if they knew the struggles faced by their therapist? Accepting this professional role carries many responsibilities, and even professional codes of ethics emphasize the need for therapists to function in a healthy way. These expectations may contribute to the potentially false idea therapists are able to manage better than others with the losses they encounter (Kouriatis & Brown, 2011). However, therapists encounter loss both in their professional and personal lives and need to develop strategies to grieve in constructive ways and to process what these losses mean to how they manage the therapeutic process. Therapists need to be careful not to engage in the myth that one has the capability to "heal" one's self (Rudick, 2012). Therapists may believe that because of their extensive knowledge about intrapsychic processes they can serve as their own counselor. Knowing the process of grief is not enough to lessen the pain of grief. Understanding the stages/phases/tasks of grief does not preclude experiencing the grief process.

Another concern relates to the stigma that might arise if a therapist admitted personal grief and loss issues to a client or colleagues and supervisors. In relation to clients, dealing with loss does not have to carry a stigma and can produce benefits but only if the therapist has made progress in addressing the loss. Cvetovac and Adame (2017) found personal experiences could facilitate empathy, yet these experiences can also create "empathic failure" (Gelso & Hayes, 2007, p. 110) when therapists over-identify with client struggles and cannot separate their own history from the clients' experiences. For therapists who are in recovery for substance use disorders (SUDs), this issue needs continued evaluation. Because recovery is an ongoing process, it may be difficult to reach a point of resolution because of the possibility of relapse. Thus, the therapist must remain vigilant about how client issues may trigger issues around substance use.

While it is a myth that therapists dealing with their own losses cannot help clients with similar issues, there is a legitimate concern about the stigma surrounding a therapist who has experienced significant personal losses. Hayes et al. (2007) found that clients perceived therapists as less empathic when the therapist was still dealing with their own loss but were more empathic when the therapist's grief had been resolved. Self-disclosure about loss proved to have therapeutic value in opening up the client to new themes and feelings that had not previously been examined (Tsai et al., 2010). But therapists can also shut down around unresolved issues and not be attuned to clients and their feelings (Kouriatis & Brown, 2011). While a therapist's personal wounds may create empathy, the therapist needs to have attended to their wounds and be engaged in self-care in order for the wounds to have value (Conchar & Repper, 2014). Not only have clients expressed concern over therapist response to grief (Hayes et al., 2007), there is also concern that colleagues and organizations may raise issues over therapists who have experienced significant mental health issues. Simpson (2013) found organizations are not always supportive of clinicians with personal losses, and there may be little room to admit one is having difficulty managing work because of being affected by grief and loss issues faced by clients. Particularly in the field of substance abuse counseling, colleagues may express concern on how the relapse of a therapist affects the organization's reputation. While client outcome is of primary importance, focus on the well-being of the therapist also needs to be considered if the organization wants therapists to be authentic about the challenges they are experiencing (Cvetovac & Adame, 2017). Being a wounded healer has many ramifications for the quality of treatment clients receive. Understanding the benefits and cautions of wounded healers as therapists is important to the well-being of both clients and clinicians.

The wounded healer

The concept of the wounded healer has been present for centuries, but was popularized by Jung in the context of therapeutic work (Conchar & Repper, 2014). It is through the therapist's own wounds that deep understanding of the client's suffering can take place, which provides space for the clients to heal themselves. This concept has been especially true in the field of substance abuse counseling since the 1930s and eventually evolved into Alcoholics Anonymous. Who can better understand the process of recovery than someone who has successfully navigated the process? Having similar loss experiences can facilitate the empathic connection.

Part of being a therapist is bringing our sense of humanity into the therapy room, which includes those aspects of us that are wounded. The therapist's personal experiences have an impact on how they work with clients. The influence of personal loss serves to inform therapeutic work (Kouriatis & Brown, 2011), and healing power can emerge from the therapist's own woundedness (Zerubavel & Wright, 2012). Therapists have reported their own personal experiences increased their understanding of others (Gilbert & Stickley, 2012), and working through personal emotional pain has led to enhanced empathy when working with clients with similar problems (Hayes et al., 2007). In the field of substance abuse counseling, therapist who are in recovery have a deep understanding of challenges faced by clients.

Does one have to be wounded in order to be an effective therapist? Being wounded itself does not produce the ability to be effective. Effectiveness is enhanced by the process of recovering from the wound (Zerubavel & Wright, 2012). Woundedness has the ability to increase understanding, but it also is important to keep in mind the key component is empathy. Therapists will not have experienced all of the issues faced by clients, but through careful listening and understanding, empathy can be conveyed. This is perhaps the ultimate goal of working with clients in their grief—the ability to care deeply for them in their loss. This process is just enhanced through the therapist's own experience with loss. However, it is also important for the therapist to recognize how each client's journey is unique and perhaps different from the therapist's own journey.

The primary issue about the impact of the therapist's personal loss on the client is related to how the therapist has addressed personal loss. Hayes et al. (2007) examined therapist-client dyads where grief was the primary focus of the therapy. The findings were quite profound in that the therapists' unresolved feelings related to their loss were inversely related to the clients' perceptions of therapist empathy. The more the therapists had resolved their grief, the more clients viewed them as empathic. Another strength that can emerge from therapists who have grown from personal experiences is gaining confidence in the client's ability to recover from their losses (Conchar & Repper, 2014). Experiencing a loss and ways one can recover from the loss contributes to the therapist's belief system about the power of therapy to heal the client. Knowing they have faced their own emotional pain and emerged from their depths of despair builds confidence their clients are capable of the same growth. Therapists who have personal experience with SUD recovery provide a reassuring role model that treatment can be effective. The presence of staff who are in recovery helps other staff be more positive about client outcomes while also keeping staff realistic about the pace and expectations of treatment. However, when recovering staff relapse, both clients and colleagues are negatively affected (Adams & Warren, 2010).

Challenges faced by wounded healers

Perhaps to some extent, all therapists are wounded healers and need to consistently be aware of how personal wounds are used in the therapeutic process (O'Brien, 2011). Unresolved grief issues can impede client progress, and therapists' personal loss may limit how receptive they are to their clients' needs around grief and loss (Garti & Bat Or, 2019). The question to be explored is "when does the therapeutic relationship become the narrative of the clinician instead of the population we serve" (Hyatt, 2014, p. 32). Of further concern is how to identify the line between therapist distress and impairment

(Zerubavel & Wright, 2012). One effect of the therapist's own wounds is becoming preoccupied with one's own losses rather than focusing on the client's experiences (Kouriatis & Brown, 2011). The result may be a therapist who is less attuned to clients as well as being more vulnerable and emotionally sensitive. When the therapist is not sufficiently recovered from personal losses, the negative impact can include a decreased ability to be emotionally present with the client, overidentification with the client's issues, projecting personal feelings onto the client, difficulty managing countertransference, and focusing on a personal agenda rather than the client's issues (Kouriatis & Brown, 2011). Even though the literature has indicated resolved grief on the part of the therapist can be beneficial (Hayes et al., 2007; O'Brien, 2011), there may be clients who do not want this information about the therapist and may be concerned the focus will shift to the therapist. In addition, clients are not bound by confidentiality, so any information shared will not stay secret, a risk that therapists may not always consider (Zerubavel & Wright, 2012).

Uncovering one's own trauma can be a traumatizing experience in itself. If the client's pain serves to reopen the therapist's wounds, there is a risk of the therapist shutting down the client (Rudick, 2012). When client issues touch upon the therapist's unresolved loss, the therapist might engage in a "protective emotional withdrawal" from the client (p. 558). At this point, the therapist may move more into the territory of being an impaired professional if boundaries become confused or violated (Zerubavel & Wright, 2012). Using the therapeutic relationship to self-comfort and gain support from the client violates the sacred relationship between client and therapist. When therapists blur the lines between their inner feelings and those of clients, there may be a need for more intense supervision as well as consideration of taking a break from client work. Therapists need to be continuously aware of how their own wounds influence the relationship with the client (Hayes et al., 2007) and know when additional personal reflection is needed. While the grief and loss experienced by the therapist can certainly enhance understanding of clients, without having achieved awareness and resolution of personal losses, therapist grief can become overwhelming to the therapeutic process. Research has shown personal wounds caused more problems when the loss was more recent, currently upsetting, or not being attended to (Cvetovac & Adame, 2017). It is most important that personal wounds do not cause the therapist to avoid difficult issues with the client or to move past these issues too quickly (St. Arnaud, 2017). Also, therapists may be tempted to direct clients to the methods that worked for themselves in dealing with their own losses without considering other approaches that might better fit the client (Cvetovac & Adame, 2017). Care needs to be taken to avoid overgeneralizing from personal experience and to maintain distinction between personal feelings and those of the client (Hayes et al., 2007). Therapists need to remain aware of how the desire to protect one's self from painful feelings may allow the client to avoid similar sorrows.

Self-disclosure

One's own grief and loss experiences can inform counseling practice in two ways. First, recognizing personal losses and the impact of these losses can increase the therapist's sensitivity to identifying the effect loss is having on the client. Using personal loss in this way may not involve any form of disclosure. Just being able to draw from one's awareness of the deep meaning of loss on all aspects of life can help the therapist see things the client may not notice. The increased empathy can build stronger connections with the client, and there can be positive effects on disclosing these experiences in therapy. Sharing one's personal losses with a client in appropriate ways can have a positive influence on the client relationship in terms of building rapport with the client and strengthening the therapeutic alliance (Henretty et al., 2014).

Self-disclosure can be unsuccessful as a result of the therapist having not resolved personal loss issues. Pinto-Coelho et al. (2018) found therapists may misread what they thought were commonalities with the client. Perhaps when a therapist is struggling with personal losses, it is easy to project one's own feeling onto the client and thus be less attuned to client needs. Therapists dealing with losses that occurred when they were active in their careers demonstrated the most difficulty functioning at work, found it hard to be present with clients, had problems with concentration, and felt overwhelmed by responsibilities (Cvetovac & Adame, 2017). Deciding how much to disclose in terms of loss as well as experiencing difficulties functioning need to become an active part of supervision.

To decide how much to disclose to clients, the therapist needs to examine personal motivation. Whose needs will be met by the disclosure? It might be helpful to try a small disclosure first to see how the client reacts. It is a good policy to only disclose if the loss has been processed and resolved (Zerubavel & Wright, 2012). Losses can be discussed in nonspecific ways, such as sharing that one has experienced similar difficult times, without going into great detail. Such an approach would show the client a willingness to deal with painful material. Keep in mind self-disclosure redistributes the power in the therapy session, which can result in a more positive relationship in which the client feels more ownership of the therapy process. A strong working alliance is needed for self-disclosure to be effective, and the working alliance will be dependent upon the therapist's ability to be focused on the client without undue intrusion of personal issues into the sessions. Unresolved grief issues of the therapist have the power to derail the client's progress when those issues separate the therapist from listening and being present with the client. Because the possibility of relapse does not totally disappear for a therapist who has experienced an SUD, maintaining healthy abstinence practices and support networks will be key to dealing with client losses related to substance abuse.

Countertransference

As much as therapists desire to maintain objectivity, it is their personal connections to clients that make a difference. Consequently, having a personal reaction to what the client shares is a natural consequence of empathy. But this type of emotional response by a therapist can interrupt the natural flow of the interaction, which is often termed the therapeutic alliance. One of the stressors experienced by therapists is the one-way caring nature of the interaction, which can be exhausting (Rudick, 2012). Constantly giving emotionally to clients can be a drain on internal resources and is often a source of burnout or compassion fatigue. *Countertransference* is a term used to describe a therapist's reaction to a client who has been impacted by the therapist's personal unresolved issues (Hayes et al., 2007). Managing countertransference was cited by therapists as an important skill to learn as a means of separating their own distressing experiences from those of the client (Cvetovac & Adame, 2017). Unprocessed trauma may create blind spots for the therapist that may prevent the therapist assisting clients in similar situations (Rudick, 2012). Because of protecting one's self from the client's pain, there is a danger of a therapist not being able to recognize the depth of the pain the client has experienced. The risk is that a therapist could shut down a client if they perceive the client's pain has the potential to reopen the therapist's own wounds. This point further emphasizes the need to address one's own grief issue in order to work effectively with client's grief issues. Because grief issues often have not been a part of treatment for substance use, therapists in recovery may need to engage in additional exploration of their own losses that may have even preceded their own abuse of substances. Otherwise, they may not be able to recognize the losses encountered by those in treatment and consequently avoid addressing these painful issues.

Role of recovery

For the substance abuse counselor who is also in recovery, the challenge will be moving from primarily focusing on the client's abstinence to looking at their losses related to substance use. This process may trigger personal issues for those clinicians in recovery who have not engaged in their own grief work. As discussed in Chapter 1, many losses precede substance use, with additional losses occurring while actively using substances. Learning to address one's addiction is of primary importance, and progress has to occur prior to addressing losses. We all have observed the pride of a client obtaining a new medallion or chip symbolizing their achievement managing addiction. But their changes do not stop with abstinence. Uncovering underlying contributors to addiction and making meaning of those losses is an ongoing process for those who deal with addiction. Because a large proportion of those who work in the field of substance abuse counseling have personal experiences with addiction, the probability of therapists recalling personal losses is high as clients share losses.

Many benefits have been cited for having counselors with personal addiction experience working in the field, which include street credibility, being a role model who makes treatment more acceptable, and providing a resource to other staff (Doukas & Cullen, 2010). It has been estimated that between 30% and 50% of addiction professionals are in recovery (Greene et al., 2019).

There may even be an expectation that personal experience with the disorder is necessary for treatment effectiveness (Zerubavel & Wright, 2012). But maintaining one's own recovery along with helping others can extol an emotional price. Greene et al. (2019) found a relapse rate of 14.7% among recovering addictions professionals and that the risk of relapse decreased with consistent involvement in mutual-aid groups and longer abstinence before entering the helping field. However, there is a great risk of exposure to trauma in working with clients who have an SUD, and these repeated stories can lead to secondary traumatic stress. Bride et al. (2009) found 75% of substance abuse counselors had at least one symptom of secondary traumatic stress in the past week and 19% met the diagnostic criteria for post-traumatic stress disorder (PTSD). Such exposure creates conditions that could lead to relapse for those recovering counselors because such stress can reactivate one's own issues (Rudick, 2012). Therapists in recovery may have not have identified all of the losses experienced during their time of substance use and will need to process emotions that are triggered when clients' stories bring up unprocessed blind spots (Rudick, 2012).

One place where the therapists' own losses become apparent is when the therapist has a family history of substance abuse, such as being an adult child of an alcoholic. These therapists may have grown up in an atmosphere of aggression and violence and been the recipient of physical and emotional abuse (Tedgård et al., 2018). They may even have taken on many of the parental roles and learned to be sensitive to the needs of others, characteristics that may have led them to the helping professions. Little research has been conducted with this population. One qualitative dissertation study (Doherty & Girault, 1992) examined women psychotherapists who were daughters of alcoholic fathers. She found patterns of survival were established early and created both difficulties and strengths. Habitual denial about their experiences was a common carryover from childhood, and even the research interviews elicited unexpected childhood memories. One-third of the participants reported becoming addicted themselves. The importance of this study is the way it illustrates how a therapist does not have to be addicted to be affected by the stories shared by clients. While there is no data showing how frequently substance abuse counselors have experienced family members who have an SUD, it is not uncommon to have those who enter the field of substance abuse counseling to share how this choice was influenced by a personal experience. The fact unexpected memories were triggered in the research setting is a caution for therapists who need to continue to be vigilant about ways in which client losses bring up memories of losses created by family or friends who abused substances.

Role of supervision

In the supervisory role, it is important to denote the line that separates distress from impairment (Zerubavel &Wright, 2012). Please note that using the term *impairment* may carry some additional burden as it relates to the Americans with Disabilities Act (ADA), which includes substance abuse issues. A more practical term may be professional competency (Brown-Rice & Furr, 2015) that can be defined behaviorally. Wheeler (2007) recommended creating a supervisory style that is "interactive, relational, and collegial" (p. 251). Such a style can aid in facilitating disclosure when the counselor becomes stuck in uncomfortable feelings. It is not the supervisor's role to become the therapist for the supervisee, yet exploring the dynamics of countertransference is a necessary part of examining the wounds the therapist brings into work with the client. A good supervisor will create space to process therapist exposure to losses and give the therapist a place to name the losses as well as acknowledge and accept these losses have occurred (Simpson, 2013).

In assessing the therapist's competency to handle emotions related to personal losses, the supervisor may need to ask directly about the supervisee's ability to manage the demands created by exposure to the client's intense emotions (Amundson & Ross, 2016). It is valid to examine how treatment of the client is affecting the supervisee. Often a parallel process will emerge where the supervisee's reaction to the supervisor is similar to the client's reaction to the supervisee. Parallel process refers to processes in the counselor/client relationship being reflected in the counselor/supervisor relationship (St. Arnaud, 2017). For example, a supervisee may be frustrated with a client who resists discussing deeper feelings, while at the same time the supervisee is refusing to explore their frustration with the supervisor. It is the supervisor's role to notice when the supervisee's wounds distort the therapy process. This approach may be particularly true in the area of grief, where the supervisee may not want to acknowledge woundedness. Although the supervisor must not turn supervision into therapy, it is the supervisor's responsibility to identify any limitations the supervisee's personal losses create in the therapeutic relationship, the impact of any blind spots on part of the supervisee, and the personal difficulties the supervisee is having with the client. The primary question becomes whether the wounds cause the supervisee to avoid bringing up difficult issues or move too quickly past issues (St. Arnaud, 2017).

One of the first approaches the supervisor can employ is teaching the supervisee about countertransference. This process can begin by the supervisor recognizing when the supervisee is having difficulty staying present when grief and loss issues emerge (Cvetovac & Adame, 2017). Using immediacy when listening to sessions can provide the opportunity for actively processing the supervisee's emotions in that moment of the session. Through this process, the supervisee can learn to separate personal distressing experiences from those of the client. O'Brien (2011) recommended using mindfulness and grounding techniques for supervisees to keep themselves centered and prevent their own emotions from getting in the way of the client's emotions. Zerubavel and Wright (2012) have suggested process questions such as "What do you experience when the client brings up. . . ?" and "How do you manage your personal reactions in session?" Ultimately, it will be the supervisee's responsibility to decide how to work through personal grief, but a sensitive and caring supervisor will create an environment where these issues are recognized and acknowledged.

Self-evaluation

Knowing one's own grief and how that grief has transformed life and choices made as a result of grief is essential for those who work with clients. The experience of grief has the power to affect one's ability to help others. Our own grief can cause us to react to our clients' grief with anger and frustration and make us uncomfortable in witnessing their pain (Worden, 2018). Rather than have our personal grief triggered, we may cut the relationship short (Hayes et al., 2007) or move to other issues rather than sit with the client's pain. Worden has identified three ways in which counselors are affected by the client's grief.

First, clients' grief makes therapists aware of their own losses. The more similar the losses, the more painful the exposure. If the therapist has not adequately resolved the loss, the intervention with the client can be affected (Worden, 2018). If the loss has been appropriately integrated into the therapist's self-understanding, it can be beneficial to the client. The key is the therapist finding a good adaptation to the loss. For example, a therapist may be in recovery for substance abuse and achieved years of sobriety but may have not addressed early life losses. When a client begins sharing painful childhood traumas, the therapist becomes aware of her own abusive childhood experiences she had blocked from memory and is taken by surprise by how vivid her memories are. For the moment, she finds herself shutting down and just going through the motions of listening. Rather than encouraging the client to explore the hurt, she moves on to other issues and may even dread seeing this client again. For the therapist to continue working effectively with the client, she would need to bring these issues to supervision and perhaps decide to reengage in her own therapy.

Another effect of working with client grief is becoming aware of one's own feared losses (Worden, 2018). It may be helpful to use the Gestalt perspective of background and foreground. Many of our feared losses reside in the background of our consciousness and may include anxieties over the possible death of a child or loss of a significant relationship. Other hidden fears could include public embarrassment, loss of employment and financial security, or loss of status and esteem. When clients enter treatment for substance abuse, they may share many traumatic losses that bring our own anxieties to the foreground, which will move our attention from the client to our own fears. It is important to bring this anxiety into consciousness and address it as a means of keeping personal fears from intruding on the clients' needs to explore the impact of loss on their substance use.

Finally, Worden (2018) described how client grief over losing a significant person can bring up death awareness related to the inevitability of one's own death. While death may not be the primary loss being discussed by clients in recovery, there needs to be a special caution for therapists who are in recovery.

When a client relapses, anxiety could be triggered for therapists who live with the knowledge relapse can occur for them. The more similar the therapist is to the client in terms of personal characteristics, the more this fear can trigger anxiety.

For these reasons, it is valuable for therapists to conduct an examination of personal losses through the life span and their experiences with the accompanying grief. How did the grief process work, and what coping strategies were used? What resources were available, including what was helpful and what was not? To begin this process, it would be helpful for you to complete the following activity. If you know there are powerful emotions associated with losses you have not yet processed, you may want to consider doing this in the context of your own counseling or at least have resources to support you if strong feelings are triggered.

A lifetime of loss activity

For this activity, you are going to draw a time line of the losses that have occurred in your life. In addition to deaths of significant people, it is important to include losses that may be material or symbolic. These may include those related to health, achievements, identity, relationships, life transitions, material possessions, spiritual beliefs, or hopes and dreams. Think of any examples where your world shifted because of a major change that caused an emotional response.

Keep in mind loss is highly specific to the individual: what is a loss to one person may not be perceived as a loss to someone else. You may make an initial list but revisit it as new recollections emerge.

5	10	15	20	25	30	35	40	45	50	55	60

While we try to avoid using the concept of closure after a loss, given that loss causes a permanent change in who we are, you will find that some losses have more lingering effects than others.

1. Your first step is to examine your time line and identify which losses you believe you have managed well. Under each of these losses, ask yourself what you did to grieve the loss and what kind of support did you have. What strengths might you have gained from dealing with this loss?
2. Next, identify those losses you were unable to grieve fully. Did you recognize it as loss when it happened? If you knew it was a

---

loss, what interfered with being able to grieve? Were you allowed to acknowledge the loss, or was it disenfranchised? Did others validate your loss, or was the loss dismissed? Were you a part of a group grieving this same loss? How does this grief still affect you, and what do you do to protect yourself from these feelings?

3. Your final step is to examine your time line and circle any loss you would identify as unfinished business. When you notice this loss, emotions are still "raw," with thoughts of wishing you had said or done something differently. Do you find yourself avoiding certain places or staying away from events or people that could remind you of the loss? Have you ever engaged in behaviors that block your feelings about the loss? What do think you still need to do to address this loss?

Worden (2018) has recommended that counselors who work with clients dealing with grief issues practice active grieving. This process involves experiencing one's own sadness and not feeling guilty about these emotions. Counselors can use this activity to identify areas of personal limitations in working with grieving clients by recognizing the types of losses that will be difficult to hear. For example, in the field of addictions counseling, many clients have suffered from sexual abuse, which could be triggering for a therapist who had similar trauma. Finally, for grief that is still difficult to process, be sure to reach out for help, which means knowing your sources of support. Colleagues, supervisors, and personal therapeutic work can all be useful resources to manage your own grief, which will help you in allowing clients to grieve in healthy ways. Expect that you will be affected by clients' loss and grief, but grief counseling with clients is not the place for the therapist to work through unfinished bereavement. Your losses can be very informative to understanding clients and can build a strong understanding of the clients' experiences. This increased empathy can be a valuable tool in building rapport and the therapeutic alliance, while unresolved grief can be a hindrance to client recovery.

References

Adams, P., & Warren, H. (2010). Responding to the risks associated with the relapse of recovering staff members within addiction services. *Substance Use & Misuse, 45*(6), 951–967. https://doi.org/10.3109/10826080903442810

Amundson, J., & Ross, M. (2016). The wounded healer: From the other side of the couch. *American Journal of Clinical Hypnosis: Emotional Disorders and the Wounded-Self, 59*(1), 114–121. https://doi.org/10.1080/00029157.2016.1163657

Bride, B., Smith Hatcher, S., Humble, M., & Bride, B. (2009). Trauma training, trauma practices, and secondary traumatic stress among substance abuse counselors. *Traumatology*, *15*(2), 96–105. https://doi.org/10.1177/1534765609336362

Brown-Rice, K., & Furr, S. (2015). Gatekeeping ourselves: Counselor educators' knowledge of colleagues' problematic behaviors. *Counselor Education and Supervision*, *54*(3), 176–188. https://doi.org/10.1002/ceas.12012

Conchar, C., & Repper, J. (2014). "Walking wounded or wounded healer?" Does personal experience of mental health problems help or hinder mental health practice? A review of the literature. *Mental Health and Social Inclusion*, *18*(1), 35–44. https://doi.org/10.1108/MHSI-02-2014-0003

Cvetovac, M., & Adame, A. (2017). The wounded therapist: Understanding the relationship between personal suffering and clinical practice. *Humanistic Psychologist*, *45*(4), 348–366. https://doi.org/10.1037/hum0000071

Doherty, S., & Girault, E. (1992). *Psychotherapists who are daughters of alcoholic fathers: Impact on self, self-in-relation, and clinical practice* (ProQuest dissertations publishing). http://search.proquest.com/docview/304030694/

Doukas, N., & Cullen, J. (2010). Recovered addicts working in the addiction field: Pitfalls to substance abuse relapse. *Drugs: Education, Prevention and Policy*, *17*(3), 216–231. https://doi.org/10.3109/09687630802378864

Garti, D., & Bat Or, M. (2019). Subjective experience of art therapists in the treatment of bereaved clients. *Art Therapy*, *36*(2), 68–76. https://doi.org/10.1080/07421656.2019.1609329

Gelso, C. J., & Hayes, J. A. (2007). *Countertransference and the therapist's inner experience: Perils and possibilities*. Erlbaum.

Gilbert, P., & Stickley, T. (2012). "Wounded healers": The role of lived-experience in mental health education and practice. *Journal of Mental Health Training, Education and Practice*, *7*(1), 33–41. https://doi.org/10.1108/17556221211230570

Greene, D., Yaffe, J., & Kopak, A. (2019). Relapse among recovering addiction professionals: Prevalence and predictors. *Journal of Social Work Practice in the Addictions*, *19*(4), 323–344. https://doi.org/10.1080/1533256X.2019.1653718

Hayes, J., Yeh, Y., & Eisenberg, A. (2007). Good grief and not-so-good grief: Countertransference in bereavement therapy. *Journal of Clinical Psychology*, *63*(4), 345–355. https://doi.org/10.1002/jclp.20353

Henretty, J., Currier, J., Berman, J., Levitt, H., & Henretty, J. (2014). The impact of counselor self-disclosure on clients: A meta-analytic review of experimental and quasi-experimental research. *Journal of Counseling Psychology*, *61*(2), 191–207. https://doi.org/10.1037/a0036189

Hyatt, E. (2014). From healer to transformed healer: Relearning lessons in grief. *Reflection: Narratives of Professional Helping*, *20*(2), 32–41. http://search.proquest.com/docview/1752186859/

Kouriatis, B., & Brown, D. (2011). Therapists' bereavement and loss experiences: A literature review. *Journal of Loss & Trauma*, *16*(3), 205–228. https://doi.org/10.1080/15325024.2010.519289

O'Brien, J. (2011). Wounded healer: Psychotherapist grief over a client's death. *Professional Psychology, Research and Practice*, *42*(3), 236–243. https://doi.org/10.1037/a0023788

Pinto-Coelho, K., Hill, C., Kearney, M., Sarno, E. Sauber, E., Baker, S., . . . Thompson, B. (2018). When in doubt, sit quietly: A qualitative investigation of experienced therapists' perceptions of self-disclosure. *Journal of Counseling Psychology, 65*(4), 440–452. https://doi.org/10.1037/cou0000288

Rudick, C. D. (2012). Therapist self-care: Being a healing counselor rather than a wounded healer. In L. Levers (Ed.), *Trauma counseling: Theories and interventions* (pp. 554–568). Springer.

Simpson, J. (2013). Grief and loss: A social work perspective. *Journal of Loss and Trauma, 18*(1), 81–90. https://doi.org/10.1080/15325024.2012.684569

St. Arnaud, K. (2017). Encountering the wounded healer: Parallel process and supervision. *Canadian Journal of Counselling and Psychotherapy, 51*(2), 131–144.

Tedgård, E., Råstam, M., & Wirtberg, I. (2018). Struggling with one's own parenting after an upbringing with substance abusing parents. *International Journal of Qualitative Studies on Health and Well-Being, 13*(1), 1435100. https://doi.org/10.1080/17482631.2018.1435100

Tsai, M., Plummer, M., Kanter, J., Newring, R., & Kohlenberg, R. (2010). Therapist grief and functional analytic psychotherapy: Strategic self-disclosure of personal loss. *Journal of Contemporary Psychotherapy, 40*(1), 1–10. https://doi.org/10.1007/s10879-009-9116-6

Wheeler, S. (2007). What shall we do with the wounded healer? The supervisor's dilemma. *Psychodynamic Practice, 13*(3), 245–256. https://doi.org/10.1080/14753630701455838

Worden, J. (2018). *Grief counseling and grief therapy: A handbook for the mental health practitioner* (5th ed.). Springer.

Zerubavel, N., & Wright, M. (2012). The dilemma of the wounded healer. *Psychotherapy, 49*(4), 482–491. https://doi.org/10.1037/a0027824

4 Understanding the Brain

Grief and Substance Abuse

Emily A. Barton

The human brain is a wonderfully complex piece of machinery, capable of perpetual remodeling through neuroplasticity. As we grow, learn, and interact with the world around us, our brains are constantly responding by reprograming synaptic connections and neural pathways. Even our own behaviors, controlled by the brain, can result in neuroplastic changes. This reciprocal relationship between the brain, behavior, and environment results in every individual being truly unique, a product of their own personal genetics, experiences, and environment. Although it may sound chaotic, the ability of our brain to constantly change in response to our behaviors and the outside world is a necessary factor in our continued survival and flourishing as a species. Through a constant stream of external input from the world around us, our brain will continuously form and break associations as it learns what it should drive us toward and steer us away from. In this way, our brain is able to guide our motivated behaviors to fulfill our physiological, psychological, and social needs.

One of our primary psychological needs is to achieve a sense of social connection and attachment (Maslow, 1943). We see evidence of the drive to form attachments starting at birth, with infants and their mothers forming immediate bonds. Interestingly, this is not a behavior unique to humans. Instead, mother–infant pair bonding is seen in nearly every mammalian species (Feldman, 2017). The fact that the drive to form attachments is conserved across so many species indicates that it must confer significant survival and reproductive benefits. It also suggests there is underlying circuitry in the brain specifically tuned to form and maintain attachments (Numan & Young, 2016). Although the original purpose of this neural circuitry may have been to initiate and promote the mother–infant bond, it appears we are now utilizing this neural system to form and maintain multiple complex social bonds and relationships (Chambers & Wallingford, 2017). This broad array of attachment targets suggests that the neurological mechanisms underlying attachment formation can be used well beyond infancy and childbirth, and in a multitude of ways. Moreover, individual differences in attachment style and outcomes demonstrate the flexibility of this neural system, and how it can become dysfunctional when attachments fail to form normally or are disrupted.

DOI: 10.4324/9781003106906-4

Although the ability to form complex social bonds has allowed us to flourish as a species, it has also made us vulnerable to disorders and dysfunction stemming from attachment (Chambers & Wallingford, 2017). Two specific examples of dysfunctional or disrupted attachment are addiction and grief. Addiction can be viewed as a pathological attachment, potentially stemming from insecure or chaotic attachment early in life (Schindler, 2019; Strathearn et al., 2019), whereas grief can be conceptualized as a broken or unresolved attachment, in which the subject of the attachment is gone, but the need for that attachment remains (Jain et al., 2019). Given their connections to dysfunction within the attachment system, it is not surprising that addiction and grief often co-occur and share similar patterns of neural activation and processes. This chapter will explore the neural processes of attachment formation, addiction, and grief. By first understanding the neural processes that motivate us to seek out and maintain attachments, we can explore how those processes can lead to the development of maladaptive attachments with substances of abuse, and how they are altered when an attachment is lost. We will also investigate the relationship between grief and addiction to understand how they may inform each other through similar neural pathways and developmental trajectories. Improving our understanding of these neural networks shared between addiction and grief can better inform the development of therapeutic practices to help clients detach from their addictions and disruptive attachments.

Neuroscience of Reward and Motivation

Reward is one of the primary motivational factors for our behavior, and it is driven by a set of structures in the brain known collectively as the reward system. These structures run on dopamine and are tasked with determining the incentive salience of stimuli and driving our associated goal-oriented behaviors. Anything you perceive as rewarding, such as the first sip of coffee in the morning to seeing a loved one's face, will cause an increase of dopamine in this system along with the sensation of reward. This system will learn to associate cues and behaviors with positive outcomes to reinforce the behaviors that brought about that spike in dopamine. Once conditioned, we will continue to engage in these behaviors even without the direct reinforcement. Through this action, the reward system is also responsible for our repeated behaviors and habit formation. Understanding how the components of the reward system interact with each other is crucial to understanding what motivates our behaviors.

Components of the Reward System

The structures comprising the reward system communicate through the mesocorticolimbic dopamine pathway. This interconnected pathway begins in the midbrain with the ventral tegmental area (VTA), one of the two main areas of dopamine synthesis in the brain. The neurons extending from the VTA send diverse dopaminergic signals throughout the limbic system and cortex that communicate reward prediction, aversive stimuli, alerting stimuli, and salience (Bromberg-Martin et al., 2010). Specific areas within this pathway include the striatum, prefrontal cortex (PFC), amygdala, and hippocampus (Love, 2014). Through this complex dopaminergic signaling and the unique functioning of the different neural areas involved, this network is able to respond to both novel and familiar stimuli and guide our motivated behavior.

The Striatum

Residing in the forebrain, the striatum is functionally divided into dorsal and ventral subregions. The dorsal striatum contains the caudate nucleus and putamen. These structures are part of a set of nuclei collectively known as the basal ganglia, which receive dopaminergic inputs from the substantia nigra (SN) and serve a fundamental role in the execution of voluntary movement (Báez-Mendoza & Schultz, 2013; Haber & Knutson, 2010). However, the nuclei of the basal ganglia also receive dopaminergic inputs from the VTA along the mesocorticolimbic pathway. This insight has led to an enhanced understanding of the roles of the basal ganglia in cognition, reward processing, and habit formation (Schultz, 2016). Specifically, the dorsal striatum appears to utilize reward information from the ventral striatum to make decisions and guide behavior based on expected reward value (Balleine et al., 2007).

Within the ventral striatum, we find a central node of the brain's reward system, the nucleus accumbens (NAc; Báez-Mendoza & Schultz, 2013). The NAc shares rich connections with other limbic structures including the amygdala, hippocampus, and PFC (Salgado & Kaplitt, 2015). As the primary functions of the limbic structures center around emotion and memory, these connections within the limbic system allow the NAc to be a major player in emotional processing. Indeed, dysfunction with the NAc is linked to several psychological disorders including mood disorders, anxiety disorders, and addiction (Kalivas & Volkow, 2005; Salgado & Kaplitt, 2015). The NAc is also the primary input of the basal ganglia, suggesting it serves as the interface between the motor and emotional systems (Salgado & Kaplitt, 2015). By having direct connections to emotions and behavior, the NAc drives goal-directed behavior and works to optimize the outcomes from motivated behavior (Turner et al., 2018). Overall, the NAc is viewed as a key mediator of motivation and incentivized behavior within the reward pathway (Salgado & Kaplitt, 2015).

The Prefrontal Cortex

Located in the frontal lobe, the PFC is a cortical region involved in complex cognitive processes including planning, impulse control, decision-making, and working memory (Fuster, 2019; Goyal et al., 2008). The PFC is functionally divided into several subdivisions, including the medial prefrontal cortex (mPFC), orbitofrontal cortex (OFC), and the anterior portion of the cingulate cortex (ACC; (Chaua et al., 2018; Murray & Rudebeck, 2018). Although all the subregions provide different functions, they work together to plan and guide motivated behavior. In this way, they are able to produce decisions based on the predicted rewards versus costs of a particular behavioral choice (Murray & Rudebeck, 2018).

The PFC also exerts important regulatory control over limbic structures, allowing for response inhibition, impulse control, and emotional regulation (Goldstein & Volkow, 2011). Through connections to the striatum, the different areas of the PFC contribute to the formation and maintenance of learned response inhibition (Meyer & Bucci, 2014). The PFC also shares connections with the amygdala, exerting top-down control to regulate emotional states, anxiety, and fear. In disorders like depression, anxiety, and post-traumatic stress disorder (PTSD) this circuit appears to be dysfunctional, leading the amygdala to be hyperresponsive with no dampening from the PFC (Fowler et al., 2017; Ironside et al., 2017; Liberzon & Abelson, 2016). Therefore, proper functioning of the PFC is needed for response regulation, optimal decision-making, and emotional regulation.

The Amygdala

Located bilaterally in the medial temporal lobe, the amygdala is well known for its involvement in emotion, reward, fear, and pain processing (Thompson & Neugebauer, 2017). One major role is providing emotional valence and context to stimuli. By receiving sensory information from the thalamus and several cortical areas, the amygdala is able to combine this information and attach emotional and affective context to it. This newly processed information is then relayed to additional areas to generate emotional and behavioral responses (Thompson & Neugebauer, 2019). The amygdala also plays a role in associative, or Pavlovian, learning. When presented with new stimuli, the amygdala encodes the initially neutral stimulus and connects it to the emotionally relevant outcomes (Fernando et al., 2013). This can be vitally important for survival and fear conditioning. However, this associative learning mediated by the amygdala is not specific to fearful stimuli. It appears that the amygdala can store both appetitive and aversive association memories (Fernando et al., 2013). Ultimately, this processing allows the amygdala to promote behaviors aimed at seeking out rewarding stimuli and avoiding unpleasant stimuli (Fernando et al., 2013; Kakarala et al., 2020).

The Hippocampus

Also located bilaterally in the medial temporal lobe, the hippocampus is a limbic structure known for its involvement in learning and declarative memory consolidation (Anand & Dhikav, 2012). Like the striatum, it is also functionally divided into dorsal and ventral subregions. The dorsal hippocampus is involved in cognitive processes including learning and memory, while the ventral hippocampus is involved in the processing of emotion, affect, and stress (Fanselow & Dong, 2010). The ventral hippocampus shares direct connections with the amygdala, which are thought to provide the emotional context to learning and memory (Thompson & Neugebauer, 2019). Additionally, the ventral hippocampus sends direct inputs to the NAc. Activation of this pathway strengthens the goal-direct behavior driven by the NAc (LeGates et al., 2018), suggesting this pathway plays an important role in regulating reward behavior.

Motivated Behavior: Forming Attachments

Our motivated behaviors are ultimately achieved through a complex signaling cascade between the PFC, amygdala, hippocampus, and areas of the striatum. One such motivated behavior, shared by both grief and addiction, is attachment formation. We are inherently social beings; having and maintaining social relationships is vital to our overall mental and physical health (Inagaki, 2018). Early in life, forming a bond with a caregiver is needed for survival. Additionally, managing to develop a secure attachment with caregivers provides a feeling of security and allows for emotional regulation and the development of healthy coping strategies (Schindler, 2019). As we grow older, continuing to have social attachments confers numerous health benefits, whereas social isolation is linked to increased health problems, increased stress, and death (Cacioppo et al., 2015; Feldman, 2017). To ensure that we seek out these needed social connections, we most likely evolved to find attachment rewarding (Eisenberger, 2015). In support of this idea, we see increased dopamine activity in the NAc of mothers watching videos of their infant children (Atzil et al., 2017) and in the VTA of adults viewing the faces of their romantic partners (Aron et al., 2005).

From Motivation to Habit: Shift in Reward Processing

There is strong support for attachments activating structures within the reward system, including the VTA, striatum, amygdala, and PFC (Haber & Knutson, 2010; Schultz, 2000). These structures work together to guide our motivated behavior by detecting the relevant cues, assessing their reward value, and guiding behavioral action. In the case of social attachment, activation of these areas motivates us to engage in social orienting, social seeking, and to maintain enduring social connections (Acevedo et al., 2012; Chevallier et al., 2012; Feldman, 2017). Interestingly, there appears to be a shift in processing as an attachment stabilizes. Initially in attachment formation, it is the NAc in the ventral striatum that drives the motivated behavior. However, as the attachment stabilizes, our motivation to maintain the attachment needs to change from reward seeking to familiarity seeking. To produce this change in behavior, the activation shifts from the NAc in the ventral striatum to the caudate and putamen in the dorsal striatum. Recall the caudate and putamen are both part of the basal ganglia, a set of nuclei involved in movement and habit formation.

Therefore, shifting from the reward-centered NAc to the habit-centered basal ganglia allows for a change in seeking out what is novel to appreciating what is familiar and stable (Feldman, 2017; Tops et al., 2014). This shift from ventral to dorsal striatal activation is seen in the automation of most of our goal-directed behaviors.

Pathological Attachment: Addiction in the Brain

Addiction and attachment share a complex and reciprocal relationship. There is strong evidence showing individuals who failed to form secure attachments early in life are more likely to develop substance use disorders (SUDs) as they grow older (Alvarez-Monjaras et al., 2019; Hiebler-Ragger & Unterrainer, 2019; Schindler, 2019). Moreover, using substances may also have a negative impact on forming subsequent attachments and relationships (Suchman & DeCoste, 2018). Given this relationship, addiction can be thought of a pathological type of attachment itself (Unterrainer et al., 2018), in which the individual has formed a detrimental attachment to the use of a substance. Conceptualizing addiction as a pathological form of attachment may aid in the understanding and treatment of addiction. Through investigating the neurodevelopmental pathways that may lead to addiction and the neural mechanisms responsible for motivation and attachment formation, we can develop a better understanding of the motivational and behavioral patterns seen in addiction.

Neurodevelopmental Pathways Connecting Attachment and Addiction

From birth, we are wired to form attachments with our parents or caregivers. Children will seek out their caregivers during times of danger or distress. If the child is met with comfort from their caregiver(s), the child will start to view their caregiver(s) as a "secure base" they can rely on. By having this security, the child is able to explore their environment, learn to regulate their feelings, and start to acquire coping strategies (Bowlby, 1969, 1973). Failing to form this secure attachment during childhood can lead individuals to have negative views of themselves, issues trusting others, and negative expectations when it comes to relationships. Individuals may also develop poor coping strategies and have issues regulating their emotions (Schindler, 2019). In an effort to "self-medicate," individuals may then seek out substances of abuse as a way to control their emotions, cope, and replace the relationships they find difficult to form (Schindler & Bröning, 2015). In addition to this psychosocial hypothesis, a complementary explanation for the increased susceptibility to developing an SUD ties in a neurodevelopmental perspective. Early life experiences shape both the oxytocin and dopamine pathways involved in motivated and social behavior (Peña et al., 2014; Strathearn et al., 2009). Alterations in these pathways during development may fundamentally alter affiliative and goal-directed behavior in adulthood.

Alterations in the Oxytocin Pathway

The neuropeptide oxytocin is an important regulator of parental, romantic, and socially affiliative behaviors (Feldman, 2012). When functioning at a normal level, the oxytocin system should promote trust, reduce stress, increase resilience, and provide protection against addiction (Tops et al., 2014). Oxytocin is hypothesized to play a role in the shift from ventral to dorsal striatal processing as behavior changes from reward seeking to an appreciation of what is familiar (Tops et al., 2014). Through this action, oxytocin should offer some protection against addiction by enhancing the salience of familiar social cues, while reducing novelty and reward seeking (Strathearn et al., 2019). However, early life adversity including trauma, insecure attachment, and other stressors can alter the development and long-term functioning of oxytocin pathways, potentially resulting in an increased vulnerability to addiction (Buisman-Pijlman et al., 2014; Strathearn et al., 2019). In rats, maternal separation (a model of early life stress) results in impaired social behavior, impaired maternal behavior, increased anxiety, and increased reward seeking (Kambali et al., 2019; Todeschin et al., 2009). Furthermore, this exposure to early life stress was shown to reduce the number of oxytocin neurons, suggesting adverse early life events can produce lasting alterations in the oxytocin pathway (Todeschin et al., 2009). Clearly, we cannot investigate the specific number of oxytocin neurons or receptors in the brains of people after experiencing early life adversity. However, there is consistent evidence showing decreased levels of circulating oxytocin in individuals who experienced childhood trauma and stress (Fries et al., 2005; Heim et al., 2009; Opacka-Juffry & Mohiyeddini, 2012). Combined with the results from animal studies, it appears early life adversity is sufficient to induce long-lasting alterations to the oxytocin system. Furthermore, these alterations contribute to behaviors linked to addiction susceptibility, including reduced social affiliation and increased reward seeking.

Alterations in the Dopamine Pathway

Early life experiences also alter the development and long-term functioning of the dopaminergic reward pathways. Maternal separation sensitizes the dopaminergic reward pathway by increasing dopamine activity in the NAc (Amancio-Belmont et al., 2020; Meaney et al., 2002). Additionally, Amancio-Belmont et al. (2020) found that rats exposed to maternal separation as pups displayed increased anxiety and alcohol consumption in adulthood. It is highly probable that the increase in anxiety contributed to the increase in alcohol preference and consumption. From these results, we can extrapolate that children who are lacking that sense of trust and security may have difficulty learning how to regulate their emotions and form healthy coping mechanisms. Moreover, that early life experience may alter the development of their dopamine and oxytocin pathways leading to a sensitized reward system, increased reward-seeking behavior, and increased anxiety. These neurological predispositions coupled with poor regulatory and coping skills create the perfect storm of conditions leading to an increased likelihood of seeking out and relying on substances of abuse later in life.

Neural Systems Contributing to the Establishment of Addiction

The etiology of addiction is highly complex, involving multiple environmental, social, genetic, and biological factors. Given this complexity, there will always be individual differences in vulnerability, expression, and degree of addiction. Despite these differences, we do see some consistencies in the effects substances of abuse exert on specific areas of the brain and how those effects allow for the establishment of an addiction. Specifically, substances of abuse appear to hijack the reward and motivational pathways to produce the compulsive drug seeking, loss of control in drug use, and drug cravings that are characteristic of addiction (Edwards & Koob, 2010; P. J. Meyer et al., 2016). These behavioral changes are hypothesized to be due to substances of abuse altering two major neural systems: (a) the striatal system responsible for initiating and stabilizing motivated behavior and (b) the frontal cortical system responsible for regulating our actions (P. J. Meyer et al., 2016).

Motivated Behavior and Conditioning: The Striatum

For a substance to have addictive potential, it must be rewarding. This means that every substance of abuse will find a way to increase dopamine transmission in the NAc (Wise, 2008). This sudden activation of the reward pathway will increase the likelihood of using the substance again, through positive reinforcement. Once an individual is addicted to a substance, however, taking the drug will fail to cause the same spike of dopamine in the NAc (Uhl et al., 2019). Instead, the spike of dopamine will occur in the dorsal striatum in response to cues associated with the drug (Volkow et al., 2006). Shifting to a cue-induced spike in dopamine will cause increased cravings and drug-seeking behaviors, driven by negative reinforcement and the basal ganglia.

Loss of Control and Executive Function: The Prefrontal Cortex

Individuals struggling with addiction fall into a cycle of continuing to use substances even though it leads to negative consequences (Crews & Boettiger, 2009). The rewarding properties of substances of abuse certainly contribute to the establishment of addiction; however, the inability to stop using despite negative outcomes suggests additional issues with cognitive and behavioral control. This has led researchers to examine the role of the frontal lobes, specifically the PFC, in addiction. Patients with damage to the PFC show a propensity for impulsive and risky behaviors and tend to favor immediate rewards over larger rewards they would have to wait for (Bialaszek et al., 2017; McHugh & Wood,

2008). These traits bear a striking similarity to behaviors we see in addiction, suggesting frontal dysfunction is involved in the addictive cycle.

Several regions of the PFC share connections with the striatum and basal ganglia through frontostriatal circuits. These circuits allow the PFC to exert top-down control over the striatum and basal ganglia, in order to control impulsive actions, inhibit responses, and drive goal-directed behaviors (Morein-Zamir & Robbins, 2015). Substances of abuse appear to have direct influence over the functioning of these connections, allowing for many of the behaviors seen in habitual drug use to develop and persist. Specifically, prolonged drug use is linked to reduced excitability of neurons in the mPFC, and experimental excitation of those neurons reduces drug-seeking behavior in rats (Chen et al., 2013). This finding suggests drugs of abuse may reduce activation of the mPFC, thereby hampering its ability to inhibit impulsive, drug-seeking behavior.

In addition to altering the connectivity between structures, prolonged substance misuse, especially of alcohol, can significantly damage the overall structure and integrity of the frontal lobes. Patients with alcohol use disorders (AUDs) will often have reduced metabolic activity and cortical atrophy in the PFC, correlating with reduced cognitive flexibility and memory impairments (Kubota et al., 2001; Pandey et al., 2018). Moreover, animal models of binge alcohol consumption show evidence of cellular dysfunction in the PFC, with reduced neuronal volume and priming of the microglia, the primary immune cells of the brain (Barton, Baker et al., 2017; Barton, Lu et al., 2017; West et al., 2019). These cellular alterations suggest a potential compounding effect of continued alcohol binges that could lead to an exaggerated immune response, neuroinflammation, and potential cell death. Ultimately, the alterations of the frontal lobes at the cellular, structural, and functional levels allow for significant alterations in behavioral and cognitive control. Given the influential role of the frontal lobes in behavioral regulation, decision-making, and impulsivity, it is hypothesized that the alcohol-induced damage to this area contributes to the "spiral of addiction," as continued alcohol intake leads to progressive neurodegeneration of the area required to make good decisions and control continued consumption of alcohol (Crews et al., 2004; Koob & Volkow, 2010). Essentially, alcohol and other substances of abuse are able to weaken the inhibitory control over the striatum and our cognitive control, allowing for continued drug seeking and use.

When Attachment Is Disrupted: Grief in the Brain

Recall that we have a biological drive to seek out and form social attachments with caregivers and those close to us. These attachments activate the reward system, producing spikes in dopamine when we see our children and romantic partners (Aron et al., 2005; Atzil et al., 2017). But what happens if we lose those close to us? What once brought a feeling of pleasure and reward now also brings sadness, longing, and a reminder of loss. This turns memories of those we have lost into both rewarding and punishing stimuli. How does our brain deal with this dichotomy and learn to regulate our emotions following the loss of a loved one? Neuroimaging studies are able to provide us a glimpse into this process. Compared to addiction, however, the neuroscientific study of grief is still fairly nascent, and is primarily focused on the more clinically significant complicated grief (CG). Therefore, this section will outline the major brain structures highlighted to date as being involved in CG.

Neural Structures Implicated in Grief

In investigating CG, neuroimaging studies are beginning to reveal a fairly consistent neural footprint, involving disruption in the neural reward center and corticolimbic pathways. The involvement of these areas and pathways certainly correlates with the intense yearning, obtrusive thoughts, preoccupation with the deceased, and issues with emotional regulation that characterize CG (Arizmendi & O'Connor, 2015). Specific neural areas that have been highlighted in the literature include the striatum, basal ganglia, ACC, OFC, and amygdala (Arizmendi et al., 2016; Fernández-Alcántara et al., 2016; Freed et al., 2009; Kakarala et al., 2020). We will dive deeper into the role these structures may play in processing grief to gain a better understanding of the potential root causes for some of the most common symptoms.

Alterations in the Reward System: Striatum, Basal Ganglia, and Orbitofrontal Cortex

Given the role the reward system plays in attachment formation and maintenance, it is not surprising that several neuroimaging studies have highlighted the reward system as being a key player in grief processing. Our attachments offer us sustained feelings of reward through activation of this pathway, but the loss of a primary attachment can cause significant psychological upheaval (Inagaki, 2018). Following a significant loss, our motivational systems have to learn to reprioritize our attachments and utilize other relationships as our primary attachment to regain balance. Failing to do so and continuing to rely on a deceased or lost attachment figure may contribute to the development of CG (LeRoy et al., 2019). Specifically, this would result in continued expectation of reward without receiving it and may underlie the intense yearning felt in CG (Kakarala et al., 2020). Interestingly, this intense yearning and persistent fixation mirrors the drug cravings seen in addiction; again, implicating the involvement of the reward system, specifically the striatum.

Initial evidence showing reward system activation while grieving came from O'Connor et al. (2008). This study demonstrated a significant increase in NAc activity in only those diagnosed with CG, compared to those experiencing noncomplicated grief, while viewing grief-related photos and words. Unfortunately, this study utilized fMRI analysis methods now known to produce a high rate of false positives (Eklund et al., 2016), and additional studies have failed to replicate this exact finding in elderly individuals experiencing grief (Kakarala et al., 2020; McConnell et al., 2018). This does not eliminate the possibility of the NAc contributing to the experience of CG, however additional research is needed to confirm its role.

Additional striatal structures have also been implicated in CG by neuroimaging studies, namely, the portion of the basal ganglia in the dorsal striatum. It is theorized that the basal ganglia structures utilize reward information from the OFC and error detection from the ACC to select the proper behavioral response in any given situation (Huey et al., 2008). However, a dysfunction in this circuit can lead to disruptions in reward processing and behavior selection. In obsessive-compulsive disorder (OCD), for example, over-activation of this circuit leads to increased error messages and incomplete reinforcement signals reaching the basal ganglia. This may lead the individual to feel certain behavioral sequences are wrong or incomplete, forming a feeling of dissonance and the basis of an obsession. The individual may then enact compulsive behaviors as a way to reduce the dissonance (Huey et al., 2008). A similar activation pattern between the OFC and basal ganglia has been see in those experiencing grief and is linked to increased rumination and intrusive thoughts about the deceased (Schneck et al., 2017, 2018). In this model, thoughts of the deceased would activate the neural reward system, however this feeling of reward coupled with the reminder of loss may cause an increase in error signals sent to the basal ganglia. To correct this feeling of dissonance from the unresolved attachment, the basal ganglia may seek out rewarding behavior, including thinking about the deceased, thus perpetuating a cycle of overactivation between the OFC and basal ganglia. Although recurring thoughts of the deceased are a typical part of the grieving process (Arizmendi & O'Connor, 2015), these obtrusive thoughts persisting for an extended amount of time may contribute to the pathological symptoms of CG.

Emotional Dysregulation: Amygdala Connectivity

Emotional experience is an integral aspect of the grieving process; during which individuals will often experience emotions including sadness, guilt, and anger (Fernández-Alcántara et al., 2020). For those who experience CG, we often see dysfunctions in emotional processing and impairments in regulating emotions across different contexts (Fernández-Alcántara et al., 2016; Gupta & Bonanno, 2011). Given the importance of emotional experience in grief, several researchers have focused their attention on the neural areas responsible for generating and regulating our emotions, namely, the limbic system. Several limbic areas have been linked to grief through neuroimaging studies (Fernández-Alcántara et al., 2020; Freed et al., 2009; Kakarala et al., 2020). One specific pattern that continues to emerge in these studies is disrupted connectivity between the amygdala and regions of the PFC, correlating strongly with the severity of grief symptoms.

As discussed previously, the amygdala plays an important role in determining emotional salience of stimuli and guiding our behavior accordingly. Additionally, the amygdala receives inhibitory signals from the PFC to further regulate emotional reactivity and behaviors. Inhibitory functional connectivity between the amygdala and PFC allows for emotional regulation (Lee et al., 2012). However, disruptions to this connectivity prevent the PFC's top-down control of the amygdala and are linked to different affective disorders including depression and anxiety (Fowler et al., 2017; Ironside et al., 2017). One study by Freed et al. (2009) found that low negative functional connectivity between the PFC and amygdala correlated with sadness intensity. These results suggest the reduced control from the PFC allowed the amygdala to bias attention toward grief-related cues. In another study by Arizmendi et al. (2016), the researchers found that individuals with CG failed to recruit frontal regions to regulate their emotions during an emotional Stroop task. Furthermore, the researchers also found reduced connectivity between the PFC and amygdala in those with CG reporting intrusive thoughts. Additional studies have also found increased activation in the amygdala while participants viewed sad and death-related images, although they did not examine the functional connectivity with the PFC (Bryant et al., 2019; Fernández-Alcántara et al., 2020). Taken together, these results suggest increased amygdala activation coupled with decreased regulation from the PFC may contribute to the disrupted emotional processing observed in CG. Moreover, the over-activation of the amygdala may specifically bias attention toward the lost attachment figure, further perpetuating the yearning and inability to move on.

Overlap Between Addiction and Grief: Clinical Implications

Many parallels exist between addiction and grief. In both, a maladaptive attachment results in intense yearning or cravings, preoccupation with the attachment target, and disruptions to daily functioning. Moreover, clinical evidence suggests the experience of one is often a risk factor for developing the other (Parisi et al., 2019). For instance, following a significant loss, individuals may turn to the use of substances to fill the lost attachment and, in turn, risk developing an SUD (Pilling et al., 2012; Stahl & Schulz, 2014). Additionally, different models attempting to explain the occurrence of CG point toward substance misuse as a risk factor (Boelen, 2006; Stroebe et al., 2006). Several links and commonalities exist between these disorders, most likely accounting for the shared risk and overlap. In terms of social and environmental experience, there is overlap between substance misuse and loss. Often those coping with SUDs have experienced loss in their lives and may even find themselves grieving the loss of the substance itself and the life they once had (Furr et al., 2015). Additionally, early life experiences and other biological predispositions may bias the functioning of reward and motivational pathways toward the development of these disorders.

Neural Similarities of Addiction and Grief

Both addiction and CG appear to stem from disfunction within the reward and motivational systems. In both disorders, cues are driving the craving or yearning for the object of attachment, at the detriment to the individual. This cue-induced craving can be traced back to dopaminergic signaling in the dorsal striatum in both addiction (Volkow et al., 2006) and grief (Schneck et al., 2017). Someone struggling with an addiction may encounter drug-related environments or paraphernalia that signal drug use, cueing the dorsal striatum to engage in drug-seeking behaviors to alleviate the cravings and conditioned compensatory response to the drug (Ramos et al., 2002). If the drug seeking is successful, the reduction of this negative state will further perpetuate drug use through negative reinforcement. During bereavement, an individual could encounter reminders of their loss through photographs, objects, environments, and activities. These reminders may act as cues, triggering the dorsal striatum to produce yearning and seeking behaviors. However, the seeking behavior may not be possible if the grief is due to loss. This could leave their negative state unresolved and drive them to seek comfort elsewhere. Some may be able to refocus this behavior to seeking out social support, which would help to facilitate reorganizing their attachment hierarchy to present individuals. For others, however, this option may not be viable or simply may not be utilized. Instead, this negative state may drive others to seek out relief through unhealthy coping mechanisms like substance use.

Another striking similarity between the neural patterns of addiction and grief is the reduced functional connectivity between the PFC and other limbic structures. Some substances of abuse, such as alcohol, specifically target and damage the PFC, allowing for impulsive behavior and reduced behavioral control. Even with substances that do not produce direct damage in the PFC, we still see reduced functional connectivity between the striatum, hippocampus, and amygdala (Chen et al., 2013; Pascoli et al., 2018). Reduced top-down control of these regions from the PFC may specifically bias drug and cue-related attention, memory, and goal-directed behavior. Moreover, reduced functional connectivity between the PFC and amygdala has also been found in individuals experiencing CG (Arizmendi et al., 2016; Freed et al., 2009). In grief, a failure of the PFC to dampen amygdala activity may create an attentional bias toward the cues and memories of the lost attachment. Just as in addiction, this may contribute to the preoccupation and craving for what the individual cannot, or should not, have. In all, both addiction and grief appear to stem from reduced inhibition of attention toward and seeking of unhealthy or absent attachments.

Combined Developmental Susceptibilities for Addiction and Grief

Similar alterations in the functioning of cortical and limbic structures are seen in both addiction and CG using neuroimaging studies. These studies, however, cannot tell us the directionality of this effect. It may be the case that changes in these structures and pathways cause the behavioral symptoms and thought patterns of both addiction and CG. However, it is also plausible that the experience of addiction and CG induces the alterations in these pathways. In truth, it is most likely a combination of both explanations. Given the ability of experience and the environment to exert profound effects on the structure and function of the brain, determining true causality can be nearly impossible. One specific period when the brain is uniquely susceptible to change in response to the environment and experiences is during early childhood. At this time period, adverse experiences are able to reshape and alter pathways in the brain that can persist into adulthood. Two pathways particularly vulnerable to the shaping effects of these events are the dopamine and oxytocin pathways involved in social, motivated, and reward behavior (Peña et al., 2014; Strathearn et al., 2009). As previously discussed, early life adversity, especially related to disrupted attachment, may predispose individuals to be more susceptible to developing SUDs. In addition, the increased anxiety, changes to the reward system, and potential development of poor coping skills could also contribute to the development of CG later in life. Moreover, children who experience loss early in life have an increased risk for developing SUDs (Høeg et al., 2017) and CG (Zisook & Shear, 2009). An early lack or loss of attachment appears to reshape how the brain responds to and seeks out reward and social affiliation, increasing the risk for an individual to develop both addiction and CG. This is not to say that early life adversity is to blame for either disorder, or that it is required to experience addiction or grief. Instead, these findings support the idea that there are shared neural pathways at the heart of both addiction and grief.

Implications for Practitioners

Whenever a client presents with a disorder like addiction, grief, or a dual diagnosis, their neural pathways will already be functioning in an altered way. This altered function could be due to early life experiences altering their developmental trajectory as well as their current experiences and behaviors reshaping their neural pathways and overall function. One culprit behind this neural rewiring may be the stress system. Both addictive substances and the initial experience of grief activate the hypothalamus-pituitary-adrenal (HPA) axis, resulting in increased levels of cortisol and other stress hormones (Lovallo, 2006; O'connor, 2012). Activation of this system is needed in life-or-death situations, however prolonged activation of the HPA axis can produce numerous detrimental effects. In the brain, the hippocampus is specifically vulnerable to the effects of stress. Prolonged exposure to stress hormones will cause cell death, an overall loss of volume, and a loss of plasticity (Kim et al., 2015). Following this loss of hippocampal neurons, or "burn-down," there may be a period of regrowth, or "build-up." In this regrowth period, new neurons would be created in the neurogenic region of the hippocampus and begin to work their way into the hippocampal circuitry. However, researchers who have tracked these neurons have found that they are functionally altered and engage in different connectivity patterns (Chambers et al., 2004; Chambers & Wallingford, 2017). These new neurons born from stress may contribute to the altered functional connectivity in both addiction and grief seen in the reward center circuitry including the hippocampus, amygdala, striatum, and PFC. Moreover, this suggests the recovery from both addiction and grief will engage similar, interconnected processes of using neuroplasticity to rewire the circuits connecting these structures (Chambers & Wallingford, 2017).

In treating patients with addiction or a dual diagnosis, it may be beneficial to view addiction recovery as a form of grief. The recovery process will require the individual to undergo emotional work that requires grieving and processing the giving up of relationships, activities, environments, and habits of their former lives (Chambers & Wallingford, 2017). In addition to reshaping their lives, those in recovery will also need to jumpstart neuroplasticity to reshape their brains. Increasing neuroplasticity can be achieved pharmacologically through traditional antidepressants like selective serotonin reuptake inhibitors (SSRIs), although it can take multiple weeks to start seeing the beneficial effects (Kraus et al., 2017). Other pharmacological options, like ketamine, may offer additional treatment options. Ketamine is much faster acting than traditional SSRIs and is thought to be beneficial in treating addiction and reducing depressive symptoms through increasing neuroplasticity and neurogenesis (Ivan Ezquerra-Romano et al., 2018). Continued research and randomized control trials are still needed to determine its safety and efficacy; however, the initial findings are encouraging. Another interesting avenue is the use of neuromodulation to retrain the addicted, or grieving, brain. Real-time functional magnetic resonance imaging neurofeedback (rtfMRI-nf) is emerging as a way for patients to learn how to self-regulate the activation and connectivity in specific areas of their brains. Researchers and clinicians are using rtfMRI-nf to help regulate brain activity for several different disorders ranging from PTSD (Zotev et al., 2018) to schizophrenia (Orlov et al., 2018). Studies utilizing rtfMRI-nf as an intervention for addiction are still very new; however, they show some promising effects with the managing of cravings (Luigjes et al., 2019; Martz et al., 2020). An intervention that combined the self-regulated neuromodulation of rtfMRI-nf with the neuroplastic boost of medication or even physical exercise (El-Sayes et al., 2019) could prove to be immensely beneficial in the neural rewiring needed to detach individuals from their addictions and facilitate the grieving process. Although all of these treatment options require further research and clinical trials, this continued research and interest in retraining the brain will hopefully yield improved treatment options.

Every person brings with them a unique blend of biological, psychological, and environmental factors that shape how their brain interprets and responds to the world around them. All these individual differences can necessitate the use of personalized therapeutic methods and recovery plans that may still fail or need revising. One commonality among all of us, however, is the ability of the brain to change. Utilizing this neuroplasticity could bring about immense changes in how individuals process and move past their addictions. Through rewiring the connections between the striatum, amygdala, hippocampus, and PFC, individuals may be able to regain regulatory control over their intrusive thoughts, cravings, and actions, thereby allowing them to break cycles of unhealthy reward seeking and successfully detach from their addictions and dysfunctional attachments.

References

Acevedo, B. P., Aron, A., Fisher, H. E., & Brown, L. L. (2012). Neural correlates of long-term intense romantic love. *Social Cognitive and Affective Neuroscience, 7*(2), 145–159. https://doi.org/10.1093/scan/nsq092

Alvarez-Monjaras, M., Mayes, L. C., Potenza, M. N., & Rutherford, H. J. V. (2019). A developmental model of addictions: Integrating neurobiological and psychodynamic theories through the lens of attachment. *Attachment and Human Development, 21*(6), 616–637. https://doi.org/10.1080/14616734.2018.1498113

Amancio-Belmont, O., Becerril Meléndez, A. L., Ruiz-Contreras, A. E., Méndez-Díaz, M., & Prospéro-García, O. (2020). Maternal separation plus social isolation during adolescence reprogram brain dopamine and endocannabinoid systems and facilitate alcohol intake in rats. *Brain Research Bulletin, 164,* 21–28. https://doi.org/10.1016/j.brainresbull.2020.08.002

Anand, K., & Dhikav, V. (2012). Hippocampus in health and disease: An overview. *Annals of Indian Academy of Neurology, 15*(4), 239–246. https://doi.org/10.4103/0972-2327.104323

Arizmendi, B. J., Kaszniak, A. W., & O'Connor, M. F. (2016). Disrupted prefrontal activity during emotion processing in complicated grief: An fMRI investigation. *NeuroImage, 124,* 968–976. https://doi.org/10.1016/j.neuroimage.2015.09.054

Arizmendi, B. J., & O'Connor, M. F. (2015). What is "normal" in grief? *Australian Critical Care, 28*(2), 58–62. https://doi.org/10.1016/j.aucc.2015.01.005

Aron, A., Fisher, H., Mashek, D. J., Strong, G., Li, H., & Brown, L. L. (2005). Reward, motivation, and emotion systems associated with early-stage intense romantic love. *Journal of Neurophysiology, 94*(1), 327–337. https://doi.org/10.1152/jn.00838.2004

Atzil, S., Touroutoglou, A., Rudy, T., Salcedo, S., Feldman, R., Hooker, J. M., Dickerson, B. C., Catana, C., & Barrett, L. F. (2017). Dopamine in the medial amygdala network mediates human bonding. *Proceedings of the National Academy of Sciences of the United States of America, 114*(9), 2361–2366. https://doi.org/10.1073/pnas.1612233114

Báez-Mendoza, R., & Schultz, W. (2013). The role of the striatum in social behavior. *Frontiers in Neuroscience, 7,* 233. https://doi.org/10.3389/fnins.2013.00233

Balleine, B. W., Delgado, M. R., & Hikosaka, O. (2007). The role of the dorsal striatum in reward and decision-making. *Journal of Neuroscience, 27*(31), 8161–8165. https://doi.org/10.1523/JNEUROSCI.1554-07.2007

Barton, E. A., Baker, C., & Leigh Leasure, J. (2017). Investigation of sex differences in the microglial response to binge ethanol and exercise. *Brain Sciences, 7*(10). https://doi.org/10.3390/brainsci7100139

Barton, E. A., Lu, Y., Megjhani, M., Maynard, M. E., Kulkarni, P. M., Roysam, B., & Leasure, J. L. (2017). Binge alcohol alters exercise-driven neuroplasticity. *Neuroscience, 343.* https://doi.org/10.1016/j.neuroscience.2016.11.041

Bialaszek, W., Swebodzinski, B., & Ostaszewski, P. (2017). Intertemporal decision making after brain injury: Amount-dependent steeper discounting after frontal cortex damage. *Polish Psychological Bulletin, 48*(4), 456–463. https://doi.org/10.1515/ppb-2017-0052

Boelen, P. (2006). Cognitive-behavioral therapy for complicated grief: Theoretical underpinnings and case descriptions. *Journal of Loss and Trauma, 11*(1), 1–30. https://doi.org/10.1080/15325020500193655

Bowlby, J. (1969). *Attachment and loss*. Basic Books.

Bowlby, J. (1973). *Attachment and loss: Volume 2. Separation, anxiety and anger.* Basic Books.

Bromberg-Martin, E. S., Matsumoto, M., & Hikosaka, O. (2010). Dopamine in motivational control: Rewarding, aversive, and alerting. *Neuron, 68*(5), 815–834. https://doi.org/10.1016/j.neuron.2010.11.022

Bryant, R. A., Andrew, E., & Korgaonkar, M. S. (2019). Distinct neural mechanisms of emotional processing in prolonged grief disorder. *Psychological Medicine*. https://doi.org/10.1017/S0033291719003507

Buisman-Pijlman, F. T. A., Sumracki, N. M., Gordon, J. J., Hull, P. R., Carter, C. S., & Tops, M. (2014). Individual differences underlying susceptibility to addiction: Role for the endogenous oxytocin system. *Pharmacology Biochemistry and Behavior, 119*, 22–38. https://doi.org/10.1016/j.pbb.2013.09.005

Cacioppo, J. T., Cacioppo, S., Capitanio, J. P., & Cole, S. W. (2015). The neuroendocrinology of social isolation. *Annual Review of Psychology, 66*, 733–767. https://doi.org/10.1146/annurev-psych-010814-015240

Chambers, R. A., Potenza, M. N., Hoffman, R. E., & Miranker, W. (2004). Simulated apoptosis/neurogenesis regulates learning and memory capabilities of adaptive neural networks. *Neuropsychopharmacology, 29*(4), 747–758. https://doi.org/10.1038/sj.npp.1300358

Chambers, R. A., & Wallingford, S. C. (2017). On mourning and recovery: Integrating stages of grief and change toward a neuroscience-based model of attachment adaptation in addiction treatment. *Psychodyn Psychiatry, 45*(4), 451–473. https://doi.org/10.1521/pdps.2017.45.4.451

Chaua, B. K. H., Jarvisc, H., Lawa, C. K., & Chongc, T. J. (2018). Dopamine and reward: A view from the prefrontal cortex. *Behavioural Pharmacology, 29*(7), 569–583. https://doi.org/10.1097/FBP.0000000000000424

Chen, B. T., Yau, H. J., Hatch, C., Kusumoto-Yoshida, I., Cho, S. L., Hopf, F. W., & Bonci, A. (2013). Rescuing cocaine-induced prefrontal cortex hypoactivity prevents compulsive cocaine seeking. *Nature, 496*(7445), 359–362. https://doi.org/10.1038/nature12024

Chevallier, C., Kohls, G., Troiani, V., Brodkin, E. S., & Schultz, R. T. (2012). The social motivation theory of autism. *Trends in Cognitive Sciences, 16*(4), 231–239. https://doi.org/10.1016/j.tics.2012.02.007

Crews, F. T., & Boettiger, C. A. (2009). Impulsivity, frontal lobes and risk for addiction. *Pharmacology Biochemistry and Behavior, 93*(3), 237–247. https://doi.org/10.1016/j.pbb.2009.04.018

Crews, F. T., Collins, M. A., Dlugos, C., Littleton, J., Wilkins, L., Neafsey, E. J., Pentney, R., Snell, L. D., Tabakoff, B., Zou, J., & Noronha, A. (2004). Alcohol-induced neurodegeneration: When, where and why? *Alcoholism: Clinical and Experimental Research, 28*(2), 350–364. https://doi.org/10.1097/01.ALC.0000113416.65546.01

Edwards, S., & Koob, G. F. (2010). Neurobiology of dysregulated motivational systems in drug addiction. *Future Neurology, 5*(3), 393–410. https://doi.org/10.2217/fnl.10.14

Eisenberger, N. I. (2015). Social pain and the brain: Controversies, questions, and where to go from here. *Annual Review of Psychology, 66*(1), 601–629. https://doi.org/10.1146/annurev-psych-010213-115146

Eklund, A., Nichols, T. E., & Knutsson, H. (2016). Cluster failure: Why fMRI inferences for spatial extent have inflated false-positive rates. *Proceedings of the National Academy of Sciences, 113*(28), 7900–7905. https://doi.org/10.1073/pnas.1602413113

El-Sayes, J., Harasym, D., Turco, C. V., Locke, M. B., & Nelson, A. J. (2019). Exercise-induced neuroplasticity: A mechanistic model and prospects for promoting plasticity. *Neuroscientist, 25*(1), 65–85. SAGE. https://doi.org/10.1177/1073858418771538

Fanselow, M. S., & Dong, H. W. (2010). Are the dorsal and ventral hippocampus functionally distinct structures? *Neuron, 65*(1), 7–19. https://doi.org/10.1016/j.neuron.2009.11.031

Feldman, R. (2012). Oxytocin and social affiliation in humans. *Hormones and Behavior, 61*(3), 380–391. https://doi.org/10.1016/j.yhbeh.2012.01.008

Feldman, R. (2017). The neurobiology of human attachments. *Trends in Cognitive Sciences, 21*(2), 80–99. https://doi.org/10.1016/j.tics.2016.11.007

Fernández-Alcántara, M., Cruz-Quintana, F., Pérez-Marfil, M. N., Catena-Martínez, A., Pérez-García, M., & Turnbull, O. H. (2016). Assessment of emotional experience and emotional recognition in complicated grief. *Frontiers in Psychology, 7*, 126. https://doi.org/10.3389/fpsyg.2016.00126

Fernández-Alcántara, M., Verdejo-Román, J., Cruz-Quintana, F., Pérez-García, M., Catena-Martínez, A., Fernández-Ávalos, M. I., & Pérez-Marfil, M. N. (2020). Increased amygdala activations during the emotional experience of death-related pictures in complicated grief: An fMRI study. *Journal of Clinical Medicine, 9*(3), 851. https://doi.org/10.3390/jcm9030851

Fernando, A. B. P., Murray, J. E., & Milton, A. L. (2013). The amygdala: Securing pleasure and avoiding pain. *Frontiers in Behavioral Neuroscience, 7*(DEC). https://doi.org/10.3389/fnbeh.2013.00190

Fowler, C. H., Miernicki, M. E., Rudolph, K. D., & Telzer, E. H. (2017). Disrupted amygdala-prefrontal connectivity during emotion regulation links stress-reactive rumination and adolescent depressive symptoms. *Developmental Cognitive Neuroscience, 27*, 99–106. https://doi.org/10.1016/j.dcn.2017.09.002

Freed, P. J., Yanagihara, T. K., Hirsch, J., & Mann, J. J. (2009). Neural mechanisms of grief regulation. *Biological Psychiatry, 66*(1), 33–40. https://doi.org/10.1016/j.biopsych.2009.01.019

Fries, A. B. W., Ziegler, T. E., Kurian, J. R., Jacoris, S., & Pollak, S. D. (2005). Early experience in humans is associated with changes in neuropeptides critical for regulating social behavior. *Proceedings of the National Academy of Sciences of the United States of America, 102*(47), 17237–17240. https://doi.org/10.1073/pnas.0504767102

Furr, S. R., Johnson, W. D., & Goodall, C. S. (2015). Grief and recovery: The prevalence of grief and loss in substance abuse treatment. *Journal of Addictions and Offender Counseling, 36*(1), 43–56. https://doi.org/10.1002/j.2161-1874.2015.00034.x

Fuster, J. M. (2019). The prefrontal cortex in the neurology clinic. In *Handbook of clinical neurology* (Vol. 163, pp. 3–15). Elsevier B.V. https://doi.org/10.1016/B978-0-12-804281-6.00001-X

Goldstein, R. Z., & Volkow, N. D. (2011). Dysfunction of the prefrontal cortex in addiction: Neuroimaging findings and clinical implications. *Nature Reviews Neuroscience*, *12*(11), 652–669. https://doi.org/10.1038/nrn3119

Goyal, N., Siddiqui, S., Chatterjee, U., Kumar, D., & Siddiqui, A. (2008). Neuropsychology of prefrontal cortex. *Indian Journal of Psychiatry*, *50*(3), 202. https://doi.org/10.4103/0019-5545.43634

Gupta, S., & Bonanno, G. A. (2011). Complicated grief and deficits in emotional expressive flexibility. *Journal of Abnormal Psychology*, *120*(3), 635–643. https://doi.org/10.1037/a0023541

Haber, S. N., & Knutson, B. (2010). The reward circuit: Linking primate anatomy and human imaging. *Neuropsychopharmacology*, *35*(1), 4–26. https://doi.org/10.1038/npp.2009.129

Heim, C., Young, L. J., Newport, D. J., Mletzko, T., Miller, A. H., & Nemeroff, C. B. (2009). Lower CSF oxytocin concentrations in women with a history of childhood abuse. *Molecular Psychiatry*, *14*(10), 954–958. https://doi.org/10.1038/mp.2008.112

Hiebler-Ragger, M., & Unterrainer, H. F. (2019). The role of attachment in poly-drug use disorder: An overview of the literature, recent findings and clinical implications. *Frontiers in Psychiatry*, *10*, 579. https://doi.org/10.3389/fpsyt.2019.00579

Høeg, B. L., Appel, C. W., von Heymann-Horan, A. B., Frederiksen, K., Johansen, C., Bøge, P., . . . Bidstrup, P. E. (2017). Maladaptive coping in adults who have experienced early parental loss and grief counseling. *Journal of Health Psychology*, *22*(14), 1851–1861. https://doi.org/10.1177/1359105316638550

Huey, E. D., Zahn, R., Krueger, F., Moll, J., Kapogiannis, D., Wassermann, E. M., & Grafman, J. (2008). A psychological and neuroanatomical model of obsessive-compulsive disorder. *Journal of Neuropsychiatry*, *20*(4), 390–408. https://doi.org/10.1176/appi.neuropsych.20.4.390

Inagaki, T. K. (2018). Opioids and social connection. *Current Directions in Psychological Science*, *27*(2), 85–90. https://doi.org/10.1177/0963721417735531

Ironside, M., Browning, M., Ansari, T. L., Harvey, C. J., Sekyi-Djan, M. N., Bishop, S. J., . . . O'Shea, J. (2017). Prefrontal cortex regulates amygdala response to threat in trait anxiety. *BioRxiv*, 215699. https://doi.org/10.1101/215699s

Ivan Ezquerra-Romano, I., Lawn, W., Krupitsky, E., & Morgan, C. J. A. (2018). Ketamine for the treatment of addiction: Evidence and potential mechanisms. *Neuropharmacology*, *142*, 72–82. https://doi.org/10.1016/j.neuropharm.2018.01.017

Jain, F. A., Connolly, C. G., Moore, L. C., Leuchter, A. F., Abrams, M., Ben-Yelles, R. W., . . . Iacoboni, M. (2019). Grief, mindfulness and neural predictors of improvement in family dementia caregivers. *Frontiers in Human Neuroscience*, *13*. https://doi.org/10.3389/fnhum.2019.00155

Kakarala, S. E., Roberts, K. E., Rogers, M., Coats, T., Falzarano, F., Gang, J., . . . Prigerson, H. G. (2020). The neurobiological reward system in prolonged grief disorder (PGD): A systematic review. *Psychiatry Research—Neuroimaging*, *303*. https://doi.org/10.1016/j.pscychresns.2020.111135

Kalivas, P. W., & Volkow, N. D. (2005). The neural basis of addiction: A pathology of motivation and choice. *American Journal of Psychiatry*, *162*(8), 1403–1413. https://doi.org/10.1176/appi.ajp.162.8.1403

Kambali, M. Y., Anshu, K., Kutty, B. M., Muddashetty, R. S., & Laxmi, T. R. (2019). Effect of early maternal separation stress on attention, spatial learning and social interaction behaviour. *Experimental Brain Research*, *237*(8), 1993–2010. https://doi.org/10.1007/s00221-019-05567-2

Kim, E. J., Pellman, B., & Kim, J. J. (2015). Stress effects on the hippocampus: A critical review. *Learning and Memory*, *22*(9), 411–416. https://doi.org/10.1101/lm.037291.114

Koob, G. F., & Volkow, N. D. (2010). Neurocircuitry of addiction. *Neuropsychopharmacology*, *35*(1), 217–238. https://doi.org/10.1038/npp.2009.110

Kraus, C., Castrén, E., Kasper, S., & Lanzenberger, R. (2017). Serotonin and neuroplasticity—Links between molecular, functional and structural pathophysiology in depression. *Neuroscience and Biobehavioral Reviews*, *77*, 317–326. https://doi.org/10.1016/j.neubiorev.2017.03.007

Kubota, M., Nakazaki, S., Hirai, S., Saeki, N., Yamaura, A., & Kusaka, T. (2001). Alcohol consumption and frontal lobe shrinkage: Study of 1432 non-alcoholic subjects. *Journal of Neurology Neurosurgery and Psychiatry*, *71*(1), 104–106. https://doi.org/10.1136/jnnp.71.1.104

Lee, H., Heller, A. S., van Reekum, C. M., Nelson, B., & Davidson, R. J. (2012). Amygdala-prefrontal coupling underlies individual differences in emotion regulation. *NeuroImage*, *62*(3), 1575–1581. https://doi.org/10.1016/j.neuroimage.2012.05.044

LeGates, T. A., Kvarta, M. D., Tooley, J. R., Francis, T. C., Lobo, M. K., Creed, M. C., & Thompson, S. M. (2018). Reward behavior is regulated by the strength of hippocampus-nucleus accumbens synapses HHS Public Access. *Nature*, *564*(7735), 258–262. https://doi.org/10.1038/s41586-018-0740-8

LeRoy, A. S., Knee, C. R., Derrick, J. L., & Fagundes, C. P. (2019). Implications for reward processing in differential responses to loss: Impacts on attachment hierarchy reorganization. *Personality and Social Psychology Review*, *23*(4), 391–405. https://doi.org/10.1177/1088868319853895

Liberzon, I., & Abelson, J. L. (2016). Context processing and the neurobiology of post-traumatic stress disorder. *Neuron*, *92*(1), 14–30. https://doi.org/10.1016/j.neuron.2016.09.039

Lovallo, W. R. (2006). Cortisol secretion patterns in addiction and addiction risk. *International Journal of Psychophysiology*, *59*(3), 195–202. https://doi.org/10.1016/j.ijpsycho.2005.10.007

Love, T. M. (2014). Oxytocin, motivation and the role of dopamine. *Pharmacology Biochemistry and Behavior*, *119*, 49–60. https://doi.org/10.1016/j.pbb.2013.06.011

Luigjes, J., Segrave, R., de Joode, N., Figee, M., & Denys, D. (2019). Efficacy of invasive and non-invasive brain modulation interventions for addiction. *Neuropsychology Review*, *29*(1), 116–138. https://doi.org/10.1007/s11065-018-9393-5

Martz, M. E., Hart, T., Heitzeg, M. M., & Peltier, S. J. (2020). Neuromodulation of brain activation associated with addiction: A review of real-time fMRI neurofeedback studies. *NeuroImage: Clinical*, *27*, 102350. https://doi.org/10.1016/j.nicl.2020.102350

Maslow, A. H. (1943). A theory of human motivation. *Psychological Review*, *50*(4), 370–396. https://doi.org/10.1037/h0054346

McConnell, M. H., Killgore, W. D. S., & O'Connor, M.-F. (2018). Yearning predicts subgenual anterior cingulate activity in bereaved individuals. *Heliyon*, *4*(10), e00852. https://doi.org/10.1016/j.heliyon.2018.e00852

McHugh, L., & Wood, R. L. (2008). Using a temporal discounting paradigm to measure decision-making and impulsivity following traumatic brain injury: A pilot study. *Brain Injury*, *22*(9), 715–721. https://doi.org/10.1080/02699050802263027

Meaney, M. J., Brake, W., & Gratton, A. (2002). Environmental regulation of the development of mesolimbic dopamine systems: A neurobiological mechanism for vulnerability to drug abuse? *Psychoneuroendocrinology, 27*(1–2), 127–138. https://doi.org/10.1016/S0306-4530(01)00040-3

Meyer, H. C., & Bucci, D. J. (2014). The contribution of medial prefrontal cortical regions to conditioned inhibition. *Behavioral Neuroscience, 128*(6), 644–653. https://doi.org/10.1037/bne0000023

Meyer, P. J., King, C. P., & Ferrario, C. R. (2016). Motivational processes underlying substance abuse disorder. *Current Topics in Behavioral Neurosciences, 27*, 473–506. https://doi.org/10.1007/7854_2015_391

Morein-Zamir, S., & Robbins, T. W. (2015). Fronto-striatal circuits in response-inhibition: Relevance to addiction. *Brain Research, 1628*(Pt A), 117–129. https://doi.org/10.1016/j.brainres.2014.09.012

Murray, E. A., & Rudebeck, P. H. (2018). Specializations for reward-guided decision-making in the primate ventral prefrontal cortex. *Nature Reviews Neuroscience, 19*(7), 404–417. https://doi.org/10.1038/s41583-018-0013-4

Numan, M., & Young, L. J. (2016). Neural mechanisms of mother-infant bonding and pair bonding: Similarities, differences, and broader implications. *Hormones and Behavior, 77*, 98–112. https://doi.org/10.1016/j.yhbeh.2015.05.015

O'connor, M. F. (2012). Immunological and neuroimaging biomarkers of complicated grief. *Dialogues in Clinical Neuroscience, 14*(2), 141–148. https://doi.org/10.31887/dcns.2012.14.2/mfoconnor

O'Connor, M. F., Wellisch, D. K., Stanton, A. L., Eisenberger, N. I., Irwin, M. R., & Lieberman, M. D. (2008). Craving love? Enduring grief activates brain's reward center. *NeuroImage, 42*(2), 969–972. https://doi.org/10.1016/j.neuroimage.2008.04.256

Opacka-Juffry, J., & Mohiyeddini, C. (2012). Experience of stress in childhood negatively correlates with plasma oxytocin concentration in adult men. *Stress, 15*(1), 1–10. https://doi.org/10.3109/10253890.2011.560309

Orlov, N. D., Giampietro, V., O'Daly, O., Lam, S. L., Barker, G. J., Rubia, K., . . . Allen, P. (2018). Real-time fMRI neurofeedback to down-regulate superior temporal gyrus activity in patients with schizophrenia and auditory hallucinations: A proof-of-concept study. *Translational Psychiatry, 8*(1), 46. https://doi.org/10.1038/s41398-017-0067-5

Pandey, A. K., Ardekani, B. A., Kamarajan, C., Zhang, J., Chorlian, D. B., Byrne, K. N. H., . . . Porjesz, B. (2018). Lower prefrontal and hippocampal volume and diffusion tensor imaging differences reflect structural and functional abnormalities in abstinent individuals with alcohol use disorder. *Alcoholism: Clinical and Experimental Research, 42*(10), 1883–1896. https://doi.org/10.1111/acer.13854

Parisi, A., Sharma, A., Howard, M. O., & Blank Wilson, A. (2019). The relationship between substance misuse and complicated grief: A systematic review. *Journal of Substance Abuse Treatment, 103*, 43–57. https://doi.org/10.1016/j.jsat.2019.05.012

Pascoli, V., Hiver, A., Van Zessen, R., Loureiro, M., Achargui, R., Harada, M., . . . Lüscher, C. (2018). Stochastic synaptic plasticity underlying compulsion in a model of addiction. *Nature, 564*(7736), 366–371. https://doi.org/10.1038/s41586-018-0789-4

Peña, C. J., Neugut, Y. D., Calarco, C. A., & Champagne, F. A. (2014). Effects of maternal care on the development of midbrain dopamine pathways and reward-directed behavior in female offspring. *European Journal of Neuroscience, 39*(6), 946–956. https://doi.org/10.1111/ejn.12479

Pilling, J., Konkolÿ Thege, B., Demetrovics, Z., & Kopp, M. S. (2012). Alcohol use in the first three years of bereavement: A national representative survey. *Substance Abuse: Treatment, Prevention, and Policy, 7*(1), 3. https://doi.org/10.1186/1747-597X-7-3

Ramos, B. M. C., Siegel, S., & Bueno, J. L. O. (2002). Occasion setting and drug toler-ance. *Integrative Physiological and Behavioral Science, 37*(3), 165–177. https://doi.org/10.1007/BF02734179

Salgado, S., & Kaplitt, M. G. (2015). The nucleus accumbens: A comprehensive review. *Stereotactic and Functional Neurosurgery, 93*(2), 75–93. https://doi.org/10.1159/000368279

Schindler, A. (2019). Attachment and substance use disorders—theoretical models, empirical evidence, and implications for treatment. *Frontiers in Psychiatry, 10*, 727. https://doi.org/10.3389/fpsyt.2019.00727

Schindler, A., & Bröning, S. (2015). A review on attachment and adolescent substance abuse: Empirical evidence and implications for prevention and treatment. *Substance Abuse, 36*(3), 304–313. https://doi.org/10.1080/08897077.2014.983586

Schneck, N., Haufe, S., Tu, T., Bonanno, G. A., Ochsner, K. N., Sajda, P., & Mann, J. J. (2017). Tracking deceased-related thinking with neural pattern decoding of a cortical-basal ganglia circuit. *Biological Psychiatry: Cognitive Neuroscience and Neuroimaging, 2*(5), 421–429. https://doi.org/10.1016/j.bpsc.2017.02.004

Schneck, N., Tu, T., Michel, C. A., Bonanno, G. A., Sajda, P., & Mann, J. J. (2018). Attentional bias to reminders of the deceased as compared with a living attachment in grieving. *Biological Psychiatry: Cognitive Neuroscience and Neuroimaging, 3*(2), 107–115. https://doi.org/10.1016/j.bpsc.2017.08.003

Schultz, W. (2000). Multiple reward signals in the brain. *Nature Reviews Neuroscience, 1*(3), 199–207. https://doi.org/10.1038/35044563

Schultz, W. (2016). Reward functions of the basal ganglia. *Journal of Neural Transmission, 123*(7), 679–693. https://doi.org/10.1007/s00702-016-1510-0

Stahl, S. T., & Schulz, R. (2014). Changes in routine health behaviors following late-life bereavement: A systematic review. *Journal of Behavioral Medicine, 37*(4), 736–755. https://doi.org/10.1007/s10865-013-9524-7

Strathearn, L., Fonagy, P., Amico, J., & Montague, P. R. (2009). Adult attachment pre-dicts maternal brain and oxytocin response to infant Cues. *Neuropsychopharmacology, 34*(13), 2655–2666. https://doi.org/10.1038/npp.2009.103

Strathearn, L., Mertens, C. E., Mayes, L., Rutherford, H., Rajhans, P., Xu, G., . . . Kim, S. (2019). Pathways relating the neurobiology of attachment to drug addiction. *Frontiers in Psychiatry, 10*, 737. https://doi.org/10.3389/fpsyt.2019.00737

Stroebe, M. S., Folkman, S., Hansson, R. O., & Schut, H. (2006). The predic-tion of bereavement outcome: Development of an integrative risk factor frame-work. *Social Science and Medicine, 63*(9), 2440–2451. https://doi.org/10.1016/j.socscimed.2006.06.012

Suchman, N. E., & DeCoste, C. L. (2018). Substance abuse and addiction: Implications for early relationships and interventions. *Zero to Three, 38*(5), 17–22. www.ncbi.nlm.nih.gov/pubmed/30662145

Thompson, J. M., & Neugebauer, V. (2017). Amygdala plasticity and pain. *Pain Research and Management, 2017*. https://doi.org/10.1155/2017/8296501

Thompson, J. M., & Neugebauer, V. (2019). Cortico-limbic pain mechanisms. *Neuro-science Letters, 702*, 15–23. https://doi.org/10.1016/j.neulet.2018.11.037

Todeschin, A. S., Winkelmann-Duarte, E. C., Jacob, M. H. V., Aranda, B. C. C., Jacobs, S., Fernandes, M. C., . . . Lucion, A. B. (2009). Effects of neonatal han-dling on social memory, social interaction, and number of oxytocin and vasopressin neurons in rats. *Hormones and Behavior, 56*(1), 93–100. https://doi.org/10.1016/j.yhbeh.2009.03.006

Tops, M., Koole, S. L., Ijzerman, H., & Buisman-Pijlman, F. T. A. (2014). Why social attachment and oxytocin protect against addiction and stress: Insights from the dynamics between ventral and dorsal corticostriatal systems. *Pharmacology Biochemistry and Behavior*, *119*, 39–48. https://doi.org/10.1016/j.pbb.2013.07.015

Turner, B. D., Kashima, D. T., Manz, K. M., Grueter, C. A., & Grueter, B. A. (2018). Synaptic plasticity in the nucleus accumbens: Lessons learned from experience. *ACS Chemical Neuroscience*, *9*(9), 2114–2126. https://doi.org/10.1021/acschemneuro.7b00420

Uhl, G. R., Koob, G. F., & Cable, J. (2019). The neurobiology of addiction. *Annals of the New York Academy of Sciences*, *1451*(1), 5–28. https://doi.org/10.1111/nyas.13989

Unterrainer, H. F., Hiebler-Ragger, M., Rogen, L., & Kapfhammer, H. P. (2018). Addiction as an attachment disorder. *Nervenarzt*, *89*(9), 1043–1048. https://doi.org/10.1007/s00115-017-0462-4

Volkow, N. D., Wang, G. J., Telang, F., Fowler, J. S., Logan, J., Childress, A. R., . . . Wong, C. (2006). Cocaine cues and dopamine in dorsal striatum: Mechanism of craving in cocaine addiction. *Journal of Neuroscience*, *26*(24), 6583–6588. https://doi.org/10.1523/JNEUROSCI.1544-06.2006

West, R. K., Wooden, J. I., Barton, E. A., & Leasure, J. L. (2019). Recurrent binge ethanol is associated with significant loss of dentate gyrus granule neurons in female rats despite concomitant increase in neurogenesis. *Neuropharmacology*, *148*. https://doi.org/10.1016/j.neuropharm.2019.01.016

Wise, R. A. (2008). Dopamine and reward: The anhedonia hypothesis 30 years on. *Neurotoxicity Research*, *14*(2–3), 169–183. https://doi.org/10.1007/BF03033808

Zisook, S., & Shear, K. (2009). Grief and bereavement: What psychiatrists need to know. *World Psychiatry*, *8*(2), 67–74. https://doi.org/10.1002/j.2051-5545.2009.tb00217.x

Zotev, V., Phillips, R., Misaki, M., Wong, C. K., Wurfel, B. E., Krueger, F., . . . Bodurka, J. (2018). Real-time fMRI neurofeedback training of the amygdala activity with simultaneous EEG in veterans with combat-related PTSD. *NeuroImage: Clinical*, *19*, 106–121. https://doi.org/10.1016/j.nicl.2018.04.010

5 Women, Substance Use, and Grief

Susan R. Furr

What image comes to mind when you think of women and addiction? Do you flash on a group of women friends having a martini at lunch? Or do you immediately think of the sex worker "turning tricks" to pay for her drug habit? Alcohol and drug use among women takes on many different looks; however, for much of history substance use in women has been accompanied by a sense of shame from society. Betty Ford shocked the world in 1978 when she announced she was entering treatment for addiction to alcohol and pain medication. She did not make this decision easily; in fact, it took a family intervention for her to realize the seriousness of her addiction. She later wrote, "My makeup wasn't smeared, I wasn't disheveled, I behaved politely, and I never finished off a bottle, so how could I be alcoholic?" (Brody, 2011, p. 1).

History of women and substance use

There is a long history in the United States addressing women and substance use, which is often tied to physician involvement in prescribing medications to relieve symptoms rather than dealing with underlying, psychological issues. In the 1800s, women with serious substance use problems could be committed to asylums, lose their children, or have involuntary hysterectomies (Carter, 1997). Social stigma for the use of alcohol increased during the mid-1800s as the temperance movement became more powerful. Drinking became hidden within the home, with women often using a number of alcohol-based medicines. Opiate addiction also was prevalent during this time, with affluent women even disguising syringes as jewelry to be worn on clothing (White & Kilbourne, 2006). Opium was viewed as a "convenient sort of respectable intoxication" (Morgan, 1981, p. 27). In fact, most opiate addicts at this time were women (Kandall & Petrillo, 1996), with opium called "God's own medicine" (Morgan, 1981, p. 4).

Moving into the 20th century, women began to drink more openly and rebelled against traditional patriarchal attitudes by drinking in public (Carter, 1997). Their actions, however, continued to be linked to promiscuity and neglect of their parental responsibilities. Even during Prohibition, young women "embraced alcohol and cigarettes as symbols of liberation" (White &

DOI: 10.4324/9781003106906-5

Kilbourne, 2006, p. 4); however, these women still faced stigmatization from society's views of women and drinking. The Great Depression reduced employment opportunities for women and moved them back into the home. Coupled with the temperance movement, these two events provided some incentive for women to abstain from alcohol use. World War II was perhaps one of the biggest turning points for women because of increased employment opportunities. Although some of these work options were lost when the soldiers returned, women continued to resist gender expectations by increasing their use of alcohol. While a drunk male was seen as the life of the party, a drunk female was still viewed as loose. The public continued to see alcoholism in women as more shameful than in men. This bias may even have created discomfort for health care providers in discussing substance use with women (Padayachee, 1998). Treatment strategies emerged for males, whereas females were ignored in the research, which typically just generalized the findings about males to females (Carter, 1997).

The 1960s brought a new wave of medical treatment options for anxiety that unleashed a new type of addiction. The development of benzodiazepines (e.g., Librium, Valium) was seen as a medical miracle in the reduction of anxiety. These drugs soon became the most widely prescribed class of drugs on the market, with nearly 90 million bottles dispensed yearly (Herzberg, 2006), and were twice as likely to be prescribed to women, although their addictive properties were not recognized immediately. The use of the drug was so extensive that books such as Barbara Gordon's *I'm Dancing as Fast as I Can* (1979) and songs such as *Mother's Little Helper* by the Rolling Stones reflected this trend.

What made this trend gain attention was the focus on a legal drug that involved White, middle-class women and was supplied by physicians. The idea of addiction as a disease rather than criminal action gained new support in treatment. The recognition that drugs used to treat symptoms could create additional problems gained credence along with the idea that anyone could become an addict. Society had to grapple with the cultural split between the view of the "accidental middle class addict" and the illicit drug user (Herzberg, 2006, p. 87). One's affluent neighbor could be just as addicted as the urban poor. Yet the image of the addict has continued to be one that reflected the urban poor more than the upper strata of society.

But perhaps the most powerful evolution in response to the Valium panic was the voice of feminists in highlighting the reasons women were prescribed the drugs to begin with. These feminist voices criticized the prescribing of drugs for the psychological distress women experienced. The feminist view shifted the conversation to focus on the distress created by the constraints placed on women by political and social systems (Herzberg, 2006). One positive consequence of this shift was women were not viewed as being at fault for their addiction given that they were ignorant of the risks and were not seeking a "high" from the drug; they were just seeking relief and were provided with that relief by their physician. In addition, the sources of women's grievances with current social structures were beginning to be recognized. This was still a period of time when women were expected to support the spouse's career to the detriment of their own interests. Depression and loneliness were often ignored as contributors to their unhappiness. These feminist views were being translated into treatment programs that focused on healing the total individual rather than only promoting abstinence. The focus of addiction changed from the negative characteristics of the addict to the hardships faced by the user (Herzberg, 2006). Ironically, some of the deeper traumas experienced by women still were not addressed in relation to addiction until much later.

Women specific issues

Women's issues related to substance use often went undetected because of less visibility. Men were perceived to have higher rates of substance use disorder (SUD) due to consequences such as accidents, work problems, and drug-related crimes (Velasquez et al., 2017). Even today, young males often view drinking as a way to prove masculinity and to belong to a peer group. Risk-taking is a part of this culture and increases the chance of substance use problems being recognized. One's manhood often has been defined in terms of how "one could hold one's liquor," and alcohol use has often been praised rather than stigmatized.

However, gender differences have been found in how men and women are first exposed to substance use. Females often are introduced to alcohol use through the opposite sex yet also are taught more shame-based restraint because of concerns about vulnerability to sexual risks. In Western culture, types of drugs used also differ in that men are more likely to use illicit drugs, whereas women are more likely to become dependent on psychotherapeutic drugs that are used nonmedically (Cormier et al., 2004). Research has shown women are more likely than men to be prescribed opioids and are more likely to abuse opioids after being prescribed them for legitimate purposes (McHugh et al., 2015). In the national study on comorbidity with substance use, women were more likely to display anxiety and depressive symptoms while men more frequently displayed conduct disorders and antisocial disorders (Khan et al., 2013; McHugh et al., 2015). For women in this study, a traumatic event was significantly more likely to happen prior to the onset of the substance use problem with these women using substances to reduce negative affect.

Although a gender gap has existed in men exhibiting SUDs at a higher rate than women, this gap appears to be decreasing. The ratio of male to female alcohol abuse has decreased over time from 7:1 to 2:1 (Keyes et al., 2008), with women becoming increasingly likely to experience an SUD. These authors noted changes in gender-based norms around drinking, which reflect a more general acceptance of women engaging in alcohol use. For college students, socialization has been strongly related to the use of alcohol (Capone et al., 2007), with evidence that drinking rates increase significantly over time in college for both females and males (Brown-Rice et al., 2015). While changes in patterns of female substance use are recognized, what seems to be missing is the complexity of motivations for substance use. For clinicians, it is important to understand both the vulnerabilities that substance use creates for women and how women use substances as ways to connect as well as to cope.

Biological differences

Gender bias has been the norm in medicine throughout history, meaning the "normal" standard is assumed to be male (Hamberg, 2008). This bias has carried over to research where the typical population for clinical trials has been White males, with results generalized to whole populations. This phenomenon also has been found in the field of addiction counseling, where treatment programs have been geared to the needs of males. A distinction is needed between *gender differences*, which are defined as "socially determined roles that vary across culture and over time" (McHugh et al., 2018, p. 12), and *sex differences*, which result from biological factors that affect how the body responds to ingestion of substances. These two areas can interact to create even more complexity (National Institute on Drug Abuse [NIDA], 2018). One area of sex differences between females and males is the biological differences in response to alcohol use. Females metabolize alcohol differently from males, which results in higher blood alcohol concentrations even when equivalent amounts of alcohol are consumed (McHugh et al., 2018). Because of the metabolic difference, females reach a greater level of intoxication in relation to males when ingesting the same amount of alcohol. Even though women begin use of substances at a later age then men, they more rapidly progress to problems with substances and then rapidly move from problems to treatment seeking. This process is referred to as "telescoping" (McHugh et al., 2018, p. 14) and has been found for women using alcohol, marijuana, cocaine, and prescription opioids. The research cited in this chapter refers to cisgender individuals; research examining the biological effects of SUDs among the transgender population is rare, although high levels of SUDs have been found, with 10% of the participants reporting having received treatment for SUDs and 47% reporting binge drinking in the past three months (Keuroghlian et al., 2015). The studies reported in this chapter focus on cisgender women.

In terms of overall health issues related to alcohol use, women are more susceptible to liver disease due to women's small amount of total body water and lower level of the enzyme that metabolizes alcohol, which results in a larger proportion of alcohol being absorbed (Ait-Daoud & Bashir, 2011). Concern has been expressed over the impact of alcohol on the brains of women who meet the criteria for an SUD. Using MRIs, women identified as alcoholic had lost about 11.1% of their gray matter compared to healthy women, whereas men identified as alcoholic lost about 5.6% of their gray matter. These diagnosed women also lost about 8.2% of their white matter compared to diagnosed men, who lost about 5.3% of their white matter (Wuethrich, 2001).

Another critical difference is in the area of alcohol cravings, which have been seen as a major cause of relapse (Mo & Deane, 2016). Detoxification has been shown to be a key time for reducing both negative emotions and craving, which have been shown to be related (Petit et al., 2017). These researchers demonstrated the connection between emotions and craving was only present for men at the beginning of detoxification but continued to be present for women throughout the detoxification period. The findings indicated a need for specific treatment for depressive symptoms for women who are undergoing detoxification. Understanding this association is crucial for women in recovery. Women who are not able to see improvement in their ability to manage cravings may conclude they are failing in their recovery attempts, which is another source of loss for them. Men in treatment may view women as less capable of managing their recovery and come across as critical of women's recovery efforts. Paired with the research that indicates depression in males dissipates when sobriety is achieved but remains in females (Ait-Daoud & Bashir, 2011), women may be viewed as just needing to try harder to stay sober or dwelling too much on their feelings. The focus of the recovery program needs to shift to include approaches to manage the differences in biology.

Trauma and addiction

Which comes first: substance misuse, mood disorder, or victimization? For women, there is a complex interaction of negative life events, concurrent mental health problems, and use of substances (Cormier et al., 2004). Does one aspect lead to another, or is there a clear triggering event? What is known is as many as two-thirds of women with an SUD also have a current mental health problem such as post-traumatic stress disorder (PTSD), depression, eating disorder, or panic disorder (Zilberman et al., 2003). Women with SUDs present with these comorbid disorders at higher rates than men with SUDs. Depression is a primary diagnosis for women, whereas with men, this diagnosis is often secondary to the SUD. For women, depression is more likely to precede alcoholism and anxiety. For men, when the SUD is treated, the depression tends to subside. However, depression is a concomitant disorder for women and needs to be treated separately (Ait-Daoud & Bashir, 2011).

In a seminal study on the relationship between substance use and assault, researchers found active illicit drug use (excluding alcohol) increased the likelihood of a new violent assault for women, and that assault also led to increased risk of substance use (Kilpatrick et al., 1997). This two-year longitudinal study demonstrated the reciprocal effect between assault and substance use for women. Substance use became both a precursor to assault and a consequence of experiencing violence. Additional research has shown that women exposed to trauma with or without developing PTSD were at elevated risk for alcohol dependence, with those who developed PTSD at even greater risk for an alcohol use disorder (Sartor et al., 2010).

In examining the history of women who were in treatment for substance abuse, one study discovered that over 85% of the women surveyed in treatment centers had been victimized. Types of victimization included adult physical abuse (56.1%), childhood sexual abuse (56.3%), childhood physical abuse (56.1%), and adult sexual abuse (45.4%; Cormier et al., 2004). In an extensive review of the research literature, Simpson and Miller (2002) found in the general population that 27% of women and 16% of men reported experiencing some type of childhood sexual situation. One of the difficulties of determining these rates is related to how broadly childhood sexual abuse is defined, and the numbers previously listed included any unwanted sexual experience occurring prior to the age of 18. In comparison, the rates of childhood sexual abuse found among individuals in treatment for substance abuse have been found to be 60.9% for adolescent girls and 44.5% for adult women. However, the rates of childhood sexual abuse for males in treatment was 16% for adult males and 16.2% for adolescent males, similar to the rate in the general population. Another factor examined in this analysis was childhood physical abuse. Adult women in treatment for substance abuse had an average rate of 38.7% compared to a rate of 21% in the general population, whereas adolescent females in treatment had a rate of 46.2% compared to a 21% rate in the general population. The rate for adult males in treatment was almost identical to the rate for males in the general population (31%) but was higher for adolescent males (44.7%). While these studies cannot indicate that childhood sexual abuse and physical abuse are causes of an SUD, these authors concluded these are likely etiological factors that contribute to substance misuse (Simpson & Miller, 2002). Other studies have shown the greater the degree of lifetime trauma and the more severe the sexual abuse in childhood, the greater the likelihood substances would be used as a coping mechanism (Ullman et al., 2013).

Traumatic experiences for women do not end in childhood. Intimate partner violence (IPV) is experienced by nearly 1 in 3 women (32.9%) with nearly 1 in 10 women being raped by an intimate partner (Breiding et al., 2014). The response to IPV may be substance use, particularly for White and Latina women (Nowotny & Graves, 2013). Lacey and colleagues (2013) found women experiencing any type of abuse were at greater odds for substance use and for experiencing depressive symptoms. Adverse effects were found for specific types of abuse in that women who experienced physical abuse encountered more issues with alcohol abuse while women who were psychologically abused were more likely to experience depressive symptoms and substance use. These authors proposed that experiencing violent acts might lead to depressive symptoms resulting in alcohol and substance use being employed as coping methods. Cumulative IPV appears to create subsequent risk for PTSD, depression, delinquency, and binge drinking among adolescents (Ullman et al., 2013), which illustrates the impact of trauma through different ages. If early victimization is not addressed, there is the possibility women will continue to face mental health issues, including those associated with addiction (Salisbury & Van Voorhis, 2009). This type of trauma often leads to depression and other internalized mood disorders, which may lead to drug use as a form of self-medicating.

Loss, grief, and recovery

Often grief is only thought of in terms of dealing with death. Yet any loss, whether a physical or symbolic loss, can trigger feelings of grief. For women, many losses accompany victimization and sexual trauma, and a strong relationship has been found between grief that is unexpressed and relapse (Sanders, 2011). When sexual trauma occurs early in life, there is a loss of safety and innocence. Victims may not believe they have any power to control their own lives, thus shaping how they view future relationships. When interpersonal traumas occur, there may be a corresponding loss in the ability to trust others (Ullman et al., 2013). For example, in the face of IPV, the woman may hide this abuse from her support network, thus cutting off a coping resource. Often the partner perpetrating the violence has contributed to this loss of connection to others as well, therefore taking away all sources of support through isolating the victim by limiting contact, controlling financial resources, or restricting mobility.

As mentioned earlier, interpersonal traumas not only lead to PTSD but also to using substances to cope (Ullman et al., 2013). As discussed in Chapter 1, many losses for women precede the use of substances. While we cannot establish trauma as a causative factor due to the limits of research, a strong link has been identified between those who have experienced trauma and higher SUD rates. Women who report experiencing more types of gender-based violence have an increased risk (1.7–4.8 times higher) for psychopathology and SUD (Walsh et al., 2014).

Although not all grief meets the criteria for trauma, trauma almost always has an element of grief and loss. Sanders (2011) recommended providing a period of mourning in therapy when dealing with clients who have an SUD. Grief seems to reemerge when someone stops using (Sanders, 2011). If substance use was engaged as a means of self-medicating the pain, entering treatment takes away a primary coping mechanism. During the time period of using, many other losses may occur, such as losing custody of children, job loss, or loss of a primary relationship through separation or divorce. If sexual trauma early in life was behind the substance abuse, the victim may have been forced into premature entry into adulthood, which means a lost childhood. Recovery will need to include acknowledging and mourning the losses of the past. While there are the primary losses associated with sexual abuse, there can also be secondary losses that follow as a consequence of the primary loss. These losses can include loss of self-esteem, sense of safety, dreams associated with future relationships, and even loss of faith.

How women grieve

There is no one right way to grieve, and in many ways contemporary culture is a "mourning-avoidant culture" (Wolfelt, 2007, p. 23). Mourning is an outward expression of grief that allows the loss to be integrated into one's life. While it is natural to initially desire to push away the strong emotions of a loss, only by encountering the reality of the loss can one heal from the loss and integrate its meaning into life. In response to loss, women are more likely to seek out support groups of those with similar losses as a way to find support for their loss (Neimeyer et al., 2014). Traditionally, women have been given a healthier path to deal with grief because they have permission for emotional expression (Buckingham & Howard, 2017). More recently, there has been more emphasis on women showing strength and not being dictated by emotions. However, suppression of grief may lead to delayed reactions or unhealthy coping mechanisms such as substance use.

There has been a movement to discuss grieving differences, not in terms of female or male but in terms of intuitive and instrumental grieving. Along this continuum, intuitive grievers tend to engage in exploring and expressing the powerful emotions of loss, whereas instrumental grievers gravitate toward action-oriented ways of responding. Many individuals display a blended pattern that draws from both reactions, yet women have a greater tendency to engage in the intuitive pattern while the instrumental pattern is typical of the way males grieve (Doka & Martin, 2010). These authors emphasized that "patterns are *influenced* by gender but not *determined* by it" (p. 4). They also have found that individuals will tend to be more intuitive or more instrumental rather than a balance of the two.

Intuitive grievers will gain comfort from sharing their emotional experiences with others, particularly others who are grieving. Affect is valued above cognitions, and these grievers will openly experience the grief others are feeling and share burdens with each other. Often, terms like "working through" are used to explain the process of the intuitive griever (Doka & Martin, 2010, p. 60). While instrumental grievers do experience feelings, their feelings may not be as intense as those experienced by the intuitive griever. The instrumental griever may deal with feelings by redirecting their energy toward actions and cognitive efforts. They may be less inclined to participate in support groups but need planned actions to channel emotional energy and solve problems resulting from the loss.

Given there is a greater possibility of women being intuitive grievers and men being instrumental grievers, what might happen in a group dominated by one gender? It is not uncommon in programs that include both males and females for males to outnumber females. If the majority of group members are males, females maybe reluctant to share their painful feelings around loss for fear of being seen as overly emotional. Doka and Martin (2010) have identified the harm that may come from having to adopt a **dissonant pattern** of grieving. They view it as particularly harmful for intuitive grievers to suppress their feelings associated with the loss and believe such actions can contribute to substance abuse. It is unclear about the contribution of gender role socialization in women's ability to share emotional experiences, but it is important for treatment programs to be sensitive to the differences that may be present when males and females are assigned to the same groups. Traditional socialization practices have contributed to the acceptability of women forming strong emotional attachments and expressing their grief over losing these attachments through crying. Men have been socialized to not display their emotions for fear of being weak (Buckingham & Howard, 2017). Although men may have a need to express grief through crying, their own anxieties about doing so publicly may lead to them shutting down these emotions in women as well as in themselves.

Need for woman-focused treatment

Women entering treatment for alcohol addiction often feel undeserving of support (Gunn & Canada, 2015). Stigma is associated with women who abuse substances, in that they are seen as violating "the norms of femininity" and failing to meet the expectations of being "the good mother" (Gunn & Canada, 2015, p. 282). These issues are further compounded by the intersection of addiction with promiscuity and engagement in sex work. Stigmatization is even greater for women of color and women who have been incarcerated. Facing rejection from family and friends, women with addictions are more likely to find support from peer groups experiencing similar issues and who are more likely to provide affirmation (Sanders, 2014).

There have been mixed results with gender-specific treatment programs. While one study found no differences in retention between women-only versus mixed groups (Condelli et al., 2000), other studies have indicated women-only programs had higher retention rates, greater reduction in substance use at six-month follow-up, and greater satisfaction with the gender-specific group than those in mixed groups (Greenfield et al., 2007). Furthermore, women with low self-efficacy have shown improved treatment outcomes when assigned to women-only groups compared to those in mixed groups (Greenfield et al., 2010). Based on these results, Greenfield (2016) developed an empirically based treatment protocol that included women-specific topics related to loss such as violence and abuse.

When women enter treatment, they are also more likely to encounter treatment barriers, some of which are related to losses such as dealing with family and meeting their responsibilities for care of children. However, it can be difficult to find a program that accepts mothers and children. Financial barriers increase as the mother entering treatment tries to find care that is affordable and safe. Also, there may be a fear of children being taken from them (Cormier et al., 2004), a stigma not often encountered by men. Mothers who lose custody rights experience another challenge to self-esteem (Padayachee, 1998). In addition, the stigma of abusing substances is particularly salient for women who are pregnant, and use during pregnancy may lead to punishment rather than treatment (Velasquez et al., 2017). Not only do women fear loss of children, but women who have been in abusive relationships also fear losing the relationship because of seeking treatment (Greenfield & Grella, 2009). Even though the relationship may not have been healthy, women still may need to grieve the loss of this attachment. Programs that have primarily focused on treating men may not be attuned to address the multiple losses women experience upon entering treatment.

Although women-only programs may seem like a panacea to the issues related to being in treatment with men, the issue is not a simple one. Evidence points to the complexity of women-only treatment that needs to be more fully explored. In a qualitative study of a women-only program, participants expressed anxiety about this type of treatment in that they may not get along with the other women and feared they would not be able to hide their true feelings given the perceptive nature of women (Neale et al., 2018). Many of these women also expressed past bullying experiences with females and having previous experiences with competition with other females when engaging in sex work. In many instances, these women reported relating better to men and not trusting other women. This study focused more on client perspectives as opposed to actual outcomes. Outcome-based studies have shown participants in women-only programs had significantly less substance use and lower criminal activity a year after completion of the program compared to women in a mixed-gender program (Prendergast et al., 2011). While the women-only treatment approach provided space for discussing losses particular to women, dynamics that interfere with trust may reduce some the treatment efficacy.

Treatment needs to be tailored to the female client's needs. As discussed previously, individuals entering treatment may not be ready to delve into earlier life losses that might been the initial trigger for substance use. When first working toward abstinence, losses need to be acknowledged, but the emotional impact must be managed in a way that does not trigger more trauma. Zuckoff et al. (2006) developed a treatment strategy for complicated grief that was applied to clients with an SUD. Complicated grief is similar to PTSD, but complicated grief focuses on loss of a life-sustaining person, whereas PTSD results from exposure to a life-threatening event. They suggested treatment should first focus on developing healthy coping skills and that the counselor needs to be cautious when using provocative treatment strategies with a client with an SUD. Clients need to proceed at a pace they feel they can handle. The counselor needs to assess for the client's ability to manage the complex trauma and teach coping skills to support the client's ability to manage the immediate emotions without delving into the psychic pain until emotional strengths are built.

One treatment issue is the use of medications for conditions such as depression and anxiety. There has been a strong tendency in Alcoholics Anonymous (AA) to avoid use of prescription medications given the risks faced by alcoholics to misuse medications. However, AA has produced materials for physicians as guidelines about how to responsibly prescribe medications that can help manage these underlying conditions (AA, 2011). Given the high rates of these conditions for women with SUDs, it is important to work with a physician who is knowledgeable about the treatment of individuals with an SUD. Chambers and Wallingford (2017) have advocated for pharmacotherapies to be the norm in addiction recovery. They believe psychiatric medications help facilitate the cognitive and emotional stability needed to participate in psychotherapy.

Women enter substance abuse treatment with a myriad of losses that differ from the losses experienced by men. Their progression to addiction may be quicker, yet the recognition and support for treatment may contain more stigma. Although both men and women enter treatment to reduce the negative effects of continued substance use and to attain abstinence, a woman's path to this achievement may need to address the losses related to depression and anxiety that might have been the trigger for their substance use. Only by including emotional space for grieving can women address the losses that underlie the substance use.

References

Ait-Daoud, N., & Bashir, M. (2011). Women and substance abuse: Health considerations and recommendations. *CNS Spectrums, 16*(2), 37–47. https://doi.org/10.1017/S1092852912000168

Alcoholics Anonymous. (2011). *The AA member—medications and other drugs*. www.aa.org/pages/en_US/aa-member-medications-and-other-drugs

Breiding, M. J., Chen, J., & Black, M. C. (2014). *Intimate partner violence in the United States—2010*. National Center for Injury Prevention and Control, Centers for Disease Control and Prevention.

Brody, M. (2011, July 21). Editorial: Betty Ford transformed public perception of addiction. *Clinical Psychiatry News*. www.mdedge.com/psychiatry/article/36679/pain/editorial-betty-ford-transformed-public-perception-addiction/page/0/1

Brown-Rice, K., Furr, S., & Jorgensen, M. (2015). Analyzing Greek members alcohol consumption by gender and the impact of alcohol education interventions. *Journal of Alcohol & Drug Education, 59*(1).

Buckingham, R., & Howard, P. (2017). *Understanding loss and grief for women: A new perspective on their pain and healing*. Praeger, an imprint of ABC-CLIO, LLC.

Capone, C., Wood, M. D., Borsari, B., & Laird, R. D. (2007). Fraternity and sorority involvement, social influences, and alcohol use among college students: A prospective examination. *Psychology of Addictive Behaviors, 21*, 316–327. https://doi.org/10.1037/0893-164X.21.3.316

Carter, C. (1997). Ladies don't: A historical perspective on attitudes toward alcoholic women. *AFFILIA, 12*(4), 471–485.

Chambers, R., & Wallingford, S. (2017). On mourning and recovery: Integrating stages of grief and change toward a neuroscience-based model of attachment adaptation in addiction treatment. *Psychodynamic Psychiatry, 45*(4), 451–473. https://doi.org/10.1521/pdps.2017.45.4.451

Condelli, W., Koch, M., & Fletcher, B. (2000). Treatment refusal/attrition among adults randomly assigned to programs at a drug treatment campus: The New Jersey substance abuse treatment campus, Secaucus, NJ. *Journal of Substance Abuse Treatment, 18*(3), 395–407. http://search.proquest.com/docview/217343364/

Cormier, R., Dell, C., & Poole, N. (2004). Women and substance abuse problems. *BMC Women's Health, 4*(Suppl 1), S8–S8. https://doi.org/10.1186/1472-6874-4-S1-S8

Doka, K., & Martin, T. (2010). *Grieving beyond gender: Understanding the ways men and women mourn* (2nd ed.). Brunner-Routledge.

Gordon, B. (1979). *I'm dancing as fast as I can.* Harper & Row.

Greenfield, S. (2016). *Treating women with substance use disorders: The women's recovery group manual.* Guilford Press.

Greenfield, S., Back, S., Lawson, K., & Brady, K. (2010). Substance abuse in women. *Psychiatric Clinics of North America, 33*(2), 339–355. https://doi.org/10.1016/j.psc.2010.01.004

Greenfield, S., & Grella, C. (2009). Alcohol & drug abuse: What is "women-focused" treatment for substance use disorders? *Psychiatric Services, 60*(7), 880–882. https://doi.org/10.1176/appi.ps.60.7.880

Greenfield, S., Trucco, E., McHugh, R., Lincoln, M., & Gallop, R. (2007). The women's recovery group study: A stage I trial of women-focused group therapy for substance use disorders versus mixed-gender group drug counseling. *Drug and Alcohol Dependence, 90*(1), 39–47. https://doi.org/10.1016/j.drugalcdep.2007.02.009

Gunn, A., & Canada, K. (2015). Intra-group stigma: Examining peer relationships among women in recovery for addictions. *Drugs: Education, Prevention and Policy, 22*(3), 281–292. https://doi.org/10.3109/09687637.2015.1021241

Hamberg, K. (2008). Gender bias in medicine. *Women's Health, 4*(3), 237–243. https://doi.org/10.2217/17455057.4.3.237

Herzberg, D. (2006). "The pill you love can turn on you": Feminism, tranquilizers, and the valium panic of the 1970s. *American Quarterly, 58*(1), 79–103. https://doi.org/10.1353/aq.2006.0026

Kandall, S., & Petrillo, J. (1996). *Substance and shadow: Women and addiction in the United States.* Harvard University Press.

Keuroghlian, R. (2015). Substance use and treatment of substance use disorders in a community sample of transgender adults. *Drug and Alcohol Dependence, 152,* 139–146. https://doi.org/10.1016/j.drugalcdep.2015.04.008

Keyes, K., Grant, B., & Hasin, D. (2008). Evidence for a closing gender gap in alcohol use, abuse, and dependence in the United States population. *Drug and Alcohol Dependence, 93*(1–2), 21–29. https://doi.org/10.1016/j.drugalcdep.2007.08.017

Khan, S., Okuda, M., Hasin, D., Secades-Villa, R., Keyes, K., Lin, K., . . . Blanco, C. (2013). Gender differences in lifetime alcohol dependence: Results from the national epidemiologic survey on alcohol and related conditions. *Alcoholism: Clinical and Experimental Research, 37*(10), 1696–1705. https://doi.org/10.1111/acer.12158

Kilpatrick, D., Acierno, R., Resnick, H., Saunders, B., & Best, C. (1997). A 2-year longitudinal analysis of the relationships between violent assault and substance use in women. *Journal of Consulting and Clinical Psychology, 65*(5), 834–847. https://doi.org/10.1037/0022-006X.65.5.834

Lacey, K. K., McPherson, M. D., Samuel, P. S., Powell Sears, K., & Head, D. (2013). The impact of different types of intimate partner violence on the mental and physical health of women in different ethnic groups. *Journal of Interpersonal Violence, 28*(2), 359–385. https://doi.org/10.1177/0886260512454743

McHugh, R., Nielsen, S., & Weiss, R. (2015). Prescription drug abuse: From epidemiology to public policy. *Journal of Substance Abuse Treatment, 48*(1), 1–7. https://doi.org/10.1016/j.jsat.2014.08.004

McHugh, R., Votaw, V., Sugarman, D., & Greenfield, S. (2018). Sex and gender differences in substance use disorders. *Clinical Psychology Review, 66,* 12–23. https://doi.org/10.1016/j.cpr.2017.10.012

Mo, C., & Deane, F. P. (2016). Reductions in craving and negative affect predict 3-month post-discharge alcohol use following residential treatment. *International Journal of Mental Health Addiction* (14), 761–774.

Morgan, H. W. (1981). *Drugs in America: A social history 1800–1880*. Syracuse University Press.

National Institute on Drug Abuse. NIDA. (2018, July 12). *Substance use in women.* Retrieved January 10, 2020, from www.drugabuse.gov/publications/research-reports/substance-use-in-women

Neale, J., Tompkins, C., Marshall, A., Treloar, C., & Strang, J. (2018). Do women with complex alcohol and other drug use histories want women-only residential treatment? *Addiction, 113*(6), 989–997. https://doi.org/10.1111/add.14131

Neimeyer, R., Klass, D., & Dennis, M. (2014). A social constructionist account of grief: Loss and the narration of meaning. *Death Studies, 38*(8), 485–498. https://doi.org/10.1080/07481187.2014.913454

Nowotny, K., & Graves, J. (2013). Substance use and intimate partner violence victimization among White, African American, and Latina Women. *Journal of Interpersonal Violence, 28*(17), 3301–3318. https://doi.org/10.1177/0886260513496903

Padayachee, A. (1998). Hidden health burden: Alcohol-abusing women, misunderstood and mistreated. *International Journal of Drug Policy, 9*(1), 57–62. https://doi.org/10.1016/S0955-3959(97)00013-3.

Petit, G., Luminet, O., Cordovil de Sousa Uva, M., Monhonval, P., Leclercq, S., Spilliaert, Q., . . . de Timary, P. (2017). Gender differences in affects and craving in alcohol-dependence: A study during alcohol detoxification. *Alcoholism, Clinical and Experimental Research, 41*(2), 421–431. https://doi.org/10.1111/acer.13292

Prendergast, M., Messina, N., Hall, E., & Warda, U. (2011). The relative effectiveness of women-only and mixed-gender treatment for substance-abusing women. *Journal of Substance Abuse Treatment, 40*(4), 336–348. https://doi.org/10.1016/j.jsat.2010.12.001

Salisbury, E., & Van Voorhis, P. (2009). Gendered pathways: A quantitative investigation of women probationers' paths to incarceration. *Criminal Justice and Behavior, 36*(6), 541–566. https://doi.org/10.1177/0093854809334076

Sanders, M. (2011). *Slipping through the cracks: Intervention strategies for clients with multiple addictions and disorders*. Health Communications.

Sanders, J. (2014). *Women in narcotics anonymous: Overcoming stigma and shame*. Palgrave Macmillan.

Sartor, C., McCutcheon, V., Pommer, N., Nelson, E., Duncan, A., Waldron, M., . . . Heath, A. (2010). Posttraumatic stress disorder and alcohol dependence in young women. *Journal of Studies on Alcohol and Drugs, 71*(6), 810–818. https://doi.org/10.15288/jsad.2010.71.810

Simpson, T., & Miller, W. (2002). Concomitance between childhood sexual and physical abuse and substance use problems: A review. *Clinical Psychology Review, 22*(1), 27–77. https://doi.org/10.1016/S0272-7358(00)00088-X

Ullman, S., Relyea, M., Peter-Hagene, L., & Vasquez, A. (2013). Trauma histories, substance use coping, PTSD, and problem substance use among sexual assault victims. *Addictive Behaviors, 38*(6). https://doi.org/10.1016/j.addbeh.2013.01.027

Velasquez, M. M., Sirrianni, L., & Stotts, A. L. (2017). Substance use disorders in women. In M. Kopala & M. Keitel (Eds.), *Handbook of counseling women* (pp. 470–504). Sage.

Walsh, K., Keyes, K., Galea, S., Grant, B., & Hasin, D. (2014). Gender-based violence, psychopathology, and substance use disorder in a national sample of women. *Drug and Alcohol Dependence*, *140*(1), e236–e237. https://doi.org/10.1016/j.drugalcdep.2014.02.654

White, W., & Kilbourne, J. (2006). American women and addiction: A cultural double bind. *Counselor*, *7*(3), 46–51. www.williamwhitepapers.com/pr/2006AmericanWomen%26Addiction.pdf

Wolfelt, A. (2007). *Living in the shadow of the ghosts of grief step into the light.* Companion Press.

Wuethrich, B. (2001). Neurobiology: Does alcohol damage female brains more? *Science*, *291*(5511), 2077–2079. https://doi.org/10.1126/science.291.5511.2077

Zilberman, M., Tavares, H., Blume, S., & El-Guebaly, N. (2003). Substance use disorders: Sex differences and psychiatric comorbidities. *Canadian Journal of Psychiatry*, *48*(1), 5–13. https://doi.org/10.1177/070674370304800103

Zuckoff, A., Shear, K., Frank, E., Daley, D., Seligman, K., & Silowash, R. (2006). Treating complicated grief and substance use disorders: A pilot study. *Journal of Substance Abuse Treatment*, *30*(3), 205–211. https://doi.org/10.1016/j.jsat.2005.12.001

6 Men, Substance Use, and Grief

Mark S. Woodford

There is no grief like the grief that does not speak.
—Henry Wadsworth Longfellow

As addiction recovery deepens, individuals for the first time may begin to face the emotional impact from significant losses in their life. Unprocessed grief from the death of a loved one (Creighton et al., 2013) or relationship losses from breakups, estrangement, or divorce (Baum, 2004) can begin to surface as the numbing effects of substance use leave the body. There are also losses related to the impact of changing one's "people, places, and things" to support sustained recovery. If substance use has become a way to avoid dealing with painful life experiences (Creighton et al., 2016), then facing difficult emotions without using alcohol and other drugs may be overwhelming for individuals identifying as male who have been socialized to "take it like a man" and bear the pain of grief and loss in silence.

Given approximately two-thirds of individuals aged 12 and older admitted for the treatment of substance use disorders in the United States identify as male (Substance Abuse and Mental Health Services Administration, 2017), practitioners in the field of addiction counseling can benefit from gaining an understanding about the intersection between treatment and recovery processes and clients' notions about masculinity. More to the point, the encounters with grief and loss issues boys and men may face in treatment are inseparable from gender and cultural socialization processes (Adams, 2001). Therefore, a broader lens of "masculinities" (Seidler et al., 2018, p. 93) informed by an assessment process sensitive to the multiple ways males are taught to "be a man" in their family and culture is needed to understand the often hidden levels of loss that may begin to surface for males in recovery from substance use disorders. Understanding masculinities in this way will include being intentionally curious about the intersectionality of ethnic, familial, multicultural, racial, and sexual identities and how these points of reference include experiences with gender role conflict and oppression (O'Neil, 2015) as well as marginalization in response to their expressions of grief and loss (Zinner, 2000).

DOI: 10.4324/9781003106906-6

The ability to grieve is not a masculine or a feminine trait. Individuals—those who identify as male, female, or gender-fluid—grieve in many different ways. Some are described as "intuitive" (having adaptive ways to ventilate their feelings) and others as "instrumental" (describing their grief in more physical, behavioral, or cognitive terms), whereas some grief is described as "complicated" (Masferrer et al., 2017). Some of these behavioral patterns have been described as being related to gender but not determined by it (Doka & Martin, 2001, 2010). As Doka and Martin described in *Grieving Beyond Gender* (2010), differences in grieving behaviors are not deficiencies, rather "each pattern, depending on the way that it is utilized—as well as the societal expectations about grief—can complicate or facilitate the grieving process" (p. 202).

In this chapter, the recovery process (from grief and/or problematic substance use) is conceptualized as a *journey*. Within this metaphorical framework, there are notions about the lived experiences clients may go through as well as the role a counselor may play in the process of being a helper on the road of recovery. Related to the latter, the role of the addiction counselor can be conceptualized as a supportive *companion* on the journey (Altmaier, 2011) who can help the client to find their bearings as they encounter their grief in recovery. In this regard, the counselor can think of their work metaphorically as reflecting two relevant meanings of the word "bearing": (a) *bearing weight* (i.e., helping the client to recognize the weight they are bearing as a result of unrecognized grief) and (b) *bearing witness* (i.e., creating the space for clients to see themselves more clearly and to be seen more fully in the therapeutic relationship).

Bearing the Weight of Grief and Loss

As the song goes, "Boy you're gonna carry that weight/Carry that weight a long time" (The Beatles, 1969). Grief can be physically excruciating and exhausting. It can appear as physical effects that may show up as stiffness and pain in the head, neck, and shoulders or lower back or in a general feeling of fatigue, described in a matter of fact way by a man as "just stress." Carrying loss emotionally can manifest as if one were physically bearing the weight of the world like Atlas on one's shoulders and back. Unfortunately, traditional male socialization processes in Western culture teach boys and men to "carry that weight" and to downplay the emotional pain and suffering by remaining stoic and silent as a way to show their strength to others. Although this is not the case in every family, this burden can create a desolate, lonely landscape to begin the journey of grieving (Doka & Martin, 2010; Ossefort-Russell, 2018).

As a companion on the journey, a counselor can listen closely for the reactions in the client's body to the physical manifestations of loss that can be sometimes subtle and at other times intense, leaving one feeling out of control. Counselors can normalize these physiological reactions as an entry point into the experience of feeling grief and loss in the body. However, creating the space to normalize the somatic markers of grief and loss with boys and men is more than just a counseling technique. It takes knowledge, skills, and self-awareness to foster a welcoming gender- and culturally responsive therapeutic environment that recognizes the challenges of moving through the layers of a male client's learned, internal narratives that say things like, "Asking for help is a sign of weakness in a man."

Help-seeking behaviors are deeply influenced by gender and cultural narratives that contribute to the stigma associated with asking for help for addiction and other mental health issues (Seidler et al., 2020). Because of stigma, seeking help for problematic substance use is a challenge in and of itself, even before facing such gender-specific messages as the male cultural edict to "just suck it up" (referring to the active suppression of emotions related to grief and loss) and impulsively use alcohol (Pilling et al., 2012) or other drugs to try to forget about one's problems and temporarily alleviate suffering. This combination of barriers is the perfect storm to inhibit voluntary help seeking to cope with loss. At best, clients in this situation are ambivalent about asking for help.

Help-Seeking Behaviors: "I Am Grateful for It Now. . . . It Got Me Through the Door"

Stages of Change and Motivational Interviewing

Counselors trained in addiction treatment should be familiar with the stages of change (SOC) model and its use within the motivational interviewing (MI) counseling approach (Connors et al., 2013; Miller & Rollnick, 2013; SAMHSA, 2019). Fortunately, the SOC model and MI approach can be adapted to address ambivalent feelings or thoughts males may have related to seeking help for grief and loss. A full discussion about MI principles and practices is beyond the scope of this chapter. However, for those who are not trained in MI or the SOC models, the Substance Abuse and Mental Health Services Administration (SAMHSA) provides a Treatment Improvement Protocol (TIP 35) called *Enhancing Motivation for Change in Substance Use Disorder Treatment* (SAMHSA, 2019; downloadable at https://store.samhsa.gov). This is an excellent resource for understanding how to effectively address a client's feelings of ambivalence about seeking help in counseling for substance use disorders.

The SOC and MI models often are used in tandem to address the ambivalence clients may have about seeking help in general for various issues. Importantly, they recognize the back-and-forth pattern of inner conflict characteristic of ambivalence ("I want to, but I don't want to") as being a normal process involved in seeking help. Counselors can use MI to meet their clients at this contemplation stage of change to help them resolve their inner conflict related to seeking help from a professional. Asking the simple, open-ended question, "What brought you in the door?" will help to reveal where they are in relation to various points of clinical interest. They will likely be at very different stages of change with each clinical challenge. The emotional weight of their grief may be the furthest from their conscious awareness of why they are seeking help at this time in their life.

Consider the following stages of change of a man who may be coming to counseling to "get them off my back" (referring to his concerned significant others or coworkers). This client may be at different stages of change related to substance use versus grief. Even though you may have gleaned information from collateral contacts about a recent loss he has experienced in his life, he may be at the *precontemplation* stage of change with his grief compared to the *contemplation* stage of change for his substance use. Being in the *precontemplation* stage with his grief means he may have never considered he is having difficulties after the loss or that his losses may be affecting his substance use. He may be at the *contemplation* stage of change in relation to his substance use, meaning he is ambivalent about changing, but he has thought about reducing his alcohol use before. Focusing prematurely on the loss may create tension in the therapeutic relationship.

Importantly, the initiation of help seeking may have been the result of his loved ones' concerns about his physical health; his impatient, aggressive, or violent behaviors with others; and/or their complaints that he is "burying himself in work" instead of dealing with his grief and loss. In short, he may be in the *preparation* stage of change related to trying to do something to "get them off of my case." In this scenario, starting with what he is prepared to talk about at present will help with the beginning stages of building the counselor-client connection. In this case, it is not the pain related to the grief of loss that he is prepared to talk about in counseling. However, with patience and attention to his readiness to change, he has a chance at moving through surface-level challenges to address the underlying, unresolved feelings of grief and loss.

Each of these challenges at any stage of change may be related to what has been referred to in the psychology of boys and men as dysfunctional aspects of traditional male socialization, which is an overfocus on success, power, and competition; placing work before family relationships; or seeing emotional expression as being a solely feminine quality, reserved only for women or gay men (just to name a few examples; Adams, 2001; Clayton, 2015; Englar-Carlson et al., 2010; O'Neil, 2015). Therefore, focusing prematurely on his grief and loss, his problematic substance use, or on any other behavior labeled as "dysfunctional" by professionals or concerned significant others in his life may unintentionally evoke pushback and lessen the chances this man will return for help in counseling. The key is to listen closely and accurately reflect what specifically brought him physically in the door (or onto the telehealth screen) and to affirm and support his courage and actions thus far in reaching out.

Additionally, counselors may with all good intentions focus solely on the assessment process and on evaluating and labeling behaviors, particularly related to the client's stage of grief and/or his substance use or other mental health diagnoses. This focus will likely create a tension in the therapeutic relationship, which is a clinical indication the counselor is focusing prematurely on assessing an area that may need more "seasoning" in terms of building rapport and developing of a trusting therapeutic relationship. Focusing too heavily on evaluations and labeling patterns of grief can create an intrinsically threatening environment (Ossefort-Russell, 2018). Alternatively, a client-paced, male-sensitive approach can lay the foundation for healing and growth by fostering movement through the grief work in due time with compassionate attention to meeting the client "where they are" in the counseling process.

Importantly, related to help-seeking behaviors (or the lack thereof), using the SOC and MI models effectively with men honors their lived experiences and their readiness to face various areas of their life, including grief and loss. This approach respects the client's autonomy and freedom of choice in the counseling process and honors a "healthy dose of self-reliance," which is a position supported by the positive psychology approach to working with boys and men (Kiselica et al., 2016, p. 127).

Moving through grief in this way can be conceptualized as part of a larger gender role journey where "gender role socialization, sexism, and other forms of oppression" (O'Neil, 2015, p. 251) can be more closely examined. Importantly, with a gender-responsive counseling lens, counselors can employ the SOC and MI approaches to help a man resolve his ambivalence about seeking help. Subsequently, he may move through his own gender role journey and be able to say about the emotional, psychological, and interpersonal challenges that brought him into counseling: "I am grateful for it now. . . . it got me through the door."

Socially Constructed Masculine Ideals and Grieving: "Take It Like a Man"

Cognitive-Behavioral Therapy

A second addiction counseling approach that can be adapted for male-responsive grief work is cognitive-behavioral therapy (CBT), which in the substance use disorder treatment field is often used for either helping to maintain abstinence or reduce substance use. In this capacity, CBT has been commonly referred to as "relapse prevention" (Larimer et al., 1999; Marlatt & Gordon, 1985), although there are calls to retire this phrase as it inaccurately implies only dichotomous outcomes of either "success or failure, perfection or disaster" (Miller et al., 2019, p. 333).

CBT is particularly helpful when clients have just moved into the preparation and action stages of change in the earliest phases of recovery and need to identify high-risk situations for lapsing into problematic substance use. Identifying high-risk situations that may need to be avoided for a time can bring up feelings of loss related to changing people, places, and things in recovery. These discussions in counseling can create a dilemma: on the one hand, they create a vulnerable state of mind, whereas on the other hand, they can be an opening for beginning grief work. For example, CBT interventions focus on two specific categories of factors that can lead to a lapse back to problematic substance use: covert antecedents and immediate determinants. Examples of covert antecedents are urges and cravings. An urge is a sudden, often unexpected, behavioral impulse to use, while a craving is a desire to reexperience the effects of the substance. Covert antecedents can accompany experiences with immediate determinants of a lapse, which are those internal (emotional states) or external (people, places, or things) factors identified as high-risk situations that may lead to a lapse if one is not conscious of them and has a sudden unexpected urge or craving to use. Being sad, anxious, frustrated, or angry are just a few of the affective states associated with the grieving process (Doka & Martin, 2010) that may be included in the category of immediate determinants. These types of unacknowledged internal, emotional states can trigger thoughts of substance use.

Altmaier (2011) identified domains of grieving that may be helpful to explore as immediate determinants of a lapse into problematic substance use. For example, grief and loss and early addiction recovery share two of these important domains: (a) cognitive difficulties related to remembering, learning, or thinking; and (b) not accepting one's loss (or addictive behaviors), often with responses that manifest as numbness or shock. These challenges come with a range of internal feelings related to the loss (e.g., sadness, fear, shame) that may appear in men as anger directed at the injustice of their losses. These feelings may be accompanied by thoughts they "don't deserve to be treated this way," or they may have shattered ideals about their manhood and/or the world as a whole as they are faced with unexpected and unfamiliar territory in counseling.

Affective and cognitive responses such as these may be connected to what the psychology of boys and men call gender role schema (O'Neil, 2006), which are belief systems intricately tied to one's familial and cultural definitions of maleness and femaleness. Belief systems can guide a person's perceptions and notions about masculinity and femininity, which are often based on traditional, culturally based sex and gender roles. Importantly, gender role schema influences an individual's self-concept and therefore is used in self-evaluations related to one's adequacy in comparison to other males or females. Consequently, if one does not "meet the demands" of traditional gender roles in one's family or culture, then the learned schema creates internal "strain and conflict," which during significant gender role transitions, such as dealing with a major loss, can put pressure on boys and men to "demonstrate, resolve, reevaluate, and integrate masculinity" (O'Neil, 2015, p. 99) during the grieving process.

If counselors are paying attention to gender role schema, then various themes may begin to emerge in counseling that demonstrate places where notions about masculinity may be inhibiting the grieving process. For example, imagine the consequences of a man's thoughts (schema) related to the following themes that may emerge in grief counseling: "I should never show weakness" (strength); "Emotions are for women" (emotionality); "I have to always be in control to feel secure" (control); "I can never fail as a man" (competence); and/or "I don't need anybody, I can do everything on my own" (independence;

O'Neil, 2015). What may result from this male gender role schema is an emotional inexpressiveness that can be detrimental to the grieving process. Fortunately, Wong and Rochlen (2005) provide a five-step model for understanding how to support emotional expression in boys and men (originally proposed by Kennedy-Moore & Watson, 1999; cited in Wong & Rochlen, 2005).

Bearing Witness to Grief and Loss

Five-Step Model for Emotional Expression

Step One of the Wong and Rochlen (2005) model starts by building awareness of affective arousal in the body. One does not need to be deeply trained in mindfulness meditation to facilitate this process. It can simply be a matter of asking a man to notice what he is sensing in his body as he relates stories from his life. For example, if he is talking about the anger he has toward others whom he feels have forced him to come into counseling for help, then actively reflect his anger while affirming and supporting his courage to come into counseling despite these feelings. Asking him to notice where he is feeling the tension and stress in his body will begin the process of self-awareness related to the affective arousal in his autonomic nervous system.

Although a full discussion about polyvagal theory (Porges, 2011, 2018) is beyond the scope of this chapter, a brief caveat about how it can inform our work as counselors is in order. Specifically, it is important to understand that the delivery of an "intervention" in grief work with men will depend heavily on the strength of the therapeutic relationship, which is based on human interactions informed by our own and our client's neurophysiological states. Polyvagal theory provides a physiological basis for cultivating a healing relationship that can offer a counterpoint to unhelpful gender- and culture-specific grief responses. In short, with care and compassion, counselors can create a therapeutic environment in addiction counseling settings based on neurophysiological states where clients can sense they are being seen, heard, and felt, and they are not alone in bearing the weight of the grieving process.

As Porges (2011) describes in polyvagal theory, our own autonomic nervous system physically connects our facial expressions and the prosody of our voice through the vagal nerve with our heart, gut, and other visceral organs involved in multiple bodily systems (e.g., cardiovascular, endocrine, respiratory, musculoskeletal). These systems can cause physical distress when we are emotionally and psychologically upset about something. Having the ability to notice our own physiological responses has the effect of calming our own and our client's autonomic response (i.e., through mutual regulation). Finding ways to discuss this mutual regulation process with men may help them to understand the mechanics of their body and its need for social interactions. In particular, men will benefit from understanding our affective appraisal systems that help us determine with our mind, heart, and guts whether something or someone is "positive" or "negative" in terms of our overall well-being.

A deeper explanation of how the mechanics of the brain can be described to men in relation to neuroscience, addiction, and the capacity for being emotionally intimate is found in Woodford (2012).

In Step One, by "just noticing" their autonomic nervous system responses (e.g., heart rate, breathing, body temperature, tightness in various muscle groups), clients can become aware of their internal states of arousal, some of which may be fight, flight, or freeze responses in relation to "being forced into counseling." Awareness of this process on the counselor's part can help facilitate the settling down of an otherwise emotionally reactive stance into a more mutually regulated, emotionally responsive affective state. Understanding polyvagal theory and its implications for the counseling relationship can help to normalize intense physical and emotional grief responses and can provide a blueprint for creating restorative, therapeutic environments, which can be a counterpoint to ineffective cultural grief responses (see Ossefort-Russell, 2018, for an explanation of how polyvagal theory recognizes the importance of the autonomic nervous system responses in grief counseling).

Step Two of this process involves paying close attention to any gender-related automatic reactions that may be surfacing as a consequence of noticing the affective arousal in the body, particularly cognitions in which "masculine grievers are more comfortable" (Doka & Martin, 1998, p. 150). This process should be familiar to counselors trained in CBT. Listening for the gender role schema themes mentioned above and being curious about these belief systems (Breen et al., 2019) and their consequences can be helpful at this step. For example, noticing such thoughts as "I don't know why they think that I need help with this" can indicate an underlying male-specific traditional belief system related to holding on to a sense of "strength" and "independence" while avoiding appearing "weak" and "emotional" to others.

Exploring the sense of what it means to be a strong and independent man can lead to discussions about where these beliefs originated (e.g., family and culturally specific role models) and the workability of them in terms of dealing with the current concerns of the people who matter to him in his life. What can come from a discussion that honors the importance of strength and independence is a more nuanced definition of what it means "to be a strong man in the face of hardship." Ultimately, this can provide space for examining and redefining one's concepts of masculinity, and possibly even in a broader sense, reexamining one's humanity in finding the emotional strength to face one's grief and loss without the numbing effects of substance use and/or the deadening silence of male stoicism.

Step Three involves helping the man in this scenario find the words to express what he is experiencing (i.e., sensing, feeling, and thinking). As "some men have difficulty identifying and describing what they feel and are thus unable to express their emotions" (Wong & Rochlen, 2005, p. 64), counselors may need to use creative activities in individual or group counseling (Ogrodniczuk & Oliffe, 2009) that involve video clips, role-plays, and other experiential exercises designed to build skills in identifying and labeling emotional states.

Particularly helpful are short videos and role-play scenarios that involve individuals who identify as male attempting to deal effectively (or not) with their emotions in relation to others.

Within the realm of grief work, if a high level of trust and rapport has been developed in the individual or group counseling context, consider using situations that may represent a range of intensity related to men experiencing relatively common themes of loss, for example, scenes of defeat in athletics, relationship endings, job loss, or funerals (including pre- and post-gatherings). Often, scenes portraying male figures facing grief and loss in television and movies involve substance use, which can be helpful in exploring the connections between masculinity, alcohol and other drug use, and grief. Even scenes that depict the loss of the human–animal bond between a man and his canine companion may have profound significance for some clients (Bartone & Blazina, 2016).

Importantly, counselors will need to be cognizant of the fact these scenes related to grief and loss can be triggering for both intense emotional reactions and thoughts of using substances. This may be particularly true for scenes related to losses from war or terrorism (Christ et al., 2011). Therefore, counselors should speak openly about the potential triggering effects of the scene before showing it and use the trust and rapport that has been built to process the sensations, feelings, and thoughts that may arise during this experiential activity. Remember clients are not immune to these types of triggers in their home and community environments. Having emotional reactions and accurately identifying and labeling them in a nonthreatening, therapeutic environment can strengthen one's coping skills and abilities to face these challenges in the real world, a place that may be less forgiving of a man's tears or emotional outbursts.

As emotions begin to be accurately labeled, then Step Four warns the counselor that a man may "evaluate certain emotions as negative" (Wong & Rochlen, 2005, p. 64). For example, feelings of fear, shame, or vulnerability, all emotions that in traditional gender role schema and male socialization processes are seen as unacceptable, may produce an additional layer of thoughts and feelings that point to other cognitive themes (schema) related to competence, control, and/or the rejection of emotionality as being feminine, just to name a few.

In both Step Three and Step Four, MI can be used to work with any ambivalence that may be surfacing about exploring emotional awareness and expression in this context, particularly in the presence of other men in group work, which may create the context for gender role conflict. The concept of gender role conflict (O'Neil, 1981, 2006, 2015) has decades of research describing its behavioral, cognitive, and emotional clinical implications. In short, problems arise in contexts where men

(a) deviate from or violate gender role norms (Pleck, 1981); (b) try to meet or fail to meet gender role norms of masculinity; (c) experience discrepancies between their real and ideal self-concepts, based on gender role stereotypes (Garnets & Pleck, 1979); (d) personally devalue, restrict, or violate themselves (O'Neil et al., 1995); experience personal devaluations, restrictions, or violations from others; and (f) personally devalue, restrict, or violate others because of gender role stereotypes (O'Neil et al., 1995).

(Englar-Carlson, 2006, p. 19)

Remembering the potential for gender role conflict in this situation and addressing it with curiosity and empathy through MI can help with exploring the male socialization processes that are contributing to the inner conflict and ambivalence about finding the words to say what one is experiencing.

As a result of addressing the challenges faced in Steps One through Four, there should be some degree of increased awareness developing related to one's emotional state of grief. Subsequently, Step Five is about increasing the awareness of "appropriate" (i.e., culturally sanctioned) *contexts* for the expression of one's emotions to others. Where is it appropriate to express one's thoughts and feelings of grief and loss as a male? If one asks men what emotions they are allowed to express in most social contexts, they are likely to reply, "anger and pride."

One of the most challenging "external determinants" of a lapse to substance use is *other people*, specifically, how other people react to the changes in behavior that one is making in recovery (e.g., a man expressing emotions other than anger and pride). As described in previous steps, gender role conflict (both internally and with other people) is a real possibility. Therefore, related to *context*, males will need to carefully consider where and to whom they can safely confide their feelings of grief and loss and act accordingly.

Counselors can be explicit about the context of the work that has been done in a trusting counseling environment. Being explicit means openly discussing and assessing where in their lives they have experienced limited acceptance related to the expression of a full range of human emotions, including sadness and vulnerability. In this process, it is helpful to directly address how unique the counseling context is compared to other male-specific environments (e.g., at work, with family and friends, and in other male-dominated social environments). The bottom line is these men are learning how and when to identify people in their lives who will support this new process of living with a full range of human emotions versus "demanding" (overtly or covertly) they suffer in silence and continue to just "take it like a man."

In summary, in order to help a man address his problematic substance use and to find his bearings in the midst of unexpressed sorrow, counselors can (a) create the container that can help him recognize the weight of the grief and loss that he is carrying and (b) assist him as a companion (Altmaier, 2011) and a witness (Caverhill, 1997) on his journey of recovery and self-discovery. As Sam Cochran (2006), a seasoned, male-responsive clinician, aptly puts it: "The therapy relationship becomes a vessel for reclaiming, holding, and learning to contain the lost sadness and grief that a man has carried throughout his life" (p. 92). This work is strengthened by recognizing the multitude of masculinities that are possible, given the wide variety of familial, ethnocultural, and gender-specific socialization processes and intergenerational patterns that have shaped how men work and play, eat and relax, and deal with joys and sorrows—with or without substances.

As men have learned in counseling how to manage emotions and thoughts differently, may they recognize any positive changes about themselves that may be a result of the experience of facing their grief and loss. May they find the wisdom to keep rituals that either safely celebrate and honor accomplishments or compassionately mourn illness and death. May they experiment with new ways of being that are flexible and more fully human and that challenge the seemingly ingrained notions of what it means to "be a man" in this world.

References

Adams, D. (2001). The grief of male children and adolescents and ways to help them cope. In D. A. Lund (Ed.), *Men coping with grief* (pp. 273–308). Baywood.

Altmaier, E. M. (2011). Best practices in counseling grief and loss: Finding benefit from trauma. *Journal of Mental Health Counseling, 33*(1), 33–45. https://doi.org/10.17744/mehc.33.1.tu9wx5w3t2145122

Bartone, A., & Blazina, C. (2016). Exploring how the human-animal bond affects men in a relational way: Attachment, loss, and gender role conflict in middle-aged and young-men. In C. Blazina & L. R. Kogan (Eds.), *Men and their dogs: A new understanding of man's best friend* (pp. 231–256). Springer International.

Baum, N. (2004). On helping divorced men to mourn their losses. *American Journal of Psychotherapy, 58*(2), 174–185.

The Beatles. (1969). "Carry that weight." *Abbey Road*. EMI.

Breen, L. J., Croucamp, C. J., & Rees, C. S. (2019). What do people really think about grief counseling? Examining community attitudes. *Death Studies, 43*(10), 611–618. https://doi.org/10.1080/07481187.2018.1506527

Caverhill, P. A. (1997). Bereaved men: How therapists can help. *Psychotherapy in Private Practice, 16*(4), 1–16.

Christ, G. H., Kane, D., & Horsley, H. (2011). Grief after terrorism: Toward a family-focused intervention. In R. A. Neimeyer, D. L. Harris, H. R. Winokuer, & G. F. Thornton (Eds.), *Grief and bereavement in contemporary society: Bridging research and practice* (pp. 203–221). Routledge/Taylor & Francis Group.

Clayton, R. E. (2015). Men in the triangle: Grief, inhibition, and defense. *Journal of College Student Psychotherapy, 29*(2), 94–110. https://doi.org/10.1080/87568225.2015.1008361

Cochran, S. V. (2006). Struggling for sadness: A relational approach to healing men's grief. In M. Englar-Carlson & M. A. Stevens (Eds.), *In the room with men: A casebook of therapeutic change* (pp. 91–107). American Psychological Association.

Connors, G. J., DiClemente, C. C., Velasquez, M. M., & Donovan, D. M. (2013). *Substance abuse treatment and the stages of change: Selecting and planning interventions* (2nd ed.). Guilford Press.

Creighton, G., Oliffe, J. L., Butterwick, S., & Saewyc, E. (2013). After the death of a friend: Young men's grief and masculine identities. *Social Science & Medicine, 84,* 35–43. https://doi.org/10.1016/j.socscimed.2013.02.022

Creighton, G., Oliffe, J., Matthews, J., & Saewyc, E. (2016). "Dulling the edges": Young men's use of alcohol to deal with grief following the death of a male friend. *Health Education & Behavior, 43*(1), 54–60. https://doi.org/10.1177/1090198115596164

Doka, K. A., & Martin, T. (2001). Take it like a man: Masculine response to loss. In D. A. Lund (Ed.), *Men coping with grief* (pp. 37–47). Baywood.

Doka, K. J., & Martin, T. L. (1998). Masculine responses to loss: Clinical implications. *Journal of Family Studies, 4*(2), 143–158. https://doi.org/10.5172/jfs.4.2.143

Doka, K. J., & Martin, T. L. (2010). *Grieving beyond gender: Understanding the ways men and women mourn* (rev ed.). Routledge/Taylor & Francis Group.

Englar-Carlson, M. (2006). Masculine norms and the therapy process. In M. Englar-Carlson & M. Stevens (Eds.), *In the room with men: A casebook of therapeutic change* (pp. 13–47). American Psychological Association.

Englar-Carlson, M., Stevens, M. A., & Scholz, R. (2010). Psychotherapy with men. In J. Chrisler & D. McCreary (Eds.), *Handbook of gender research in psychology* (Vol. 2, pp. 221–252). Springer.

Kiselica, M. S., Benton-Wright, S., & Englar-Carlson, M. (2016). Accentuating positive masculinity: A new foundation for the psychology of boys, men, and masculinity. In Y. J. Wong & S. R. Wester (Eds.), *APA handbook of men and masculinities* (pp. 123–143). American Psychological Association.

Larimer, M. E., Palmer, R. S., & Marlatt, G. A. (1999). Relapse prevention: An overview of Marlatt's cognitive-behavioral model. *Alcohol Research & Health, 23*(2), 151–160.

Marlatt, G. A., & Gordon, J. R. (Eds.). (1985). *Relapse prevention: Maintenance strategies in the treatment of addictive behaviors.* Guilford Press.

Masferrer, L., Garre-Olmo, J., & Caparrós, B. (2017). Is complicated grief a risk factor for substance use? A comparison of substance-users and normative grievers. *Addiction Research & Theory, 25*(5), 361–367. https://doi.org/10.1080/16066359.2017.1285912

Miller, W. R., Forcehimes, A., & Zweben, A. (2019). *Treating addictions: A guide for Professionals* (2nd ed.). Guilford Press.

Miller, W. R., & Rollnick, S. (2013). *Motivational interviewing: Helping people change* (3rd ed.). Guilford Press.

Ogrodniczuk, J. S., & Oliffe, J. L. (2009). Grief and groups: Considerations for the treatment of depressed men. *Journal of Men's Health, 6*(4), 295–298. https://doi.org/10.1016/j.jomh.2009.07.005

O'Neil, J. M. (1981). Patterns of gender role conflict and strain: Sexism and fear of femininity in men's lives. *Personnel and Guidance Journal, 60,* 203–210.

O'Neil, J. M. (2006). Helping Jack heal his emotional wounds: The gender role conflict diagnostic schema. In M. Englar-Carlson & M. Stevens (Eds.), *In the room with men: A casebook of therapeutic change* (pp. 259–284). American Psychological Association.

O'Neil, J. M. (2015). *Men's gender role conflict: Psychological costs, consequences, and an agenda for change.* American Psychological Association.

Ossefort-Russell, C. (2018). Grief through the lens of Polyvagal Theory: Humanizing our clinical response to loss. In S. W. Porges & D. Dana (Eds.), *Clinical applications of the polyvagal theory: The emergence of polyvagal-informed therapies* (pp. 317–338). W. W. Norton.

Pilling, J., Konkolÿ Thege, B., Demetrovics, Z., & Kopp, M. S. (2012). Alcohol use in the first three years of bereavement: A national representative survey. *Substance Abuse Treatment, Prevention, and Policy, 7*(3). https://doi.org/10.1186/1747-597X-7-3

Porges, S. W. (2011). *The polyvagal theory: Neurophysiological foundations of emotions, attachment, communication, and self-regulation.* W. W. Norton.

Porges, S. W. (2018). Polyvagal theory: A primer. In S. W. Porges & D. Dana (Eds.), *Clinical applications of the polyvagal theory: The emergence of polyvagal-informed therapies* (pp. 50–69). W. W. Norton.

Seidler, Z. E., Rice, S. M., Kealy, D., Oliffe, J. L., & Ogrodniczuk, J. S. (2020). What gets in the way? Men's perspectives of barriers to mental health services. *International Journal of Social Psychiatry, 66*(2), 105–110. https://doi.org/10.1177/0020764019886336

Seidler, Z. E., Rice, S. M., River, J., Oliffe, J., & Dhillon, H. (2018). Men's mental health services: The case for a masculinities model. *Journal of Men's Studies, 26*(1), 92–104. https://doi.org/10.1177/1060826517729406

Substance Abuse and Mental Health Services Administration. (2017). *Center for behavioral health statistics and quality. Treatment episode data set (TEDS): 2005–2015.* National Admissions to Substance Abuse Treatment Services. BHSIS Series S-91, HHS Publication No. (SMA) 17–5037. Rockville, MD: Substance Abuse and Mental Health Services Administration.

Substance Abuse and Mental Health Services Administration. (2019). *Enhancing motivation for change in substance use disorder treatment.* Treatment Improvement Protocol (TIP) Series No. 35. SAMHSA Publication No. PEP19-02-01-003. Rockville, MD: Substance Abuse and Mental Health Services Administration.

Wong, Y. J., & Rochlen, A. B. (2005). Demystifying men's emotional behavior: New directions and implications for counseling and research. *Psychology of Men and Masculinity, 6*(1), 62–72. https://doi.org/10.1037/1524-9220.6.1.62

Woodford, M. S. (2012). *Men, addiction, and intimacy: Strengthening recovery by fostering the emotional development of boys and men.* Routledge.

Zinner, E. S. (2000). Being a man about it: The marginalization of men in grief. *Illness, Crisis, & Loss, 8*(2), 181–188. https://doi.org/10.1177/105413730000800206

7 African Americans

Substance Use, Grief, and Loss

Connie T. Jones and Gillian R. Galdy

> It is important to keep in mind that slaves did not come to the Americas from a social or religious void, and thus they brought with them highly evolved patterns of drug and alcohol use for religious, social, and medical purposes.
>
> (James & Johnson, 1996, p. 1)

Early African American Substance Use

African American people are descendants of Africans. They are descendants of empires—of kings and queens, warriors and healers. When Africans were forced into slavery, removed from their homeland, their families, and their freedom, they were still people—people with culture, traditions, and history. As we consider substance use among today's African Americans or Black Americans, we must remember substance use—and substance use does not equate addiction—existed among African people before they were enslaved in the United States and the intergenerational trauma of enslavement has a real and true effect on African Americans today (James & Johnson, 1996).

In Africa, beer and other substances were used for religious and social ceremonies, social purposes, and medicine (James & Johnson, 1996). James and Johnson (1996) note that due to limited medical treatment, African Americans relied on their traditional methods, including the use of alcohol, for religious and healing purposes. Historical writing does imply that slave owners did encourage drinking among those enslaved during holidays and other special occasions.

> These holidays serve as conductors, or safety valves, to carry off the rebellious spirit of enslaved humanity. . . . When a slave was drunk, the slave holder had no fear that he would plan an insurrection; no fear that he would escape to the north. It was the sober, thinking slave who was dangerous, and needed the vigilance of his master to keep him a slave.
>
> (Douglass, 1855, p. 256)

DOI: 10.4324/9781003106906-7

Substance use, coupled with the respite from enslaved labor, had lasting effects on African Americans and the patterns associated with alcohol and other illicit drugs.

Substance Use and Systemic Racism

After the Emancipation Proclamation, free African Americans established communities in Southern cities and migrated to the north to start a new life (James & Johnson, 1996). The "urbanization" of African Americans to include the mass migration north and into cities marks the transition of limited alcohol use to regular use to self-medicate in response to the emotional trauma of racism and poverty (James & Johnson, 1996).

Many laws have since proved to be inherently detrimental to the Black community. For example, Prohibition was used as a way to limit the ability of African American men from drinking or selling alcohol, under the guise that African American men were dangerous and should not be trusted (James & Johnson, 1996). From the 1930s through World War II, the African American community suffered a massive spike in narcotic use in urban areas (James & Johnson, 1996). Heroin addiction was on the rise after World War II, as many soldiers had become addicted to opioids as a form of physical pain relief during the war (Ray & Ksir, 1990). The homecoming experience for African Americans was stark. African Americans were met with few employment options and disparate treatment compared to returning White veterans, which furthered the cycle of poverty for African Americans. Within this context, African American veterans dispersed throughout the country, and heroin use—an inexpensive alternative to the opioids used during wartime—followed them (James & Johnson, 1996).

The 1960s introduced a more liberal use of marijuana, hallucinogens, and other recreational drugs across socioeconomic status (SES) and social classes within the African American community (James & Johnson, 1996). While heroin certainly plagued the African American urban community, alcohol was more detrimental on rural and urban Black communities alike. As we will discuss later in this chapter, the African American church preached abstinence, and as it were, conservative African Americans did not constructively acknowledge the rise in alcohol dependence and use of heroin among their community (James & Johnson, 1996). The high levels of alcohol dependence were seen as a standard, albeit horrific, side effect of poverty and racism.

In the 1950s and 1960s, treatment for substance use was predominantly available to White Americans. Due to the limited access African Americans had for treatment, community-based health programs were on the rise. While the African American church in the 1960s was at the center of the Civil Rights Movement and the fight for African American liberation, it often ignored the heroin epidemic. Exceptions included the New York African American Presbyterian and Baptist churches, along with programs out of Harlem Hospital and the New York Urban League. These establishments engaged in "historic efforts" to help those who were addicted in urban areas; however, due to a lack of funding and knowledge of addiction, these programs did not achieve a positive or lasting impact (James & Johnson, 1996). The heroin epidemic continued well into the 1970s and ultimately transitioned into the crack cocaine epidemic of the 1980s and 1990s, despite the efforts of community-based organizations, activists, social workers, and doctors. In part, this was due to the lack of acknowledgment of the epidemic, and thus a lack of preparation or action, by African American religious and political leaders.

The political and legal response to the heroin and crack cocaine drug epidemics was a continuation of well-established systemic racism that affects the African American community today, as evidenced by the following examples. Richard Nixon's 1971 declaration of the "war on drugs" militarized the police force against African American communities, a political movement that directly and disproportionately affects African Americans today. In 1973, New York City passed legislation, now known as the Rockefeller Laws, which sought "mandatory life sentences for selling or conspiring to sell any quantity of hard drugs; the elimination of plea-bargaining and suspended sentences; and the elimination of treatment under 'youthful offender' laws for those between the ages of sixteen and nineteen" (James & Jordan, 2018, p. 410). As James and Jordan (2018) explain, despite the intention to target drug kingpins, the majority of the people affected were those incarcerated for nonviolent, first-time offenses that disproportionately affected African Americans. Similarly, Ronald Reagan's 1986 Anti-Drug Abuse Act, which received bipartisan support, including from members of the Black Congressional Caucus, established federal sentencing of crack cocaine 100 times more severe than powder cocaine, thus incarcerating an overwhelming number of African American men (James & Jordan, 2018; Murch, 2015). In 1994, Bill Clinton's Violent Crime Control and Law Enforcement Act accelerated the mass incarceration of African Americans. We witness the continuation of Nixon's war on drugs in the expansion of the criminal correction system, now known as the New Jim Crow (Alexander, 2010), the school-to-prison pipeline, and racist military reactions to the Black Lives Matter movement (Southern Poverty Law Center, n.d.).

Cultural Considerations

Biological, Cultural, and Social Differences

It is imperative that we emphasize the importance of understanding the concept of "race." Race is a social construct (Appiah & Gutmann, 1996). Race is not genetic or biological. As we discuss the "biological" differences of the effects of substances among African Americans in comparison to other races (i.e., predominantly compared to White Americans), it is in conjunction with ethnic cultural opinions of substance use and substance use trends. These differences also exist within the context of a systemically racist response and repercussions of the government, law enforcement, and health care workers to African American substance use and addiction.

According to the Substance Abuse and Mental Health Services Administration (SAMHSA, 2020b), 6.5 million African Americans were diagnosed with a mental illness or a substance use disorder in 2019: 17.3% of African Americans over the age of 18 were diagnosed with a mental illness, 7.6% were diagnosed with a substance use disorder, and 3.2% were diagnosed with a combination of the two. Of those diagnosed with a substance use disorder, 43.8% used illicit drugs and 67.4% used alcohol (11.1% used both illicit drugs and alcohol; SAMHSA, 2020b). In 2019, 46.2% of African Americans who used illicit drugs and 32.7% of those who binged on alcohol had a serious mental illness (SMI). SAMHSA (2020a) defines an SMI as a "diagnosable mental, behavioral, or emotional disorder that an adult has experienced in the past year that causes [them] serious functional impairment that substantially interferes with or limits at least one major life activity." Of all African Americans who had a substance use disorder, 90% did not receive any treatment in 2019 (SAMHSA, 2020b).

Pedersen and McCarthy (2013) found in their study that African Americans are more sensitive to the effects of alcohol than White Americans. They found that African Americans experience a larger increase of effects, such as stimulation (i.e., needing less drinks to feel intoxicated) or sedation, as their blood alcohol levels increase compared to White Americans. The biological differences between ethnicities are more than likely due to social and cultural differences such as lower rates of alcohol consumption, thus more affected when they do consume, and stress (Pedersen & McCarthy, 2013). In each respective study, it was found that the likelihood of developing an alcohol-related illness is exacerbated depending on SES (Mulia et al., 2009), the experience of perceived discrimination and racism (Mulia et al., 2008), and other social consequences such as legal and financial troubles (Jones-Webb et al., 1995). African Americans suffer social consequences from substance use at a higher rate compared to White Americans, including financial, interpersonal, and dependency issues (Jones-Webb et al., 1995; Mulia et al., 2009). Mulia et al. (2009) found that African Americans who reported low to moderate levels of drinking were three times more likely to experience workplace and legal consequences than White Americans.

Across the board, African Americans use illicit substances at a lower rate than White Americans (SAMHSA, 2020b), so why are the legal ramifications disproportionately higher for the Black community? One explanation for the unjust disparity of incarceration of African Americans over mental health and substance use treatment is due to the racist response to the heroin epidemic of the late 1960s and 1970s and the crack cocaine epidemic of the 1980s and 1990s, which disproportionately affected the Black community (James & Jordan, 2018; Murch, 2015; James & Johnson, 1996; Hart, 2017). During the opioid epidemic of the 1960s and 1970s, "the face of the heroin addict in the media was Black, destitute and engaged in repetitive petty crimes to feed his or her habit" (Hart, 2017, p. 11). This description depicts African Americans who use substances as criminals and not as individuals who need support and treatment.

The United States finds itself in the middle of a deadly opioid epidemic once again, except this time the faces of the epidemic are White. The reaction to the problem is to treat it as a public health emergency (CDC, 2019). White Americans are using opioids at a much higher rate than African Americans, yet the African American death rate due to opioids, specifically due to heroin overdoses, has doubled since 2000 (James & Jordan, 2018). This reality is missing from the national conversation:

> [African American] deaths have been largely overlooked by the media, and non-white victims of the opioid epidemic are conspicuously absent from political discourse. To attribute this lack of discussion entirely to the low relative frequency of non-white deaths offers an incomplete explanation at best and a wholly inaccurate one at worst. Rather, the marginalization of Black people is highly consistent with a pattern of framing addiction affecting people of color as a pathological shortcoming to be answered by militarized policing and involvement of the criminal justice system, in lieu of treatment.
>
> (James & Jordan, 2018, p. 404)

African Americans have historically been incarcerated at severely higher rates than their White counterparts and make up close to half of all prisoners incarcerated for more than a year for a drug-related offense (Carson & Sabol, 2012; Rosenberg et al., 2017). The harrowing reality of racism and prejudice is evident by the numbers: according to the 2015 Bureau of Justice Statistics report on drug offenders in federal prison, 80% of convicted heroin traffickers were Black or Latino, despite the reality that White Americans buy drugs from within their race and use opioids at a higher rate (Taxy et al., 2015). Five percent of drug users are Black, yet 29% of those who are arrested for drug offenses and 33% of those in state prison for drug offenses are Black (NAACP, 2021).

Despite evidence that White Americans are more likely to use heroin, in 2015 only 13% of those incarcerated for heroin were White, while 39% were Black (Taxy et al., 2015). Fifty-three percent of those in federal prison for drug charges were imprisoned for powder or crack cocaine offenses. Of those imprisoned for powder or crack cocaine, 88% were Black; it is intriguing that research shows that White Americans are more likely to report lifetime cocaine use than Black Americans (James & Jordan, 2018), yet the numbers for those incarcerated send an entirely different message. The answer is in the law. For example, crack cocaine, which is more likely to be used by African Americans, carries a prison sentence 18 times as long as that for powder cocaine (James & Jordan, 2018).

Socioeconomic Status

SES affects education, access to fresh food, jobs (i.e., income), and health care. If one lives within a lower SES, then one has less access to resources (Feisthamel & Schwartz, 2009). Researchers indicate a lower SES contributes to a higher rate of mental illness (Hudson, 2005; Williams & Williams-Morris, 2000). The disparate and inequitable mental health care access for those most in need is problematic. As it stands, access to treatment for substance use is difficult in the United States across ethnicities. It is exponentially more diffi- cult for the Black community (James & Jordan, 2018). African Americans are less than two times as likely than White Americans to have access to treatment for substance use disorders—or any other mental health care service, for that matter (Wells et al., 2001). African Americans living below the poverty line must rely on public health insurance, a major contributing factor to why many African Americans do not receive mental health care (James & Jordan, 2018). Just over one-third of African Americans relied on public health insurance in 2019, and 14.3% did not have insurance at all (Cohen et al., 2020), yet only 60% of U.S. counties' substance use disorder outpatient services accept Med- icaid (Cummings et al., 2014), and counties that are rural, have underinsured residents, and/or are predominantly African American are even less likely to have these services (James & Jordan, 2018).

When we discuss substance use among the African American community, we must consider the effects of SES. SES, mental health, and substance use are interconnected. Although it would be convenient to simplify the connec- tion between substance use and SES, it would be inaccurate to do so. Racism on individual, institutional, and systemic levels contributes to a lower SES, which leads to dangerous levels of stress and heightens the risk of substance use (Stevens-Watkins et al., 2012). Additionally, poverty leads to an increased vulnerability to racism, thus some African Americans may become trapped in an insidious and institutionalized cycle of poverty, mental illness, substance use, and violence (Feisthamel & Schwartz, 2009). A study conducted by Stevens-Watkins et al. (2012) found that the effects of racism transcend SES when it comes to substance use. This is not to suggest poverty and racism do not have compounding effects but rather to highlight that substance use due to racism is not solely a poverty-related issue and cuts across SES.

The Intersection of Sexual Violence and Substance Use in the African American Community

Kimberlé Crenshaw, a law professor at Columbia and the University of California, Los Angeles, introduced the term *intersectionality* (Crenshaw, 1989) as a way to explain how racism and sexism do not operate indepen- dently but rather compound to further marginalize Black women (Crenshaw, 1991). Intersectionality is now defined in the Merriam-Webster (n.d.) diction- ary as "the complex, cumulative way in which the effects of multiple forms of discrimination (e.g., racism, sexism, and classism) combine, overlap, or intersect especially in the experiences of marginalized individuals or groups." Intersectionality is pivotal to our understanding of substance use within the African American community, the ways that substance use and treatment differ in origin and need among women, as well as those of the LGBTQIA+ community.

African American Women

African American women have been subjected to sexual assault and violence for centuries (Bryant-Davis et al., 2010). As enslaved peoples, sexual assault was used to dominate and oppress (Talty, 2003; Tillman et al., 2010). As private home workers (i.e., nannies and maids; Neville & Pugh, 1997), African American women were constant victims to their employers (Tillman et al., 2010). Post-Emancipation, U.S. law did not recognize African American women as victims of rape (West & Johnson, 2006). It is evident that transgenerational trauma (Bryant-Davis et al., 2010) and violent stereotypes of African American women being unrapable (Donovan & Williams, 2002) perpetuates sexual assault against African American women and girls today.

Living in poverty has a direct impact on the likelihood of sexual assault among African American women (Bryant-Davis et al., 2010). Communities with high rates of violence and substance use increase African American women's likelihood of sexual assault (Bryant-Davis et al., 2010). Researchers show a bidirectional relationship between sexual assault and income (Monnier et al., 2002). Women who live below the poverty level are at an increased risk for sexual assault and vice versa (Byrne et al., 1999). Researchers show that substance use leads to assault, and assault leads to substance use (Kilpatrick et al., 1997). Bryant-Davis et al. (2010) found that poverty was positively correlated to substance use.

Exposure to community violence, including simply being aware of sexual assault in their neighborhood, has severe mental health impacts on African American women (Jenkins, 2002). The cumulative stressors of poverty and sexual assault would make it imperative for African American women to receive resources such as mental health care. Unfortunately, African American women living in poverty are less likely to have access to resources including mental health care (Bryant-Davis et al., 2010). The lack of mental health care increases the likelihood for more severe and long-lasting psychological trauma, which leads to consequences such as substance use, post-traumatic stress disorder (PTSD), depression, and suicide (Bryant-Davis et al., 2010).

Later in this chapter, we will discuss the need for African American–focused mental health and substance use treatment, but for now we would be remiss not to mention a few of the many reasons that impoverished African American women may not seek out treatment. Beyond access to quality care in their community, there is the cost of services without insurance, the lack of transportation and/or childcare, poor quality of services from a previous provider who did not practice cultural competence, and the stigma around mental health care

(Brown, 2008). For women who have less access to health care, researchers indicate they are more likely to use illicit substances (Wu et al., 2008). In a study of substance-dependent African American women in a transitional home, Ehrmin (2002) discovered that all key participants began using alcohol and drugs as a way to "numb painful feelings" (p. 784). Common painful experiences the women identified were the death of a parent (i.e., loss), racism and rejection on an individual and societal level, physical assault by a loved one, sexual assault, and incest (Ehrmin, 2002).

African American LGBTQIA+

As intersectionality suggests, the more intersecting marginalized identities that make up an individual's identity and experience, the more systemic and social oppression they may face (Crenshaw, 1991). African Americans in the LGBT-QIA+ community not only deal with racism and sexism but also homophobia and transphobia inside and outside of their race (Hailey et al., 2020; Schuler et al., 2020). The African American LGBTQIA+ population suffers from psychological, physical, and sexual trauma in and outside of their families, racism within the LGBTQIA+ community, and rejection from their communities, all of which can be traumatizing and have long lasting mental health repercussions (Hailey et al., 2020; Akerlund & Cheung, 2000). Homophobic rejection from their families and racist rejection from the LGBTQIA+ community leaves many Black LGBTQIA+ persons feeling like they have to choose between cultures (Akerlund & Cheung, 2000). The estrangement or rejection from one's family and friends can be conceptualized as a loss and in turn lead to grief, as the individual is experiencing a shift in the relationship (Dodgson, 2020). The compounding oppression and stress of daily life would put LGBTQIA+ racial and ethnic minorities at higher risk for mental illness and substance use (Bauer, 2014; Bowleg, 2008). Unfortunately, there are still very few studies that focus on the African American LGBTQIA+ community and substance use to make any definitive conclusions about the rates of substance use based on sexual and gender identity and race (Schuler et al., 2020).

As we will discuss later in the chapter, the church and religiosity typically act as preventative factors for substance use and depression and as a source of strength and support for the African American community (Cater et al., 2012; Gibbs & Goldbach, 2015; Jang et al., 2005; Stevens-Watkins et al., 2012). However, the church has traditionally held negative views toward the LGBT-QIA+ community (Akerlund & Cheung, 2000; Rowatt et al., 2009). Those who are raised in the church experience internalized homophobia and discrimination (Barnes & Meyer, 2012; Harris et al., 2008; Shilo & Savaya, 2012) and/or feel the need to choose between their religion and their gender or sexual identity (Akerlund & Cheung, 2000). The traditional church's negative view of the LGBTQIA+ community has a direct negative impact on the African American gender and sexual minorities (GSM), who are more likely to attend church and thus be exposed to homophobic rhetoric (Barnes & Meyer, 2012). In a study by Ryan et al. (2010), researchers found that religious and lower SES families were less likely to accept their LGBTQIA+ youth. This lack of acceptance can lead to grief, as it can be viewed as an institutional loss (Dodgson, 2020).

Gender and sexual minority youth (GSMY) are at a higher risk for substance use than heterosexual youth, and the consequences may continue on into their young adulthood (Marshal et al., 2009). Rejection from their family is a predictive factor of substance use among GSMY (Ryan et al., 2010). GSMY are more likely to engage in risky sexual behaviors and attempt or complete suicide when rejected by their parents (Ryan et al., 2010). Even perceived rejection from their families when coming out is a predictor for substance use among GSMY (Rosario et al., 2012). GSMY are at an incredibly high risk for homelessness (SAMHSA, 2011), which significantly increases the possibility of substance use (Rosario et al., 2012).

African American Adolescents

African American adolescents use alcohol and illicit substances at a lower rate than most other ethnic groups (SAMHSA, 2020b). In the last four years, there has been a significant decrease in alcohol and opioid use among African Americans between the ages of 12 and 17, while marijuana use has remained fairly steady (SAMHSA, 2020b). In the last year, 0.05% of African American adolescents used methamphetamine, and 0.1% used cocaine. It is important to note that these numbers are only reflective of those who reported use. For those who do engage in substance use, there is a correlation between substance use and a major depressive episode (MDE) among African American adolescents (SAMHSA, 2020b). In 2019, SAMHSA (2020b) reported that 26.5% of 12- to 17-year-olds who used illicit drugs experienced an MDE. Researchers suggests that interpersonal distress and depression can lead to drug use, and perceived racial discrimination can lead to interpersonal distress and depression (Brook & Pahl, 2005).

The consequences of drug use are at a disproportionately higher rate for African American adolescents than any other ethnic adolescent group (Clark et al., 2008). The startling disparity of alcohol-related issues in the African American community is further emphasized by the fact that across age and gender, African Americans typically begin drinking at a later age (Johnson et al., 2005) and drink less than White Americans (Watt, 2005). African Americans, generally speaking, have a much more conservative view of alcohol use than White Americans (Wallace & Muroff, 2002). African American parents keep less alcohol, if any, in their homes (Zapolski et al., 2014), are reported to be more strict with their children about alcohol use, and keep a close monitor on where their children are and whom they are with (Wallace & Muroff, 2002).

How African Americans Grieve

Moore et al., 2020, states:

> because of the oral tradition passing down narratives of the slave experience from generation to generation, we contend that Black Americans live

in a perpetual state of grief and that this grief is seldom acknowledged or addressed by those within the helping professions.

(p. 1)

Thus, "it is essential that clinicians understand that death, dying, and grief takes place within the historical context of systemic racism" (Moore et al., 2020, p. 9). The United States as a nation demands that African Americans rise above and quickly recover from centuries of enslavement, oppression, relentless retraumatization from the news and social media, and the daily injustices of systemic racism. As Black bodies continue to be assaulted, and Black life is seen as *less than*, there will always be a burden of grief carried among them.

For many African Americans, family does not necessarily mean someone in the nuclear family (Schoulte, 2011). While a broader sense of kinship among the African American people offers power and support, it also means that the loss of extended kin may be felt as deeply as one would feel the loss of an immediate family member (Laurie & Neimeyer, 2008). The loss of a Black life, no matter if it were that of a sibling or a stranger, contributes to an overarching grief among African American people. In a similar light, African Americans turn to extended kin for support when dealing with addiction, loss, and grief (Schoulte, 2011).

African Americans, religious or not, often utilize religion and spirituality as means to cope with grief and loss (Schoulte, 2011). Religion, specifically Christianity and the idea of the afterlife, offers a source of comfort and meaning (Cooper-Lewter & Mitchell, 1986) to the unanswerable questions that arise from loss, addiction, and trauma. Death is seen as the way to heaven, which is free of the trauma and injustices of life (Cooper-Lewter & Mitchell, 1986). The spirit does not disappear with death but rather it continues, offering a new beginning in the afterlife. African Americans find comfort that their loved ones are not really gone; the spirit of whom has passed still lingers around the living, maintaining a connection even in their death (Laurie & Neimeyer, 2008).

In addition to religion and the comfort that comes from spirituality, the church offers community. The "church family" (Moore et al., 2020) provides support in times of grief and suffering. Through gatherings at the church or in homes of those in the congregation, family members, immediate and extended, come together to support those who are grieving. Prayer, singing, reminiscing, and sharing stories are all ways that the community honors those who have passed (Moore et al., 2020). Community and spirituality are two tenets of Afrocentric philosophy (Mbiti, 1969) or the African American worldview (Morris, 2001; Randolph & Banks, 1993).

It is important to recognize that not all Black people in the United States are African American, nor are African Americans monolithic. All African Americans are not raised with the same worldview, values, or religious beliefs; yet delving into religious or family systems is paramount to the study of grief, loss, and recovery (Laurie & Neimeyer, 2008). Not all African Americans grieve the same way, but research has identified several ways that the African American community seeks comfort and support. When it comes to grief, addiction, and/ or the loss of a loved one, African Americans do not typically turn to professional mental or behavioral health treatment. A history of malpractice, misdiagnosis, systemic racism, and the lack of culturally competent counseling has negatively affected the willingness of many African Americans to seek professional help. Instead, many African Americans reach out to their family, extended kin, and the church to receive support in times of grief (Schoulte, 2011). Without negating the need for culturally competent counseling and other helping professionals, the reality is that African Americans report similar levels of perceived support from their community as White Americans who receive mental health care (Schoulte, 2011).

Preventative Factors and Strengths

The strength that spirituality, religion, and the church offer the African American community in times of sorrow serves as a protective factor from substance use. The same can be said for extended kin and, in conjunction with community, having a strong ethnic identity and pride in one's ethnic culture helps prevent African Americans from engaging in substance use (Brook & Pahl, 2005; Stevens-Watkins et al., 2012). As descendants of enslaved African people on U.S. soil, African Americans have had to find their own identity outside of White American and African cultures, thus creating a culture all their own (Stevens-Watkins et al., 2012). Quantitative researchers demonstrate that a deep connection to one's African American cultural identity can prevent African Americans from substance use (Brook et al., 1998; Caldwell et al., 2004) and mental health issues (Sellers et al., 2003). African American women specifically are able to cope with racism and sexism by connecting to their culture and heritage (Shorter-Gooden, 2004; Stevens-Watkins et al., 2012). As we recall, racism and sexism significantly increase their likelihood to misuse various substances.

A strong relationship with African American friends helps eliminate the risk of substance use among African Americans, especially among African American youth (Brook & Pahl, 2005). A deep connection to and admiration for their African American friends foster a sense of belonging, strengthening their African American identity and pride in their racial and ethnic community. A sense of belonging fosters conventionality, which is related to lower drug use (Brook & Pahl, 2005). Brook and Pahl (2005) demonstrated that high levels of ethnic and racial identity, church attendance, and a strong sense of family, nuclear and extended, were all factors in offsetting the risk of substance use and psychological stress.

The church and religion are two pillars of African American culture and identity (Jang et al., 2005). The power of religion and the church community historically have a significant impact on the African American community, especially after the Emancipation Proclamation, promoting abstinence from drinking (James & Johnson, 1996), which continues to this day. The church is a meeting place for worship, a gathering place for the community, and as researchers indicated, a major preventative factor of substance use and psychological stress for African Americans (Brook & Pahl, 2005; Cater et al., 2012; Stevens-Watkins et al., 2012). Jang et al. (2005) found that religion may strengthen African Americans social connectivity and ability to cope with the various stressors of life, including grief and loss. Additionally, African Americans having less of a connection to religion was a predictor for depression (Jang et al., 2005).

The African American church has a more conservative view on substance use and other risky behaviors (Brook & Pahl, 2005). Brook and Pahl (2005) found that family church attendance not only led to less tolerance for perceived deviant behavior but also less risky behavior in general. Due to the church being influential in African American culture, the low tolerance extends beyond the church and into the social networks of the African American people (Brook & Pahl, 2005).

Need for African American–Focused Treatment

> When four decades of research and psychological literature suggest that Black clients generally prefer Black counselors, it creates a public health dilemma when Black people are underrepresented in the mental health profession and overrepresented in populations that have mental health care disparities.
>
> (Townes et al., 2009, p. 330)

It would certainly be ideal if there was equitable representation of Black practitioners within the mental health and behavioral health professions; however, this would not eliminate the need for culturally competent counselors of all races and ethnicities to ethically and effectively treat African Americans in need of mental health and addiction treatment. To begin, it is important to emphasize *why* African Americans would prefer Black practitioners. Townes et al. (2009) defines cultural mistrust as "the theoretical level of suspiciousness and distrust Black people exhibited toward White educational systems, political activities, business interactions, and interpersonal and social contexts" (p. 331). White practitioners are seen as an extension of the racist establishment that continues to perpetuate systemic racism (Sue & Sue, 2015). For centuries, health care in the United States was guilty of horrifically dangerous and racist practices that ranged from misdiagnosis and lack of care to experimentation on African American bodies (e.g., the Tuskegee Syphilis Study). In the 18th century, what would one day become the American Psychiatric Association (APA) routinely misdiagnosed African Americans in the interest of managing enslaved people and even accepted enslaved people as payment for their services (APA, 2021b). Over the course of history, the APA continued to ignore the mental health care needs of African Americans, complied with racist social norms (i.e., segregation), misdiagnosed African Americans, and contributed to the perpetuation of systemic racism against Black and Indigenous People of Color (BIPOC).

As you may recall from our earlier section, "Substance Use and Systemic Racism," the lack of consideration or attention to the mental health care needs of African Americans continued well into the 20th century—a trend that continues to this very day. In fact, it was only in the year 2021 that the first step toward remedying the systemic injustice of poor mental health care offered to African Americans over the years has been made. On January 18, 2021, the APA formally apologized to BIPOC with a historical addendum that holds the institution accountable to the APA's role in racist practices throughout U.S. history (APA, 2021a). It comes as no surprise that African Americans would view any establishment within the United States, especially the medical and mental health care establishments, as unhelpful and unsafe at best.

African Americans may prefer Black practitioners because of the lack of culturally competent care offered to them and the racism and prejudice they perceive and experience from White practitioners (Townes et al., 2009). Studies have shown that the mistrust of White practitioners contributes to premature termination of services (Sue & Sue, 2015; Terrell & Terrell, 1984; Townes et al., 2009); the underutilization of mental health care; and lower expectations of success in treatment among African Americans (King & Canada, 2004; Watkins & Terrell, 1988). These are not small, anecdotal problems; these are systemic misfortunes that prevent African Americans from seeking and receiving the mental health and substance use treatment that they need. And most importantly, the mistrust is warranted. Researchers indicate that African Americans are disproportionately diagnosed with psychotic disorders and childhood disorders compared to White Americans (Feisthamel & Schwartz, 2009). Consequently, the misdiagnosis of a psychotic disorder is life altering and deeply impactful. African Americans are subjected to more invasive and involuntary treatment and severe mental health diagnoses, while White Americans are offered, as Feisthamel and Schwartz (2009, p. 48) put it, "cautious" diagnoses, such as mood or adjustment disorders. Researchers indicate that even identical symptoms among Black or White clients will be met with different diagnoses based on race (Feisthamel & Schwartz, 2009; Geller, 1988). Feisthamel and Schwartz (2009) further state, "Geller (1988) reported that psychiatrists who evaluated identical clinical data among persons of different races judged African Americans as less articulate, less competent and sophisticated about mental health settings, and less able to benefit from psychotherapy than other clients" (p. 52).

Restorative justice practice emphasizes that transgressors must be responsible for reparations. Those in power must earn the trust of the African American community to help remedy the disparity of mental and behavioral health care among Black and White citizens. So, where do we begin? As we acknowledged, the APA (2021a) made an official apology to BIPOC and voiced its commitment to "working together with members and patients in order to achieve the social equality, health equity, and fairness that all human beings deserve." This is where all practitioners must begin: acknowledging the disparity, any internalized racism and/or prejudice, and commit to practicing multiculturally competent and ethical services to all human beings. This is not a journey one must do or can do alone. We offer you now several integral strategies and considerations in order to provide culturally competent treatment for African Americans.

Cultural Competence and Humility

It is the authors' belief that the responsibility of providing culturally competent care to African American clients must not rest on the shoulders of Black practitioners. It is the ethical duty of all counselors, from all racial and ethnic backgrounds, to be well trained and prepared to offer culturally competent services to anyone who may walk through their office doors seeking mental health and addictions treatment (ACA, 2014). On July 25, 2015 the American Counseling Association (ACA) approved the Multicultural and Social Justice Counseling Competencies (MSJCC; Ratts et al., 2015) which revised the Multicultural Counseling Competencies (MCC) developed by Sue et al. (1992). The MSJCC "offers counselors a framework to implement multicultural and social justice competencies into counseling theories, practices, and research" (p. 3). The MSJCC lays out, visually and textually, "the dynamics of power, privilege, and oppression that influence the counseling relationship" and the "developmental domains" that reflect "the different layers that lead to multicultural and social justice competence" (p. 3). The domains are counselor self-awareness, client worldview, counseling relationship, and counseling and advocacy interventions. There are "aspirational competencies" within the first three developmental domains: attitudes and beliefs, knowledge, skills, and action. The MSJCC provides a clear and profound demand of counselors to "develop knowledge of theories that explain how their privileged and marginalized status influences their experiences and worldview" (p. 5).

It is imperative that counselors consider *their* attitudes and beliefs, knowledge, and skills about the African American community *before* they engage in a counseling relationship with an African American or Black American client. The MSJCCs asks counselors to acknowledge their own assumptions, worldviews, values, beliefs, and biases, as well as those of their clients. It is the responsibility of the counselor to develop knowledge and skills that not only help them process and understand their own privilege or marginalization, status in society, beliefs, biases, and so forth, but also to do the same for their clients. Thus, in order to be a culturally competent and humble counselor offering services to African Americans, one must understand the historical and contemporary experience of African Americans, with an emphasis on the role that the medical and mental professional fields played on upholding racism and violence against the African American community *and* do the work necessary to reckon with their own beliefs and biases about the African American community.

Hook et al. (2013) posited that the "multicultural focus on openness to the other is closely related to the concept of humility" (p. 253), specifically as explored by Davis et al. (2010), who found through their research that definitions of humility "generally included both intrapersonal and interpersonal components" (Hook et al., 2013, p. 253). Hook et al. (2013) continued:

> On the intrapersonal dimension, humble individuals have an accurate view of self. On the interpersonal dimension, humble individuals are able to maintain an interpersonal stance that is other-oriented rather than self-focused, characterized by respect for others and a lack of superiority.
>
> (pp. 253–254)

In their study, Hook et al. (2013) focused on the interpersonal aspect of humility and the effect cultural humility has on the therapeutic relationship. The researchers indicated that a client's perception of a therapist's cultural humility was positively associated with their working alliance and their perceived improvement in therapy. Furthermore, the stronger the client perceived the working alliance, the higher the likelihood the client perceived improvement in therapy. Hook et al. (2013) also found that in addition to focusing on the *intrapersonal* principles of building self-awareness, knowledge, and skills, developing an *interpersonal* stance of humility when discussing the cultural background of a client is important. This means that as wonderful as engaging with one's own humility is, it may prove to be a moot point if one does not engage with their client in a humble manner, specifically about the client's worldview and culture.

The implications that Hook et al.'s (2013) studies have on practitioners are that a practitioner should "engage with each client with an attitude of humility in relation to the client's cultural background" and "should not assume that they understand the client's cultural background or experience based on therapists' prior knowledge, experience, or training" (p. 261). Instead, one should explore the client's cultural background *with* the client and practitioners should *express* their humility (e.g., expressing curiosity about one's client's cultural background, asking questions). Finally, in relationship to the MSJCC tenet of action, cultural humility should extend to how one engages with their activism, social justice work, and involvement with community members and leaders.

Broaching

Day-Vines et al. (2007) coined the term "broaching" to "describe the counselor's effort to examine racial and cultural factors during the counseling process" (p. 401). Broaching "describes a process by which counselors can bring cultural characteristics of the client and the counselor into the room and invite clients to explore the relevance of those characteristics" (Jones & Welfare, 2017, p. 49) and "refers to the counselor's ability to consider the relationship of racial and cultural factors to the client's presenting problem, especially because these issues might otherwise remain unexamined during the counseling process" (Day-Vines et al., 2007, p. 401). In a society that seldom, if ever, acknowledges the centuries of genocide, violence, slavery, injustice, and racism inflicted upon BIPOC, broaching can be the first step toward healing the historical and racial trauma perpetuated by color-blind mental and behavioral health practitioners (Day-Vines et al., 2007; Jones & Welfare, 2017). Broaching provides "an environment of emotional safety within which the counseling relationship can transition from a level of superficiality toward a measure of intimacy that is crucial to embracing difference" (p. 402).

Jones and Branco (2020) describe broaching as cultural humility in action, as one must broach from a culturally humble stance. Broaching is an intercultural dialogue and ongoing process of openness that helps to create a safe space for a client to explore themself as well as creating an avenue by which both counselor and client can discuss race, ethnicity, and culture (Day-Vines et al., 2007; Jones & Welfare, 2017). The responsibility is on the counselor to initiate these conversations, recognizing the power dynamics that exist within the therapeutic relationship. By demonstrating a positive regard for one's client, in addition to openness and a genuine interest in the client's cultural worldview, a counselor can build a working alliance that allows for healing, a strong working alliance, and enhances the chance of positive treatment outcomes (Jones & Branco, 2020; Jones & Welfare, 2017).

Jones and Welfare (2017) focused their study on if and how licensed professional counselors broached when working with clients diagnosed with a substance use disorder, recognizing the importance of establishing a strong therapeutic relationship early in addictions counseling due to possibility of relapse and withdrawal (Merta, 2001). Jones and Welfare (2017) also took into account that nearly half of all racial and ethnic minoritized clients prematurely terminate counseling (Sue & Sue, 2015). The researchers found that counselors recognized the importance of culture in substance use assessment and treatment, even if they did not always act on it. Jones and Welfare (2017) state, "Most participants reported that the client must be offered an open invitation to discuss multicultural considerations. An open invitation sends a message to the client that the counselor is open and comfortable with discussing multicultural considerations" (p. 57). They found that there was a need to incorporate broaching into counselor training. Additionally, Jones and Welfare (2017) found counselors working with substance use disorders must advocate for the implementation of broaching as a standard practice of care on an administrative level, due to the many benefits of broaching to strengthen the therapeutic relationship.

Strengths-Based Approach

It is imperative that counselors work from a strength-based approach when working with any and all clients, especially when working with African American clients. We encourage counselors working with members of this population not to look through a deficit lens when conceptualizing the client but instead to look at the many strengths and assets that the African American population possess. Look for strengths on the macro and individual levels. The strength-based approach to counseling consists of looking at the client's strengths rather than their deficits (Burt et al., 1998). Smith (2006) states, "This perspective [strength-based approach] is founded on the belief that people are resilient, that they bounce back from life's adversities, despite what appear to be over-whelming odds" (p. 16). It is evident that the African Americans are resilient individuals with many strengths, and as counselors we have to be sure to look for and identify these strengths.

It is important to note that psychiatry, and thus the mental and behavioral health fields, were primarily designed by, studied on, and catered to White, Christian males until very recently—we still have a long way to go. One of the major misgivings of modern mental health care is the utilization of Eurocentric views of grief and healing on diverse populations (Moore et al., 2020). From the Eurocentric perspective, grief may be assumed to have a linear process with a beginning, middle, and end (Granek, 2014). Granek (2014) posits that in Western culture, grief is a psychological condition, and it is the responsibility of the griever to move through their grief and get back to normal life as soon as possible; if the griever takes too long, their grief is pathologized. The notion that it is the individual responsibility of the griever to move on is damaging to cultures that approach life from a collectivistic perspective. Moore et al. (2020) writes:

> The modernist emphasis on the self has left people deprived of what they need to effectively grieve and instead has made the individual solely responsible for healing instead of being able to rely on religion and rituals to deal with death and grief. What has resulted is a narrow-mindedness for the gradual progression of bereavement. It is therefore understandable that Black people sometimes shun counseling, especially when the counselor has different race related experiences.
>
> (p. 6)

Utilizing spirituality and communalism as an intervention is not only dem-onstrating cultural competence, but it is working from a strengths-based perspective, as we explored in our earlier section, "Preventative Factors and Strengths."

Conclusion

In this chapter, we provided a brief history of substance use within the African American community from the pre-slavery era to the present day to include the cultural and spiritual meanings of substances. We then offered an overview of the legacy of trauma resultant of slavery and enduring systemic macro and micro racism and its impact on grief for the African American community. We also describe that grief and loss is not a new phenomenon to African Americans. So, as you work with clients who identify as African American or Black American, you would be remiss not to address the grief and loss that not only occurs in substance use and recovery, but also the grief and loss due to historical and racial trauma. Preventative factors, strengths, and strengths-based counseling tenets were presented to highlight helpful practices when working with members of the African American population. To that end, tenets of cultural humility and broaching were also described.

References

Akerlund, M., & Cheung, M. (2000). Teaching beyond the deficit model: Gay and lesbian issues among African Americans, Latinos, and Asian Americans. *Journal of Social Work Education, 36*(2), 279–292. https://doi.org/10.1080/10437797.2000.10779008

Alexander, M. (2010). *The New Jim Crow: Mass incarceration in the age of colorblindness*. New Press.

American Counseling Association. (2014). *2014 ACA code of ethics*. www.counseling.org/knowledge-center

American Psychiatric Association (APA). (2021a, January 18). *APA's apology to Black, indigenous and people of color for its support of structural racism in psychiatry.* APA. www.psychiatry.org/newsroom/apa-apology-for-its-support-of-structural-racism-in-psychiatry

American Psychiatric Association (APA). (2021b, January 18). *Historical addendum to APA's apology to Black, indigenous and people of color for its support of structural racism in psychiatry.* APA. www.psychiatry.org/newsroom/historical-addendum-to-apa-apology

Appiah, K. A., & Gutmann, A. (1996). *Color conscious: The political morality of race.* Princeton University Press.

Barnes, D. M., & Meyer, I. (2012). Religious affiliation, internalized homophobia, and mental health in lesbians, gay men, and bisexuals. *American Journal of Orthopsychiatry, 82*(4), 505–515. https://doi.org/10.1111/j.1939-0025.2012.01185.x

Bauer, G. R. (2014). Incorporating intersectionality theory into population health research methodology: Challenges and the potential to advance health equity. *Social Science & Medicine, 110*, 10–17. https://doi.org/10.1016/j.socscimed.2014.03.022

Bowleg, L. (2008). When Black + lesbian + woman ≠ Black lesbian woman: The methodological challenges of qualitative and quantitative intersectionality research. *Sex Roles: A Journal of Research, 59*(5–6), 312–325. https://doi.org/10.1007/s11199-008-9400-z

Brook, J. S., Balka, E. B., Brook, D. W., Win, P. T., & Gursen, M. D. (1998). Drug use among African Americans: Ethnic identity as a protective factor. *Psychological Reports, 83*(3_suppl), 1427–1446. https://doi.org/10.2466/pr0.1998.83.3f.1427

Brook, J. S., & Pahl, K. (2005). The protective role of ethnic and racial identity and aspects of an Afrocentric orientation against drug use among African American young adults. *Journal of Genetic Psychology, 166*(3), 329–345. https://doi.org/10.3200/GNTP.166.3.329-345

Brown, L. S. (2008). *Cultural competence in trauma therapy: Beyond the flashback.* American Psychological Association.

Bryant-Davis, T., Ullman, S., Tsong, Y., Tillman, S., & Smith, K. (2010). Struggling to survive: Sexual assault, poverty, and mental health outcomes of African American women. *American Journal of Orthopsychiatry, 80*(1), 61–70. https://doi.org/10.1111/j.1939-0025.2010.01007.x

Burt, M. R., Resnick, G., & Novick, E. R. (1998). *Building supportive communities for at-risk adolescents: It takes more than services.* American Psychological Association.

Byrne, C. A., Resnick, H. S., Kilpatrick, D. G., Best, C. L., & Saunders, B. E. (1999). The socioeconomic impact of interpersonal violence on women. *Journal of Consulting and Clinical Psychology, 67*(3), 362–366. https://doi.org/10.1037/0022-006X.67.3.362

Caldwell, C. H., Sellers, R. M., Bernat, D. H., & Zimmerman, M. A. (2004). Racial identity, parental support, and alcohol use in a sample of academically at-risk African American high school students. *American Journal of Community Psychology, 34*(1–2), 71–82. https://doi.org/10.1023/B:AJCP.0000040147.69287.f7

Carson, E. A., & Sabol, W. J. (2012, December). Prisoners in 2011. U.S. Department of justice: Bureau of justice statistics. www.bjs.gov/content/pub/pdf/p11.pdfNCJ 239808

Cater, T., May, L., & Byrd, D. (2012). Dealing with hurt: An assessment of dispositional style and ethnicity in coping strategies. *Current Psychology, 31*(2), 182–194. https://doi.org/10.1007/s12144-012-9135-4

Centers for Disease Control and Prevention (CDC). (2019, January 11). *CDC's response to the opioid overdose epidemic.* www.cdc.gov/opioids/strategy.html

Clark, T. T., Belgrave, F. Z., & Nasim, A. (2008). Risk and protective factors for substance use among urban African American adolescents considered high-risk. *Journal of Ethnicity in Substance Abuse, 7*(3), 292–303. https://doi.org/10.1080/15332640802313296

Cohen, R. A., Cha, A. E., Martinez, M. E., & Terlizzi, E. P. (2020). National health interview survey early release program. *National Center for Health Statistics.* www.cdc.gov/nchs/data/nhis/earlyrelease/insur202009-508.pdf

Cooper-Lewter, N. C., & Mitchell, H. H. (1986). *Soul theology: The heart of American Black culture.* Harper & Row.

Crenshaw, K. (1989). Demarginalizing the intersection of race and sex: A Black feminist critique of antidiscrimination doctrine, feminist theory and antiracist politics. *University of Chicago Legal Forum, 1989*(1), 139–167. https://chicagounbound.uchicago.edu/uclf/vol1989/iss1/8/

Crenshaw, K. (1991). Mapping the margins: Intersectionality, identity politics, and violence against women of color. *Stanford Law Review, 43*(6), 1241–1299. https://doi.org/10.2307/1229039

Cummings, J. R., Wen, H., Ko, M., & Druss, B. G. (2014). Race/ethnicity and geographic access to Medicaid substance use disorder treatment facilities in the United States. *Jama Psychiatry, 71*(2), 190–196. https://doi.org/10.1001/jamapsychiatry.2013.3575

Davis, D. E., Worthington, E. L. J., & Hook, J. N. (2010). Humility: Review of measurement strategies and conceptualization as personality judgment. *Journal of Positive Psychology, 5*(4), 243–252. https://doi.org/10.1080/17439761003791672

Day-Vines, N. L., Wood, S. M., Grothaus, T., Craigen, L., Holman, A., Dotson-Blake, K., & Douglass, M. J. (2007). Broaching the subjects of race, ethnicity, and culture during the counseling process. *Journal of Counseling and Development, 85*(4), 401–409. https://doi.org/10.1002/j.1556-6678.2007.tb00608.x

Dodgson, L. (2020, February 16). There are many types of grief that don't involve death—Here's how to know if you're suffering from any of them. *Insider.* www.insider.com/5-types-of-grief-what-they-mean-2020-2

Donovan, R., & Williams, M. (2002). Living at the intersection: The effects of racism and sexism on Black rape survivors. *Women and Therapy, 25,* 95–105. https://doi.org/10.1300/J015v25n03_07

Douglass, F. (1855). *My bondage and my freedom.* Miller, Orton, & Mulligan.

Ehrmin, J. (2002). "That feeling of not feeling": Numbing the pain for substance-dependent African American women. *Qualitative Health Research, 12*(6), 780–791. https://doi.org/10.1177/104973230201200605

Feisthamel, K. P., & Schwartz, R. C. (2009). Differences in mental health counselors' diagnoses based on client race: An investigation of adjustment, childhood, and substance-related disorders. *Journal of Mental Health Counseling, 31*(1), 47–59. https://doi.org/10.17744/mehc.31.1.u82021637276wv1k

Geller, J. D. (1988). Racial bias in the evaluation of patients for psychotherapy. In L. D. Comas-Diaz & E. E. H. Griffith (Eds.), *Clinical guidelines in cross-cultural mental health* (pp. 112–134). Wiley.

Gibbs, J. J., & Goldbach, J. (2015). Religious conflict, sexual identity, and suicidal behaviors among LGBT young adults. *Archives of Suicide Research, 19*(4), 472–488. https://doi.org/10.1080/13811118.2015.1004476

Granek, L. (2014). Mourning sickness: The politicizations of grief. *Review of General Psychology, 18*(2), 61–68. https://doi.org/10.1037/gpr0000001

Hailey, J., Burton, W., & Arscott, J. (2020). We are family: Chosen and created families as a protective factor against racialized trauma and anti-LGBTQ oppression among African American sexual and gender minority youth. *Journal of GLBT Family Studies, 16*(2), 176–191. https://doi.org/10.1080/1550428X.2020.1724133

Harris, J. I., Cook, S. W., & Kashubeck-West, S. (2008). Religious attitudes, internalized homophobia, and identity in gay and lesbian adults. *Journal of Gay & Lesbian Mental Health, 12*(3), 205–225. https://doi.org/10.1080/19359700802111452

Hart, C. L. (2017). People are not dying because of opioids. *Scientific American, 317*(5), 11. https://doi.org/10.1038/scientificamerican1117-11

Hook, J. N., Davis, D. E., Owen, J., Worthington, E. L., & Utsey, S. O. (2013). Cultural humility: Measuring openness to culturally diverse clients. *Journal of Counseling Psychology, 60*(3), 353–366. https://doi.org/10.1037/a0032595

Hudson, C. G. (2005). Socioeconomic status and mental illness: Tests of the social causation and selection hypotheses. *American Journal of Orthopsychiatry, 75*(1), 3–18. https://doi.org/10.1037/0002-9432.75.1.3

James, K., & Jordan, A. (2018). The opioid crisis in Black communities. *Journal of Law, Medicine & Ethics, 46*(2), 404–421. https://doi.org/10.1177/1073110518782949

James, W. H., & Johnson, S. L. (1996). *Doin' drugs: Patterns of African American addiction.* University of Texas Press.

Jang, Y., Borenstein, A. R., Chiriboga, D. A., & Mortimer, J. A. (2005). Depressive symptoms among African American and white older adults. *Journals of Gerontology. Series B, Psychological Sciences and Social Sciences, 60*(6), 313–319. https://doi.org/10.1093/geronb/60.6.P313

Jenkins, E. J. (2002). Black women and community violence: Trauma, grief, and coping. *Women and Therapy, 25,* 29–44. https://doi.org/10.1300/J015v25n03_03

Johnson, P. B., Richter, L., Kleber, H. D., McLellan, A. T., & Carise, D. (2005). Telescoping of drinking-related behaviors: Gender, racial/ethnic, and age comparisons. *Substance Use & Misuse, 40*(8), 1139–1151. https://doi.org/10.1081/JA-200042281

Jones, C. T., & Branco, S. F. (2020). The interconnectedness between cultural humility and broaching in clinical supervision: Working from the multicultural orientation framework. *Clinical Supervisor*, *39*(2), 178–189. https://doi.org/10.1080/07325223.2020.1830327

Jones, C. T., & Welfare, L. E. (2017). Broaching behaviors of licensed professional counselors: A qualitative inquiry. *Journal of Addictions & Offender Counseling*, *38*(1), 48–64. https://doi.org/10.1002/jaoc.12028

Jones-Webb, R. J., Hsiao, C., & Hannan, P. (1995). Relationships between socioeconomic status and drinking problems among Black and White men. *Alcoholism: Clinical & Experimental Research*, *19*(3), 623–627. https://doi.org/10.1111/j.1530-0277.1995.tb01558.x

Kilpatrick, D., Acierno, R., Resnick, H., Saunders, B., & Best, C. (1997). A 2-year longitudinal analysis of the relationships between violent assault and substance use in women. *Journal of Consulting and Clinical Psychology*, *65*(5), 834–847. https://doi.org/10.1037/0022-006X.65.5.834

King, A. C., & Canada, S. A. (2004). Client-related predictors of early treatment drop-out in substance abuse clinic exclusively employing individual therapy. *Journal of Substance Abuse Treatment*, *26*(3), 189–195. https://doi.org/10.1016/S0740-5472(03)00210-1

Laurie, A., & Neimeyer, R. A. (2008). African Americans in bereavement: Grief as a function of ethnicity. *OMEGA—Journal of Death and Dying*, *57*(2), 173–193. https://doi.org/10.2190/OM.57.2.d

Marshal, M. P., Friedman, M. S., Stall, R., & Thompson, A. L. (2009). Individual trajectories of substance use in lesbian, gay and bisexual youth and heterosexual youth. *Addiction*, *104*(6), 974–981. https://doi.org/10.1111/j.1360-0443.2009.02531.x

Mbiti, J. S. (1969). *African religions & philosophy*. Praeger.

Merriam-Webster. (n.d.). Intersectionality. *In Merriam-Webster.com dictionary*. Retrieved March 11, 2021, from www.merriam-webster.com/dictionary/intersectionality

Merta, R. J. (2001). Addictions counseling. *Counseling and Human Development*, *33*(5), 1–24.

Monnier, J., Resnick, H., Kilpatrick, D., & Seals, B. (2002). The relationship between distress and resource loss following rape. *Violence and Victims*, *17*(1), 85–91. https://doi.org/10.1891/vivi.17.1.85.33637

Moore, S. E., Jones-Eversley, S. D., Tolliver, W. F., Wilson, B., & Harmon, D. K. (2020). Cultural responses to loss and grief among Black Americans: Theory and practice implications for clinicians. *Death Studies*, 1–11. https://doi.org/10.1080/07481187.2020.1725930

Morris, E. F. (2001). Clinical practices with African Americans: Juxtaposition of standard clinical practices and Afrocentrism. *Professional Psychology: Research and Practice*, *32*(6), 563–572. https://doi.org/10.1037/0735-7028.32.6.563

Mulia, N., Ye, Y., Greenfield, T. K., & Zemore, S. E. (2009). Disparities in alcohol-related problems among White, Black, and Hispanic Americans. *Alcoholism: Clinical & Experimental Research*, *33*(4), 654–662. https://doi.org/10.1111/j.1530-0277.2008.00880.x

Mulia, N., Ye, Y., Zemore, S. E., & Greenfield, T. K. (2008). Social disadvantage, stress and alcohol use among Black, Hispanic and White Americans: Findings from the 2005 U.S. national alcohol survey. *Journal of Studies on Alcohol and Drugs*, *69*(8), 824–833. https://doi.org/10.15288/jsad.2008.69.824

Murch, D. (2015). Crack in Los Angeles: Crisis, militarization, and black response to the late twentieth-century war on drugs. *Journal of American History*, *102*(1), 162–173. https://doi.org/10.1093/jahist/jav260

NAACP. (2021, July 10). *Criminal justice fact sheet*. www.naacp.org/criminal-justice-fact-sheet/

Neville, H. A., & Pugh, A. O. (1997). General and culture-specific factors influencing African American women's reporting patterns and perceived social support following sexual assault: An exploratory investigation. *Violence against Women, 3*(4), 361–381. https://doi.org/10.1177/1077801297003004003

Pedersen, S. L., & McCarthy, D. M. (2013). Differences in acute response to alcohol between African Americans and European Americans. *Alcoholism: Clinical & Experimental Research, 37*(6), 1056–1063. https://doi.org/10.1111/acer.12068

Randolph, S. M., & Banks, H. D. (1993). Making a way out of no way: The promise of Afrocentric approaches to HIV prevention. *Journal of Black Psychology, 19*(2), 204–214. https://doi.org/10.1177/00957984930192009

Ratts, M. J., Singh, A. A., Nassar-McMillan, S., Butler, S. K., & McCullough, J. R. (2015). *Multicultural and social justice counseling competencies*. www.counseling.org/docs/default-source/competencies/multicultural-and-social-justice-counseling-competencies.pdf?sfvrsn=20

Ray, O., & Ksir, C. (1990). *Drugs, society, and human behavior*. Times Mirror/Mosby College.

Rosario, M., Schrimshaw, E. W., & Hunter, J. (2012). Homelessness among lesbian, gay, and bisexual youth: Implications for subsequent internalizing and externalizing symptoms. *Journal of Youth and Adolescence, 41*(5), 544–560. https://doi.org/10.1007/s10964-011-9681-3

Rosenberg, A., Groves, A. K., & Blankenship, K. M. (2017). Comparing black and white drug offenders: Implications for racial disparities in criminal justice and reentry policy and programming. *Journal of Drug Issues, 47*(1), 132–142. https://doi.org/10.1177/0022042616678614

Rowatt, W. C., LaBouff, J., Johnson, M., Froese, P., & Tsang, J.-A. (2009). Associations among religiousness, social attitudes, and prejudice in a national random sample of American adults. *Psychology of Religion and Spirituality, 1*(1), 14–24. https://doi.org/10.1037/a0014989

Ryan, C., Russell, S. T., Huebner, D., Diaz, R., & Sanchez, J. (2010). Family acceptance in adolescence and the health of LGBT young adults. *Journal of Child and Adolescent Psychiatric Nursing, 23*(4), 205–213. https://doi.org/10.1111/j.1744-6171.2010.00246.x

Schoulte, J. (2011). Bereavement among African Americans and Latino/a Americans. *Journal of Mental Health Counseling, 33*(1), 11–20. https://doi.org/10.17744/mehc.33.1.r4971657p7176307

Schuler, M. S., Prince, D. M., Breslau, J., & Collins, R. L. (2020). Substance use disparities at the intersection of sexual identity and race/ethnicity: Results from the 2015–2018 national survey on drug use and health. *LGBT Health, 7*(6), 283–291. https://doi.org/10.1089/lgbt.2019.0352

Sellers, R. M., Caldwell, C. H., Schmeelk-Cone, K. H., & Zimmerman, M. A. (2003). Racial identity, racial discrimination, perceived stress, and psychological distress among African American young adults. *Journal of Health and Social Behavior: Special Issue: Race, Ethnicity, and Mental Health, 44*(3), 302–317. https://doi.org/10.2307/1519781

Shilo, G., & Savaya, R. (2012). Mental health of lesbian, gay, and bisexual youth and young adults: Differential effects of age, gender, religiosity, and sexual orientation. *Journal of Research on Adolescence, 22*(2), 310–325. https://doi.org/10.1111/j.1532-7795.2011.00772.x

Shorter-Gooden, K. (2004). Multiple resistance strategies: How African American women cope with racism and sexism. *Journal of Black Psychology, 30*(3), 406–425. https://doi.org/10.1177/0095798404266050

Smith, E. (2006). The strength-based counseling model. *Counseling Psychologist, 34*(1), 13–79. https://doi.org/10.1177/0011000005277018

Southern Poverty Law Center. (n.d.). *Criminal justice reform.* www.splcenter.org/issues/mass-incarceration.

Stevens-Watkins, D., Perry, B., Harp, K. L., & Oser, C. B. (2012). Racism and illicit drug use among African American women: The protective effects of ethnic identity, affirmation, and behavior. *Journal of Black Psychology, 38*(4), 471–496. https://doi.org/10.1177/0095798412438395

Substance Abuse and Mental Health Services Administration (SAMHSA). (2011). *Learning from the field: Programs serving youth who are LGBTQI2-s and experiencing homelessness.* www.samhsa.gov/sites/default/files/programs_campaigns/homelessness_programs_resources/learning-field-programs-serving-youth-lgbtqi2s-experiencing-homelessness.pdf

Substance Abuse and Mental Health Services Administration (SAMHSA). (2020a, October). *Adults with SMI and children/youth with SED.* www.samhsa.gov/dbhis-collections/smi

Substance Abuse and Mental Health Services Administration (SAMHSA). (2020b, November). *2019 national survey on drug use and health: African Americans.* www.samhsa.gov/data/report/2019-nsduh-african-americans

Sue, D. W., Arredondo, P., & McDavis, R. J. (1992). Multicultural counseling competencies and *standards:* A call to the profession. *Journal of Multicultural Counseling and Development, 20*(2), 64–88. https://doi.org/10.1002/j.2161-1912.1992.tb00563.x

Sue, D. W., & Sue, D. (2015). *Counseling the culturally diverse: Theory and practice* (7th ed.). Wiley.

Talty, S. (2003). *Mulatto America.* HarperCollins.

Taxy, S., Samuels, J., & Adams, W. (2015, October). *Drug offenders in federal prison: Estimates of characteristics based on linked data.* US Department of Justice: Office of Justice Programs: Bureau of Justice Statistics. www.bjs.gov/content/pub/pdf/dofp12.pdf

Terrell, F., & Terrell, S. (1984). Race of counselor, client sex, cultural mistrust level, and premature termination from counseling among Black clients. *Journal of Counseling Psychology, 31*(3), 371–375. https://doi.org/10.1037//0022-0167.31.3.371

Tillman, S., Bryant-Davis, T., Smith, K., & Marks, A. (2010). Shattering silence: Exploring barriers to disclosure for African American sexual assault survivors. *Trauma, Violence & Abuse, 11*(2), 59–70. https://doi.org/10.1177/1524838010363717

Townes, D. L., Chavez-Korell, S., & Cunningham, N. J. (2009). Reexamining the relationships between racial identity, cultural mistrust, help-seeking attitudes, and preference for a Black counselor. *Journal of Counseling Psychology, 56*(2), 330–336. https://doi.org/10.1037/a0015449

Wallace, J. M., Jr., & Muroff, J. R. (2002). Preventing substance abuse among African American children and youth: Race differences in risk factor exposure and vulnerability. *Journal of Primary Prevention, 22*(3), 235–261. https://doi.org/10.1023/A:1013617721016

Watkins, C. E., & Terrell, F. (1988). Mistrust level and its effects on counseling expectations in Black client-White counselor relationships: An analogue study. *Journal of Counseling Psychology, 35*(2), 194–197. https://doi.org/10.1037/0022-0167.35.2.194

Watt, T. T. (2005). Race/ethnic differences in alcohol abuse among youth: An examination of risk-taking attitudes as a mediating factor. *Journal of Ethnicity in Substance Abuse, 3*(3), 33–47. https://doi.org/10.1300/J233v03n03_03

Wells, K., Klap, R., Koike, A., & Sherbourne, C. (2001). Ethnic disparities in unmet need for alcoholism, drug abuse, and mental health care. *American Journal of Psychiatry, 158*(12), 2027–2032. https://doi.org/10.1176/appi.ajp.158.12.2027

West, C. M., & Johnson, K. (2006). *Sexual violence in the lives of African American women: Risk, response, and resilience.* VAWnet, a Project of the National Resource Center on Domestic Violence. https://vawnet.org/sites/default/files/materials/files/2016-09/AR_SVAAWomenRevised.pdf

Williams, D., & Williams-Morris, R. (2000). Racism and mental health: The African American experience. *Ethnicity & Health, 5*(3–4), 243–268. https://doi.org/10.1080/713667453

Wu, Z., Eschbach, K., & Grady, J. (2008). Contextual influences on polydrug use among young, low-income women: Effects of neighborhood and personal networks. *American Journal on Addictions, 17*(2), 135–144. https://doi.org/10.1080/10550490701863025

Zapolski, T. C. B., Pedersen, S. L., McCarthy, D. M., & Smith, G. T. (2014). Less drinking, yet more problems: Understanding African American drinking and related problems. *Psychological Bulletin, 140*(1), 188–223. https://doi.org/10.1037/a0032113

8 Addiction and Grief in the Latinx Community

*Daniel Gutierrez, Michelle Colon,
and Stephanie Dorais*

At almost 60 million people, individuals of Hispanic and Latinx descent make up the largest minority group in the United States. Although well spread out across many states, the largest cluster of this ethnic group resides in California with 15 million individuals; both Texas and Florida follow closely behind. Contrary to the beliefs of some, the majority of this population are U.S. citizens and have likely had long-term residency if not born in the United States (Pew Research Center, 2019). As a note, in this chapter you will find that we may use the terms "Hispanic" and "Latinx" interchangeably; however, their differences lie in the origin of language. The term "Hispanic" refers to those whose origin is from solely a Spanish speaking country such as Mexico or Spain whereas the term "Latinx" refers to descendants of Latin American countries that may speak additional languages (such as Brazil, where Portuguese is primarily spoken; Valdeón, 2013).

In an overview of the 2019 National Survey on Drug Use (Substance Abuse and Mental Health Services Administration, 2020), researchers reported that 2.9 million Hispanic adults 18 or older had a substance use disorder. Of those 2.9 million adults, 41% utilized illicit drugs, and 71.4% utilized alcohol; 13.4% struggled with both elements. The most commonly identified illicit substances included in the report were marijuana, psychotropics, hallucinogens, cocaine, inhalants, methamphetamines, and heroin. Additionally, nearly half of all Hispanic adults with a substance use disorder also had a mental illness, with an overall increase in mental illness being reported in the Hispanic population compared to the previous year. According to the Centers for Disease Control and Prevention (2018), increased use of illicit drugs statistically correlates to health disparities such as cases of HIV, hepatitis, sexually transmitted diseases, and heart disease. Substance Abuse and Mental Health Services Administration (SAMHSA) public health analysts indicate, "Many of these consequences are associated with Hispanics/Latinos being unable to access bilingual treatment programs, fear of speaking to government agencies, and lack of health care coverage" (Moore & Chau, 2019, para. 1).

Current research indicates that substance abuse in recent immigrants of Hispanic descent increases as they assimilate into the U.S. culture. While less than 1% of non-acculturated Latinx immigrants used illicit substances, 7.1% of

DOI: 10.4324/9781003106906-8

acculturated Hispanics reported illicit drug use, according to the 2018 National Survey on Drug Use and Health (SAMHSA, 2019). Leaving behind traditional family-oriented values that are less tolerant of drug and alcohol use may relate to this trend (Zamboanga et al., 2009). Several studies have indicated a relationship between substance abuse and exposure to traumatic events among the Latinx population (Allem et al., 2015; Stevens et al., 2015). Leaving one's country of origin, leaving family members unaware whether they will see each other again, and cultural norms are just a few of the losses encountered by immigrants in their transition. Additionally, unemployment and experiences of discrimination have been linked to substance use in the immigrant population.

Understanding Latinx Addiction

The Latinx community is a heterogeneous group. This means that a group of people who identify as Latinx or Hispanic could vary in skin color, citizenship status, country of origin, and possibly even the primary language spoken at home. These within-group differences can make identifying a single model to explain addiction impossible. Not surprisingly, research is scarce on theories of addiction evaluation and treatment for the Latinx community (Rojas et al., 2012). However, as research emerges and our clinical understanding of Latinx culture progresses, we are beginning to see some important factors that can help us evaluate addiction in Latinx individuals.

First, it is important to note that many Latinx individuals encounter unique stressors, such as the stress of adapting to a new culture (known as *acculturation stress*), prejudices and injustices perpetuated by a hostile political climate, navigating language barriers, and the challenge of finding competent health care providers (Cariello et al., 2020; Mays et al., 2017). They are also more likely to be caregivers, lack health insurance, experience financial stress, receive poorer quality health care treatment from providers, experience unemployment, and be affected by COVID-19 (Harkness et al., 2020; Vega et al., 2009). The process of immigration and living as an immigrant in the United States can also be very stressful and traumatizing (Chavez-Dueñas et al., 2019; Revens, 2019). Stress affects every stage of the addiction process, leading to increased cravings, relapse, and even physiological vulnerability (Koob & Schulkin, 2019). Overall, the Latinx community is known for its resilience (Cariello et al., 2020), but being aware of these notable stressors and that they present considerable risk factors for substance use and relapse is important. Many classic addiction concepts, such as the strain theory, the self-medication hypothesis, and the psychological model, describe the relationship between coping, stress, and substance use (Agnew, 2001; Cohen & Wills, 1985; Khantzian, 1985; Tomkins, 1966). Using one of these frameworks could provide a good starting point for understanding problematic substance use in Latinx populations.

Considering social models of addiction can also be helpful. By social models, we suggest taking into account that individual recovery and substance use is heavily influenced by social learning, interpersonal relationships, family, and community environment (Borkman et al., 2007; Lardier et al., 2018; Leach & Kranzler, 2013; Smith, 2021). Latinxs are a collectivistic cultural group, meaning that much of their individual identity and motivation is shaped by the group rather than individual perspectives. Collectivism in Latinxs relates to how long they engage in addiction treatment, attend recovery programs, and their likelihood of relapse (Jason et al., 2018). Additionally, a Latinx's perception of the social norm is often a strong predictor of their substance use behavior (Edwards et al., 2019; LaBrie et al., 2012).

Cultural values are a part of what shape social norms. Traditional Latinx cultural values generally protect against substance use disorders. For example, two hallmarks of Latin culture are *familismo* (the dedication and commitment to family; Hernandez et al., 2018) and *respeto* (the value of obeying and honoring one's parents or others in authority; Unger et al., 2006). Researchers have found that *familismo* and *respeto* serve as protective factors against substance use (Alvarez et al., 2007; Unger et al., 2006). However, as Latinxs begin to acculturate to life in the United States, the protective nature of these cultural values begins to weaken (Unger, 2014).

Spirituality is also deeply interwoven in Latino culture (Barden et al., 2017; Jocson et al., 2020). Approximately 90% of the Latinx community identify with a religion (Pew Research Center, 2019). *Spiritualidad*, or *espiritismo*, is a potential positive source of coping with substance use (Salas-Wright et al., 2014). Conversely, Latinx traditional perceptions of gender, which include *machismo* or standards of masculinity, often decrease the likelihood of seeking substance use treatment (Alvarez et al., 2007). Of course, understanding a culture's shared values does not offer us license to stereotype or predict their behavior, but these values do give us a more nuanced understanding of how they experience problematic substance use and the losses that are often a part of addiction recovery.

Cultural Grief and Loss

Beneath the surface of addiction often lies trapped and unresolved grief (Beechem et al., 1996). Experiencing grief itself is not dangerous but rather a natural and necessary function of the psyche. However, grief without the ability to properly mourn can lead to maladaptive coping mechanisms and risks of mental health concerns. While grief is a universal emotion, mourning rituals depend on the culture (Rosenblatt, 2008; Schoulte, 2011). It is the candle lit for the departed, the flowers placed by the grave, and the glass toasted in remembrance. Across the globe, people mourn and find catharsis through their unique cultural expressions of mourning. When people are not able to engage in their inherent cultural expressions of mourning, they must resort to alternative forms of coping to process their grief. Minority groups, particularly immigrants of low socioeconomic status, often find themselves in such a position (Schoulte, 2011). Their losses often include geographic separation from family members, economic hardship, and discrimination. Further, as a minority member, capacity to engage in cultural expressions of mourning could be lowered. For instance, for some ethnic groups, mourning includes a religious ceremony or a family reunion, both of which may not be available to them. Thus, for minority groups who are away from their natural settings and susceptible to discrimination, cultural expressions of mourning may not be permissive, accepted, or even possible.

Latin Cultural Values and Mourning

Latin culture is known for experiencing grief with acute intensity compared to other cultures. This attribute is so deeply embedded into Latinx culture that it does not appear to lessen with acculturation (Hernandez et al., 2018). To gain insight into this experience, it is important to consider again Latino cultural values. These values give insight into grief and context to their expressions of mourning. A famous painting by Puerto Rican painter Francisco Oller profoundly depicts the intersection of Latinx cultural values and mourning (https://upload.wikimedia.org/wikipedia/commons/6/67/El_Velorio_by_ Francisco_Oller.jpg).

Considered a masterpiece, Oller's (1893) *El Velorio* (translated *The Wake*) depicts a Puerto Rican family and their village at the wake of a child. If you look closely, you can see the child's body lying in the center of the table with mourners to one side and those celebrating life on the other. The room, which is a representation of a humble traditional classic home on the island, is filled with grief stricken, stoic, and cheerful faces. Individuals are playing instruments and playing games, children are running throughout, animals are lying with family, all while parents mourn their loss. You may also notice the spiritual images throughout and what appears to be a minister standing by and many of those in the house looking upward. It can be argued that the artist is telling the viewer that life, death, and faith all belong together, and that we cope with our pain best by living our lives collectively, whole-heartedly, and spiritually.

As you can see from the painting, family support is a central component in the mourning process. Within the family unit, cultural expectations will shape the grieving process for different members of the family. *Machismo* would likely prevent men from expressing the same emotional catharsis as women. Family members may not mourn the same, but they do mourn together. In the instance of bereavement, Latin family members join together to mourn of the loss of a family member. This collectivism is not confined to individual family units. Latino families often group together to mourn a loss and find catharsis collectively. As a famous example of this collective ritual, *Dia de los Muertos* (Day of the Dead) is an annual Latin holiday observed to honor the departed and mourn through celebratory remembrance. With roots in Mexico and Catholicism, *Dia de los Muertos* symbolizes a generally held Latin belief that those living are spiritually connected with the dead. The holiday characterizes the importance of *espiritismo*, which also contextualizes grief and mourning

Spiritual coping strategies are no exception to the rituals and customs Latinx members use to process their grief and are a mediating factor on the effects of religion on wellness for those grieving (Cruz-Ortega et al., 2015; Pargament, 1997). In context of loss, faith-based practices include religious services, baptism, daily prayer, and a widespread belief in healing miracles. Spirituality provides a meaning-making framework for experiencing loss. By creating a space for ritual and integrating faith practice, Latinxs can commit their loss to the trust and will of their higher power. During his father's funeral, the Castilian renaissance poet Jorge Manrique (Marino, 2011) recited his famous *Coplas a la muerte de mi padre* (verses on the death of my father). He begins this poem by highlighting the spiritual nature of human life:

Recuerde el alma dormida, (The sleeping soul remembers)
abiue el seso e despierte (the brain departs and wakes)
contemplando (thinking)
cómo se passa la vida, (this is how life is spent)
cómo se viene la muerte (this is how death comes)
tan callando. (so silent)

As the poem continues, it enters into a description of the importance of how we use our time wisely and not be overwhelmed by the hardships of grief and loss. Manrique does this by highlighting the spiritual nature of reality and the inevitability of loss. One of the most quoted lines from the piece illustrates this spiritual understanding of loss: "Nuestras vidas son los ríos que van a dar en la mar, que es el morir" (Our lives are rivers that flow down to the sea, which is death). This line is followed by a description of how royalty and those in poverty are the same at the point of death, and our focus should be on living our best life of faith, duty, and a delight in doing right because "que querer hombre vivir cuando dios quierre que meura es locura" (For wishing still to live when God wants you to die would be insane). This sentiment illustrated by Manrique is sometimes described as a *fatalismo*, or a belief that something is inevitable and out of control (Barden et al., 2017), and it is often linked to spiritual and religious cultural values. Although *fatalismo* can negatively influence Latinx's motivation to seek treatment, it can also engender acceptance for someone grieving a loss. However, spirituality and religion are also the preferred avenues of seeking help for mental health behavior in Latino culture. The Latinx community will eschew professional services in favor of spiritual guidance or faith-based rituals. Thus, in a culture that relies heavily on faith, a lack of access to an accepting religious or spiritual community or the lack of freedom to implement a faith practice could potentially decrease the ability to mourn in a healthy way.

In the event of significant loss, some Latino families may also face the challenge of finding a Spanish-speaking mass, if that is their mourning tradition. If they had to move away from family, they may long to experience the catharsis of mourning collectively as a family unit but instead may be faced with a sense of isolation. Even the psychological release that comes from celebrating a cultural holiday like *Dia de los Muertos* would be absent unless the Latin population is particularly large in a U.S. city. Overall, the absence of mourning rituals can prevent the natural and healthy processing of grief, leaving individuals susceptible to alternative coping mechanisms.

Cultural Loss

Up until this point we have emphasized grief in the context of bereavement, but Hispanics and Latinxs experience a variety of loss. For instance, as many ethnic minority group members can attest, there are major cultural losses ranging from separation from parent culture, discrimination, and other forms of collective trauma. According to a study on Latino immigration, approximately a third of immigrants underwent a trauma in the immigration process (Perreira & Ornelas, 2013). Recalling the significance of *familismo*, many people suffer from the mental health effects of indefinite separation from family members in their home countries. Losses occur both upon leaving one's country and upon entering a new country where language, employment, and community acceptance create distressing challenges. Upon arriving to the United States, many Latino immigrants face a steady wave of discrimination ranging from economic disadvantages to social isolation. Racial discrimination is considered a major stressor that influences physical and mental health (Flores et al., 2010). The losses include health disparities, separation from family and community, and various economic disadvantages. Furthermore, there is a loss of hope that occurs when after the arduous journey of immigration in pursuit of the American dream one is faced with bigotry, injustices, chronic anxiety, and fear.

Entering into substance abuse treatment and fighting addiction also come with loss. The shame and stigma associated with addiction and addiction recovery can be isolating. The mark of shame and stigma can influence their participation in social events, family events, and even make them feel exiled from their religious community. Additionally, Latinx individuals who have addiction in their families may have to choose to distance themselves from people, places, and things that are culturally significant but serve as triggers to their addiction. Given how collectivistic and how much the Latinx culture emphasizes family relationships and personal relationships, this can be a traumatic loss leading to a significant period of grief and mourning.

Intersections of Grief and Substance Use

The acculturation process of Hispanic immigrants also has a significant impact on the experiences of both grief and addiction. The magnitude of cultural transition can provide foundational losses that may create or exacerbate addiction behaviors as a way of coping (Houben, 2011). Spanish cultures tend to be very expressive in language, physical affection, and communal celebrations. However, as a part of acculturation, some of these cultural factors may become muted in efforts to adjust to societal norms and expectations in the United States. For example, there has been a tendency of stigma that those immigrants or children of immigrants who retained their fluency in the Spanish language are perceived as less educated (Espinoza, 1999). This has led to many acculturated Hispanics to utilize their fluency in the language behind closed doors or to lose their fluency altogether. These Hispanic immigrants are now faced with the task of grieving the loss of a significant part of their identity.

Consequently, the more acculturated a Hispanic immigrant becomes, the higher chance they may acquire a substance use disorder (Alvarez et al., 2007); additionally, acculturated Hispanics may be more likely to consume alcohol than non-acculturated or less acculturated individuals (National Institute on Alcohol Abuse and Alcoholism, 2015). Challenges faced by the children of immigrants can culminate in conflict with their parents' views of new cultural experiences (Miller, 2013). Mourning and stress from the acculturation process of younger Hispanics can be viewed in notably higher occurrences of substance use disorders than older generations.

A specific group of imminent risk are undocumented Hispanics in the United States. Undocumented immigrants not only experience the challenges of acculturation, but they also experience many disparities that are reduced in their naturalized peers (Cabral & Cuevas, 2020). A few areas include access to health care, housing assistance programs, government-funded educational loans, and political involvement such as voting. Additionally, many Hispanic undocumented immigrants report primary coping mechanisms of spiritual beliefs and close-knit familial relationships may become strained due to the inability of undocumented persons to travel across the border at will (Cobb et al., 2016). Reduced access to critical care, assistance, faith communities, and family support could lead to supplementary addictive behaviors in coping.

Recommendations for Treatment and Practice

A typical mistake made by new helping professionals working with Latinxs is they focus primarily on the problem and forget to acknowledge the loss, stress, and the cultural values that are so critically important to the Latinx way of life. It is important to always remember you are working with a client struggling with a substance use disorder—a person and not just a disease. One can argue this mentality is even more important when working with Latinx groups who emphasize personal relationships (*personalismo*) over professional relationships (Barden et al., 2017; Gutierrez et al., 2016). Therefore, the first step in any work you do with Latinxs is the establishing of *confianza*, which roughly translates to developing a trusting, caring, working alliance. You cannot establish *confianza* if you ignore, even if it is inadvertently, the unique experiences of your Latinx clients, which in addictions counseling includes acknowledging their cultural perspective, stress, and grief and loss.

When a new helping professional acknowledges Latinx cultural values in a stereotypical way, they end up doing more harm than good (Mosher et al., 2017). These often well-meaning helpers will hold useful knowledge about culture but end up making stereotypical assumptions about what the client needs, and ultimately continue to force treatment recommendations developed for a majority culture, due to limited culturally adapted treatment. This might be a well-intentioned attempt at cultural competence, but it is not as effective as they would expect. Effective counselors should adopt a multicultural orientation (Owen, 2013). Through humility and openness, they join with their clients empowering the natural strength in the client's cultural values through understanding and an accepting relationship.

In order to do this, the helping professional should listen closely to the client and look for opportunities to engage them in cultural dialogue (Owen, 2013). Understanding some of the common cultural values for the Latinx culture can be good starting point for dialogue (Gutierrez et al., 2016). For example, acknowledging *familismo* and talking to your Latinx client about family and family loss can be very helpful in conceptualizing treatment and recovery within the context of their family. For example, they could be especially concerned about what to do with their children or providing for their loved one if they enter into residential treatment or concerned about their loss of identity if their family and community learned they were addicted. Creating a space for them to mourn these losses and providing avenues for social support could be incredibly helpful in facilitating recovery. Furthermore, recommending family approaches to treatment can be a practical strategy for helping your clients navigate these losses.

Likewise, spirituality could be a driving force in treatment. The concept of a higher power is commonly used in mutual aid groups, and this approach is consistent with the often held *spiritualidad* of Latinxs. Additionally, understanding the role of *fatalismo* on perspectives of health (Barden et al., 2017) can help facilitate the conversation of acceptance rather than resignation. Integrating ritual and spiritual practice into addictions treatment could strengthen the client's coping, foster hope, and motivate recovery.

Finally, helping professionals should seek to understand the stress their clients experience daily and take that into account when making treatment recommendations. Latinxs demonstrate a high amount of resilience that can strengthen addictions treatment (Perreira et al., 2019). Understanding how to help them tap into that resilience and battle the stress they encounter could motivate them to seek treatment and help them find healing. However, there are practical considerations in helping this population, including helping them access culturally appropriate services often with limited financial resources, manage the discrimination they face as a result of the sociopolitical environment, and procure adequate services to process previous trauma (DeHaven et al., 2020). When a Latinx client is presented with the choices of caring for themselves with addictions treatment or earning more money that could potentially help them support their family, they will often avoid self-care and treatment for the sake of family care. When providing services, we recommend discussing these potential challenges with clients to ensure there is a concrete plan in place that is honoring their values and their health.

Final Reflections

Mexican painter Frida Kahlo once said, "Lo que no me mata, me aliementa" (What does not kill me, nourishes me). We believe this is a good sentiment to close this chapter. The Latinx people have undergone many hardships and often experience numerous losses that can lead to substance use. However, they are also known, historically, for being those who continue to persist with passion regardless of adversity. This is exemplified by the phrase coined by Cesar Chavez and Delores Huerta, "Si Se Puede!" (Yes we can!), which was later adopted by U.S. President Barack Obama. By creating a space that allows for Latinxs to tap into this resilient spirit and fostering an environment that permits them to grieve their losses, we believe that they will not only find their healing, but they will also inspire others.

References

Agnew, R. (2001). Building on the foundation of general strain theory: Specifying the types of strain most likely to lead to crime and delinquency. *Journal of Research in Crime and Delinquency, 38*(4), 319–361. https://doi.org/10.1177/0022427801038004001

Allem, J., Soto, D. W., Baezconde-Garbanati, L., & Unger, J. B. (2015). Adverse childhood experiences and substance use among Hispanic emerging adults in southern California. *Addictive Behaviors, 50*, 199–204. https://doi.org/10.1016/j.addbeh.2015.06.038

Alvarez, J., Jason, L. A., Olson, B. D., Ferrari, J. R., & Davis, M. I. (2007). Substance abuse prevalence and treatment among Latinos and Latinas. *Journal of Ethnicity in Substance Abuse, 6*(2), 115–141.

Barden, S., Gutierrez, D., Gonzalez, J., & Ali, S. (2017). Calidad de vida: An exploratory investigation of Latino breast cancer survivors and intimate partners. *Journal of Health Disparities Research and Practice, 10*(4), 1.

Beechem, M. H., Prewitt, J., & Scholar, J. (1996). Loss-grief addiction model. *Journal of Drug Education, 26*(2), 183–198. https://doi.org/10.2190/0GXH-9Q2Y-9NUG-UQ24

Borkman, T., Kaskutas, L. A., & Owen, P. (2007). Contrasting and converging philosophies of three models of alcohol/other drugs treatment: Minnesota model, social model, and addiction therapeutic communities. *Alcoholism Treatment Quarterly, 25*(3), 21–38. https://doi.org/10.1300/J020v25n03_03

Cabral, J., & Cuevas, A. G. (2020). Health inequities among Latinos/Hispanics: Documentation status as a determinant of health. *Journal of Racial and Ethnic Health Disparities, 7*, 874–879. https://doi.org/10.1007/s40615-020-00710-0

Cariello, A. N., Perrin, P. B., & Morlett-Paredes, A. (2020). Influence of resilience on the relations among acculturative stress, somatization, and anxiety in Latinx immigrants. *Brain and Behavior, 10*(12), e01863.

Centers for Disease Control and Prevention. (2018). *Diagnoses of HIV infection in the United States and dependent areas, 2018 (Updated)*. HIV Surveillance Report. www.

cdc.gov/hiv/pdf/library/reports/surveillance/cdc-hiv-surveillance-report-2018-up-dated-vol-31.pdf

Chavez-Dueñas, N. Y., Adames, H. Y., Perez-Chavez, J. G., & Salas, S. P. (2019). Healing ethno-racial trauma in Latinx immigrant communities: Cultivating hope, resistance, and action. *American Psychologist*, *74*(1), 49–63. https://doi.org/10.1037/amp0000289

Cobb, C. L., Xie, D., & Sanders, G. L. (2016). Coping styles and depression among undocumented Hispanic immigrants. *Journal of Immigrant and Minority Health*, *18*(4), 864–870. https://doi.org.ezproxy.regent.edu/10.1007/s10903-015-0270-5

Cohen, S., & Wills, T. A. (1985). Stress, social support, and the buffering hypothesis. *Psychological Bulletin*, *98*(2), 310–357. https://doi.org/10.1037/0033-2909.98.2.310

Cruz-Ortega, L. G., Gutierrez, D., & Waite, D. (2015). Religious orientation and ethnic identity as predictors of religious coping among bereaved individuals. *Counseling and Values*, *60*(1), 67–83. https://doi.org/10.1002/j.2161-007X.2015.00061.x

DeHaven, M. J., Gimpel, N. A., Gutierrez, D., Kitzman-Carmichael, H., & Revens, K. (2020). Designing health care: A community health science solution for reducing health disparities by integrating social determinants and the effects of place. *Journal of Evaluation in Clinical Practice*, *26*(5), 1564–1572. https://doi.org/10.1111/jep.13366

Edwards, K. A., Witkiewitz, K., & Vowles, K. E. (2019). Demographic differences in perceived social norms of drug and alcohol use among Hispanic/Latinx and non-Hispanic White college students. *Addictive Behaviors*, *98*, 106060.

Espinoza, F. C. (1999). LANGUAGE: Unmasking language loss in the Hispanic community. *Hispanic Outlook in Higher Education*, *10*, 19. http://eres.regent.edu/login?url=https://www-proquest-com.ezproxy.regent.edu/magazines/language-unmasking-loss-hispanic-community/docview/219285993/se-2?accountid=13479

Flores, E., Tschann, J. M., Dimas, J. M., Pasch, L. A., & de Groat, C. L. (2010). Perceived racial/ethnic discrimination, posttraumatic stress symptoms, and health risk behaviors among Mexican American adolescents. *Journal of Counseling Psychology*, *57*(3), 264–273. https://doi.org/10.1037/a0020026

Gutierrez, D., Barden, S. M., Gonzalez, J., Ali, S., & Cruz-Ortega, L. G. (2016). Perspectiva masculina: An exploration of intimate partners of Latina breast cancer survivors. *Family Journal*, *24*(3), 222–229. https://doi.org/10.1177/1066480716648690

Harkness, A., Behar-Zusman, V., & Safren, S. A. (2020). Understanding the impact of COVID-19 on Latino sexual minority men in a US HIV hot spot. *AIDS and Behavior*, *24*(7), 2017–2023. https://doi.org/10.1007/s10461-020-02862-w

Hernandez, E., Rosales, A., & Brodwin, M. (2018). Death and dying Latino/a cultural view of death. *California Association for Postsecondary Education & Disability*. www.caped.io/fall-2018/death-and-dying-latino-a-cultural-view-of-death/

Houben, L. M. (2011). *Counseling Hispanics through loss, grief, and bereavement: A guide for mental health professionals*. Springer.

Jason, L. A., Luna, R. D., Alvarez, J., & Stevens, E. (2018). Collectivism and individualism in Latino recovery homes. *Journal of Ethnicity in Substance Abuse*, *17*(3), 223–236. https://doi.org/10.1080/15332640.2016.1138267

Jocson, R. M., Alers-Rojas, F., Ceballo, R., & Arkin, M. (2020). Religion and spirituality: Benefits for Latino adolescents exposed to community violence. *Youth & Society*, *52*(3), 349–376. https://doi.org/10.1177/0044118X18772714

Khantzian, E. J. (1985). Psychotherapeutic interventions with substance abusers—the clinical context. *Journal of Substance Abuse Treatment*, *2*(2), 83–88. https://doi.org/10.1016/0740-5472(85)90031-5

Koob, G. F., & Schulkin, J. (2019). Addiction and stress: An allostatic view. *Neuroscience & Biobehavioral Reviews*, *106*, 245–262. https://doi.org/10.1016/j.neubiorev.2018.09.008

LaBrie, J. W., Atkins, D. C., Neighbors, C., Mirza, T., & Larimer, M. E. (2012). Ethnicity specific norms and alcohol consumption among Hispanic/Latino/a and Caucasian students. *Addictive Behaviors*, *37*(4), 573–576. https://doi.org/10.1016/j.addbeh.2012.01.007

Lardier Jr, D. T., Barrios, V. R., Garcia-Reid, P., & Reid, R. J. (2018). Preventing substance use among Hispanic urban youth: Valuing the role of family, social support networks, school importance, and community engagement. *Journal of Child & Adolescent Substance Abuse*, *27*(5–6), 251–263. https://doi.org/10.1080/1067828X.2018.1466748

Leach, D., & Kranzler, H. R. (2013). An interpersonal model of addiction relapse. *Addictive Disorders & Their Treatment*, *12*(4), 183–192. https://doi.org/10.1097/ADT.0b013e31826ac408

Marino, N. F. (2011). *Jorge Manrique's Coplas por la muerte de su padre: A history of the poem and its reception*. Tamesis.

Mays, V. M., Jones, A., Delany-Brumsey, A., Coles, C., & Cochran, S. D. (2017). Perceived discrimination in healthcare and mental health/substance abuse treatment among blacks, Latinos, and whites. *Medical Care*, *55*(2), 173–193. https://doi.org/10.1097/MLR.0000000000000638

Miller, L. D. (2013). "I am not who I thought I was": Use of grief work to address disrupted identity among Hispanic adolescent immigrants. *Clinical Social Work Journal*, *41*(4), 316–323. https://doi.org.ezproxy.regent.edu/10.1007/s10615-012-0410-5

Moore, R. H., & Chau, V. (2019, October 15). *Opioid and illicit drug use among the Hispanic/Latino populations*. Substance Abuse and Mental Health Services Administration. https://blog.samhsa.gov/2019/10/15/opioid-and-illicit-drug-use-among-the-hispaniclatino-populations

Mosher, D., Hook, J. N., Captari, L. E., Davis, D. E., DeBlaere, C., & Owen, J. (2017). Cultural humility: A therapeutic framework for engaging diverse clients. *Practice Innovations*, *2I*(4), 221–233. https://doi.org/10.1037/pri0000055

National Institute on Alcohol Abuse and Alcoholism. (2015). *Alcohol and the Hispanic community*.

Oller, F. (1893). *Velorio*. Smithsonian American Art Museum.

Owen, J. (2013). Early career perspectives on psychotherapy research and practice: Psychotherapist effects, multicultural orientation, and couple interventions. *Psychotherapy*, *50*(4), 496–502. https://doi.org/10.1037/a0034617

Pargament, K. I. (1997). *The psychology of religion and coping: Theory, research, practice*. Guilford Press.

Perreira, K. M., Marchante, A. N., Schwartz, S. J., Isasi, C. R., Carnethon, M. R., Corliss, H. L., & Delamater, A. M. (2019). Stress and resilience: Key correlates of mental health and substance use in the Hispanic community health study of Latino youth. *Journal of Immigrant and Minority Health*, *21*(1), 4–13. https://doi.org/10.1007/s10903-018-0724-7

Perreira, K. M., & Ornelas, I. (2013). Painful passages: Traumatic experiences and post-traumatic stress among US immigrant Latino adolescents and their primary caregivers. *International Migration Review, 47*(4), 976–1005. https://doi.org/10.1111/imre.12050

Pew Research Center. (2019). *Key facts about U.S. Hispanics and their diverse heritage.* www.pewresearch.org/fact-tank/2019/09/16/key-facts-about-u-s-hispanics/

Revens, K. E. (2019*). Understanding the factors associated with resilience in Latino immigrants.* (Doctoral dissertation). University of North Carolina at Charlotte.

Rojas, J. I., Hallford, G., Brand, M. W., & Tivis, L. J. (2012). Latino/as in substance abuse treatment: Substance use patterns, family history of addiction, and depression. *Journal of Ethnicity in Substance Abuse, 11*(1), 75–85. https://doi.org/10.1080/1533 2640.2012.652530

Rosenblatt, P. C. (2008). Grief across cultures: A review and research agenda. In M. S. Stroebe, R. O. Hansson, H. Schut, & W. Stroebe (Eds.), *Handbook of bereavement research and practice: Advances in theory and intervention* (pp. 207–222). American Psychological Association. https://doi.org/10.1037/14498-010

Salas-Wright, C. P., Hernandez, L. R., Maynard, B. Y., Saltzman, L., & Vaughn, M. G. (2014). Alcohol use among Hispanic early adolescents in the United States: An examination of behavioral risk and protective profiles. *Substance Use & Misuse, 49*(7), 864–877. https://doi.org/10.3109/10826084.2014.880725

Schoulte, J. C. (2011). Bereavement among African Americans and Latino/a Americans. *Journal of Mental Health Counseling, 33*(1), 11–20. https://doi.org/10.17744/mehc.33.1.r4971657p7176307

Smith, M. A. (2021). Social learning and addiction. *Behavioural Brain Research, 38,* 112954. https://doi.org/10.1016/j.bbr.2020.112954

Stevens, S., Andrade, R., Korchmaros, J., & Sharron, K. (2015). Intergenerational trauma among substance-using Native American, Latina, and White mothers living in the southwestern United States. *Journal of Social Work Practice in the Addictions, 15*(1), 6–24. https://doi.org/10.1080/1533256X.2014.996648

Substance Abuse and Mental Health Services Administration. (2019). *2018 national survey on drug use and health detailed tables.* www.samhsa.gov/data/report/2018-nsduh-detailed-tables

Substance Abuse and Mental Health Services Administration. (2020). *2019 national survey on drug use and health: Hispanics, Latino or Spanish origin or descent.* www.samhsa.gov/data/report/2019-nsduh-hispanics-latino-or-spanish-origin-or-desce

Tomkins, S. S. (1966). Psychological model for smoking behavior. *American Journal of Public Health and the Nation's Health, 56*(12), 17–20. https://doi.org/10.2105/ajph.56.12_suppl.17

Unger, J. B. (2014). Cultural influences on substance use among Hispanic adolescents and young adults: Findings from Project RED. *Child Development Perspectives, 8*(1), 48–53. https://doi.org/10.1111/cdep.12060

Unger, J. B., Shakib, S., Gallaher, P., Ritt-Olson, A., Mouttapa, M., Palmer, P. H., & Johnson, C. A. (2006). Cultural/interpersonal values and smoking in an ethnically diverse sample of southern California adolescents. *Journal of Cultural Diversity, 13*(1), 55–63.

Valdeón, R. A. (2013). *Hispanic* or *Latino*: The use of politicized terms for the Hispanic minority in US official documents and quality news outlets. *Language and Intercultural Communication, 13*(4), 433–449. https://doi.org/10.1080/14708477.2012.740047

Vega, W. A., Rodriguez, M. A., & Gruskin, E. (2009). Health disparities in the Latino population. *Epidemiologic Reviews*, *31*(1), 99–112. https://doi.org/10.1093/epirev/mxp008

Zamboanga, B. L., Schwartz, S. J., Jarvis, L. H., & Van Tyne, K. (2009). Acculturation and substance use among Hispanic early adolescents: Investigating the mediating roles of acculturative stress and self-esteem. *Journal of Primary Prevention*, *30*(3–4), 315–333. https://doi.org.ezproxy.regent.edu/10.1007/s10935-009-0182-z

9 Grief and Substance Use in Asian Americans

Kok-Mun Ng, Susan R. Furr, Yun Shi, and Krupali Michaels

According to the 2010 census, Asian Americans and Pacific Islanders have been the fastest growing racial group in the United States (Pew Research Center, 2015), with the vast majority being foreign born (U.S. Census Bureau, 2010). Within this growing population, there is wide ethnic diversity among Asian subgroups living in America. Yet research often aggregates all Asians into one group where differences may not be recognized (Watkins & Ford, 2011) and may lead to a "homogenized view," even though there are over 25 Asian ethnic subgroups living in the United States (Kim, Yang et al., 2001, p. 344). The name given to this group is Asian Americans and Pacific Islanders (AAPI). Even when sharing similar values, these subgroups may differ in the degree to which they endorse commonly held cultural values.

Kim, Yang et al. (2001) identified and measured Asian cultural value dimensions, including collectivism, conformity to norms, emotional self-control, family recognition through achievement, filial piety, and humility. When comparing these dimensions among Chinese, Filipino, Korean, and Japanese American college students, differences were found in how strongly each group endorsed these values, but overall the same items were endorsed more strongly in Asian American populations than in European American populations, indicating Asian subgroups held similar meaning of the dimensions (Kim et al., 1999). Interestingly, these researchers did not find differences between first, second, and third or greater generations associated with adherence to these dimensions, indicating consistency of these values over time. Despite the findings, to our knowledge, researchers have yet to compare such value dimensions across all 25 Asian ethnic subgroups living in the United States. Consequently, it is important for counselors to understand both the similarities among AAPI clients as well as the subgroup differences that may emerge. Further, when considering between-group differences, it is critical to remember within-group differences—that is, recognizing that many individuals within a group may differ significantly in their levels of endorsement of a certain value compared to the group mean. Such within-group sensitivity is needed to prevent ethnic overgeneralization and stereotyping. In term of substance use, even when values overlap among AAPI groups, the ways in which substance use affects subgroups may differ. Similarly, substance use effects and patterns may also differ

DOI: 10.4324/9781003106906-9

'within groups. This highlights a need for counselors to understand subgroup distinctions while bearing in mind individual uniqueness and difference.

Within-Group Differences

As AAPI subgroups are disaggregated, substance use patterns have been found to vary according to cultural background. Cook et al. (2013) found that among foreign-born Asian American young adults, Asian Indians had the lowest consumption of alcohol followed by Vietnamese and Chinese/Taiwanese. The highest consumption rate was found in Koreans followed by Japanese. Not only are immigrants affected by drinking patterns in the United States, but these researchers uncovered an influence from a person's country of origin (COO) that carried over to the new country. If more harmful drinking was found in the COO, an individual was found to be at higher risk for developing substance use problems in the new country (Cook et al., 2013). However, U.S.-born Asians are more likely to engage in heavy drinking than Asians who have immigrated, with those who have recently immigrated having the lowest rates (Lo et al., 2014).

Within-group differences among the AAPI populations also exist in treatment rates with Native Hawaiians and Pacific Islanders displaying higher levels of substance use than other Asian subgroups (Wu & Blazer, 2015) and having the lowest treatment rates as well as being less likely to complete treatment (Godinet et al., 2020). These authors concluded research that aggregates Asians and Native Hawaiians/Pacific Islanders will fail to capture the unique differences of each of these groups.

Substance Use Disorders in Asian American Populations

AAPI have been shown to have lower rates of co-occurring substance use and mental health disorders (2.1% lifetime) when compared to Whites (8.2%), Blacks (5.4%), and Latinx (5.8%) individuals living in the United States (Mericle et al., 2012). Watkins and Ford (2011) also found Asians had lower levels of substance use when compared to Whites and to other racial and ethnic groups, including lower rates of prescription misuse. Yet research has shown that AAPI demonstrated a greater increase in admissions for substance abuse treatment than non-AAPI from 2000 to 2012, with prescription opioid use showing the largest increase (Sahker et al., 2017). When Pacific Islanders are compared to Asian Americans, Pacific Islanders had lower treatment rates but higher rates of substance use, thus showing the importance of disaggregating groups (Godinet et al., 2020). However, counselors should not be surprised when they encounter clients of Asian descent in substance use treatment who differ from these patterns.

Co-occurring substance abuse and mental disorders have been found to be lower in Asian populations than in other populations. Based on a large national study of co-occurring substance abuse and mental health disorders, Asians were significantly less likely to indicate having a co-occurring disorder in their lifetime (Mericle et al., 2012). However, in all the ethnic groups in the study, most of the participants reported symptoms of their psychiatric disorder preceded their symptoms of substance use disorder. Given the tendency for Asian Americans to seek mental health services only when problems become severe (Kim-Goh et al., 2015; Lei & Pellitteri, 2017), Mericle et al. (2012) speculated these numbers may be lower because help seeking may be less prevalent in the AAPI community and services are less available. When comparing AAPI clients in treatment to non-AAPI clients, AAPI clients had lower use of medical and psychiatric services, but these differences did not appear to be related to differences in need. Upon admission to treatment, both groups were similar in problem severity in medical and psychiatric problems. It was unknown whether the lower rates of admission were related to inaccessibility of services or unacceptability of treatment (Niv et al., 2007). Yu et al. (2009) viewed the problem as related to culture and language barriers to seeking treatment, and when culturally appropriate services are available, service utilization rates increase.

Genetic factors have been linked with alcohol use in Asian Americans (Bujarski et al., 2015). In a meta-analysis of the literature, Li et al. (2012) found the presence of a particular genetic factor (ALDH2 504lys allele) can greatly lower the risk for alcohol addiction as well as alcohol-induced diseases in Asian populations, and this protective allele is barely found in populations of European descent. These studies also demonstrated the presence of this factor varied across Asian subpopulations. Matsushita and Higuchi (2017) found the ADH1B*2 and ALDH2*2 alleles appeared to provide some protective effects against the development of an alcohol use disorder and indicated that several studies suggested the ADH1B*2 allele was associated with a hypersensitivity to alcohol. The mechanism of how this allele is protective is through a high accumulation of acetaldehyde following drinking, which results in a number of unpleasant physiological effects from drinking, including headaches, nausea, facial flushing, and tachycardia. These authors cautioned that alleles alone cannot explain differences in alcohol use between racial and ethnic groups and consideration needs to be given to the roles played by personal and environmental factors. These factors can include peer pressure, availability, and cultural values around drinking.

Cultural Influences

Cultural expectations may become a barrier to seeking treatment. For example, family beliefs around working to contribute to the family may prohibit going to treatment (Masson et al., 2013). In addition, Asian Americans may hold a belief that substance abuse brings "shame to the family" and may choose to try and cope with the problem within the family rather than seek outside help (Niv et al., 2007, p. 313). For the clinician, it is important to become familiar with these commonly endorsed values and the cultural barriers Asian Americans may encounter when needing any type of mental health treatment (Masson et al., 2013).

Further, it is important to note Asian groups may differ in their degree of acceptance of alcohol consumption, an indicator of drinking culture. For example:

> Asian Americans who are descendants of Asian countries with high per capita alcohol consumption (e.g., South Korea and Japan) may be at higher risk of problematic alcohol use compared with individuals from ethnic drinking cultures with low per capita alcohol consumption (e.g., Malaysia).
>
> (Iwamoto et al., 2016, p. 20)

Also, many Asian cultures may consider alcohol consumption acceptable and illicit drug use unacceptable and stigmatizing, like the larger culture in the United States. However, Asians who are adherents to the Islamic faith are likely to hold a strong prohibition against both alcohol and illicit drug use. Such attitudes and beliefs may influence substance use behavior and help-seeking intentions and behavior.

Acculturation is the process by which individuals make changes in their behaviors and values as they gradually embrace the dominant culture. However, behavior changes needed for survival in the new culture will occur first, whereas there may not be a compelling reason to change one's cultural values (Kim et al., 1999). Thus, Asian cultural values may remain over time, which would have an impact on help-seeking behavior. Sodowsky et al. (1995) have pointed out that while Asian Americans may quickly embrace the behaviors of their new culture, they may remain committed to their Asian cultural values indefinitely. Relatedly, acculturation stress has been found to be associated with heavy drinking in the research (e.g., Park et al., 2014). Kim, Atkinson et al. (2001) outlined a set of propositions that relate the Asian cultural values to the counseling process. These authors stated the field of psychology evolved from individualistic cultures and may be in conflict with the values of collectivistic cultures. Unless the counselor has a good understanding of these values, establishing a therapeutic relationship will be hindered. The following list summarizes the value domains established by the research of Kim, Atkinson, et al. (2001). However, it is important to note that cultural values are dynamic variables, and their influences differ with groups and may change across a person's life span due to processes such as acculturation. Hence, the concepts listed are starting points of consideration for clinicians who are working with Asian clients in substance use treatment settings and, they should not let the list contribute to an essentialist and reductionist view of a culture.

Ability to resolve psychological problem: Value is placed on the ability to resolve one's own psychological issues through using one's own inner resources and by moderating one's own thoughts, emotions, and behaviors. Seeking outside help would be viewed as a weakness.

Avoidance of family shame: Any individual failure is viewed as reflecting badly on the family. Disgracing one's family is seen as the worst thing a person can do.

Collectivism: The group to which one belongs takes on greater value than one's personal interests and goals, with group members being interdependent with each other.

Conformity to family and social norms and expectations: Following the expectations of family and society is seen as important. It is critical not to disrupt the existing state of affairs.

Deference to authority figures: Authority figures are to be respected and not questioned. Those with higher education should receive higher respect and not be referred to by their first name.

Educational and occupational achievement: One's success in life is measured by these achievements and becomes a source of parental pride.

Filial piety: Obedience to parents is unquestioned, and children are expected to accept their authority. Parental love is not expressed openly but is understood implicitly. It is expected that adult children will take care of aging parents.

Importance of family: Family well-being takes precedence over one's own achievements: accomplishments by one family member are viewed as achievements of the family. The most important thing is family well-being, and individuals are expected to make sacrifices for the family.

Maintenance of interpersonal harmony: Maintaining harmony is viewed as more important than resolving differences. Feelings should not be expressed in any way that disrupts this harmony or would cause a person to lose face.

Placing others' needs ahead of one's own: Considering the needs of others comes first, and their needs should be anticipated. The goal is to not cause discomfort to another.

Reciprocity: The expectation is that one will repay any favor from another. However, reciprocity works both ways, in that if one gives a favor, a favor is expected in return.

Respect for elders and ancestors: Children are expected to respect the wisdom of their elders and honor their ancestors. Young people should not talk back to elders or go against their wishes.

Self-control and restraint: Controlling emotions is seen as a sign of strength, whether those emotions are positive or negative. Holding pain and suffering inside is viewed as better than expressing strong feelings.

Self-effacement: One's achievements should be minimized, and success should be attributed to the support from others. Humbleness and modesty are valued above talking about accomplishments.

As can be seen from this list, commonly accepted counseling practices in both substance abuse counseling and grief counseling may be challenged by clients holding these values. Yet the ability of the counselor to find strengths in these values rather than viewing them as a detriment to counseling will enable the counselor to form a supportive alliance with the client. Singh et al. (2015) have shown the positive impact family support has in decreasing psychological distress, so finding meaningful ways to include family as allies in treatment may provide a valuable resource. For example, linking Asian American mothers and adolescent daughters in a web-based substance use prevention program resulted both in stronger mother–daughter connections and greater self-efficacy in daughters to avoid using substances (Fang & Schinke, 2013). Asian clients often come to substance abuse treatment through school referrals (Garrison et al., 2019) or court mandates (Masson et al., 2013). When working with school referrals, finding ways to engage the strength and support of the family could help encourage program completion. By the counselor showing respect about the importance of the family unit, stronger bonds can be created. Keeping the focus on the importance of the client rather than a focus on negative legal consequences can help move the focus away from the shame the family might have encountered.

One challenge in treatment for SUDs might be the confrontational nature that often occurs in these treatment settings, particularly in groups. Such a setting could employ methods contrary to the values of many Asian clients. Directly confronting an Asian client to disclose inner conflicts would be contrary to personal values, whereas showing respect for personal boundaries could build trust. It would be particularly important to approach Asian clients in a way in which the client can save face in the presence of others. Being asked to contribute by the leader could have more positive results than using a nondirective style. Further, going over the structure, process, and expectations of group work individually with all clients, and particularly Asian clients, to assess their readiness for group work and addressing concerns they may have about their participation will likely provide an opportunity to orientate them to group work. Paying attention to and positively valuing group dynamics that may be related to cultural values may help to foster mutual respect and therapeutic working alliance among group members.

Gender Differences

In AAPI cultures, gender roles may be more distinctive because of the hierarchies established in the culture, with males and females fulfilling specific roles (Han et al., 2016). Males are expected to fulfill the role of provider, so they may feel more pressure to seek help if substance use is interfering with their role as financial provider. In a comparison of AAPI men and women who were in treatment, women reported to experience more psychological problems and encountered more problems with employment and family (Han et al., 2016).

Differences were found in treatment preferences, with females favoring an empathic counseling style and men preferring a utilitarian style. In a follow-up after treatment, females reported lower satisfaction with the attitudes of their counselors related to experiencing lower counselor empathy. Females in treatment for SUD were more likely to report dependent living status and to be living with someone who also used substances, which may indicate a need for family treatment.

Research has shown Asian American men are more likely to use substances more than Asian American women (Lum et al., 2009). We believe that Asian women's lower substance use is related to cultural values that stigmatize women who use and abuse substances more than it does their gender counter-parts. In a qualitative study, Asian American women reported feeling isolated and alone when dealing with substance use issues due to the shame and stigma associated with seeking treatment. They also reported the need to appear strong and avoid showing vulnerability (Augsberger et al., 2015).

One predictor of substance use in males is conformity to masculine norms (Liu & Iwamoto, 2007). Using regression analyses, these researchers found marijuana use was predicted by the variables *peer substance use, disdain for homosexuality, winning, playboy*, and *violence*, while *peer use and power over women* were associated with binge drinking. In this population of Asian American college men, those who reported regulating emotions and who did not endorse risk-taking were less likely to use alcohol. Avoidant coping (which includes alcohol use) and adherence to masculine norms have been associated with depression in Asian American men (Iwamoto et al., 2010). These research-ers believed their findings provide support for the self-medication theory that substance use is a method to deal with psychological issues. Iwamoto et al. (2010) postulated that Asian American men may adopt an unhealthy hyper-masculinity as a means of adapting to the White masculine identity. Because the Western media has often emasculated Asian men, these men may feel an increased need to appear more masculine, which may lead to harmful coping behaviors (SAMHSA, 2017). This intersection of racial and gender identities may result in psychological stress, leading to substance use as a means of cop-ing. One recommendation is for clinicians to discuss masculinity with Asian American clients to understand how gender roles and racial bias influence sub-stance use.

Model Minority

Mental health issues have often been overlooked among Asian Americans due to the perception they are a "model minority," in which people of Asian descent are viewed as experiencing increasing wealth accompanied by upward social mobility (Wong & Halgin, 2006, p. 38). This population is seen as free from crime and mental health issues and lauded for academic achievement. This image has been especially true for Asian Indians, who have generally achieved higher levels of education and greater proficiency in English than other immigrant groups (Rastogi & Wadhwa, 2006). Although this view appears to be positive, the model minority stereotype may increase psychological distress and in turn increase problematic drinking (Iwamoto et al., 2014). These assumptions about Asian American success can serve to minimize problems experienced and even conceal those who are encountering psychological difficulties (Mercado, 2000). Because Asian Americans underutilize mental health services, the myth they have fewer mental health and substance abuse issues may cover up actual problems. While Asian Americans generally have lower levels of alcohol use, they have a higher percentage of heavy drinkers among those who drink alcohol. Mercado goes on to state expectations of being a model minority may be tied to the stress that accompanies these high expectations.

Wong and Halgin (2006) examined Asian college students' attitudes toward the model minority label and found over 50% had a negative response to the label. Only 26.3% expressed positive feelings toward the label, and these students were likely to score high on measures of collectivism, connectedness, interdependent achievement, and work ethic scales, emphasizing connection to traditional Asian values. Those who had negative attitudes placed equal emphasis on group identity and individual self-identity and expressed they did not like having these expectations placed on them. The model minority label was seen as a form of marginalization by the larger society, where students believed they were not seen as individuals. Such expectations can result in inner conflict for students when there are differences between their own interests and parental expectations, leading to feelings of failure for not living up to this internalized model. Further, the model minority myth "has been used strategically by opponents of equal opportunity policies and programs to support the notion of meritocracy with evidence that racial discrimination does not exist" (Museus & Kiang, 2009, p. 6). Counselors who work with Asian Americans need to be cognizant of their own perceptions, which may include beliefs about this population being a model minority and examine how these beliefs may contribute to substance use and the clinicians' response to clients in this population.

Expressions of Grief in Asian Culture

Grieving and the rituals used to facilitate grief expression are culturally bound, and we can only understand them in the context of clients' beliefs and values. Most of the writings about grief and loss in Asian subgroups come from the context of grieving a death. Although there are many other sources of loss, clients may only consider grief as associated with death. Once the counselor helps clients see their grief over other types of losses, clients may be ready to explore other losses in counseling once trust is established.

In examining the meaning of death in Asian populations, beliefs can range from ancestor worship as an aspect of Confucianism to the concept of reincarnation in Buddhism, in which premature death may result in a belief someone did something bad and is being punished for this action (Braun & Nichols, 1997). Another important concept is continuing bonds with the deceased and is often shown by having an altar for honoring the ancestors (Chan et al., 2005). Younger members of a culture may move away from traditions and simplify rituals as they acculturate to the new culture. For example, one of our students from an Asian subculture shared a story about how young people may still bring food to the family altar, but it had shifted to the sharing of "fast food" as opposed to preparing food offerings. The period of rituals can extend for a week or more, and the period of mourning may extend for several years. Clients may share how they feel, hear, or see the deceased and view the deceased appearing in dreams (Chan et al., 2005). Many of these practices are changing, as those from Asian cultures move away from their more traditional practices. For the counselor, insight into a client's cultural traditions can demonstrate respect for the client and help them make sense of their losses (Braun & Nichols, 1997). Because of the communal nature of many of the important rituals, the client's substance use may have interfered with practicing meaningful rituals, and shame in facing the family may have kept them away from these important grieving ceremonies. It is important for counselors whose cultural backgrounds differ from Asian clients to be cognizant of their own expectations about grief rituals, not perceive their clients' beliefs and rituals from their own values, and actively seek to understand the meaningful practices from other cultures.

Although our clients with SUD may have unresolved grieving around death, there are many other losses prevalent in the Asian community. Immigration, racism and discrimination, trauma, and human trafficking are just some of the sources of loss experienced. These losses may result in disenfranchised grief, which results from loss not recognized as socially acceptable (Casado et al., 2010). As counselors, we need to be receptive of the cultural losses experienced by our clients who are immigrants and develop sensitivity and invitational skills to broach these issues therapeutically when necessary. Choosing to leave a country because of political, social, economic, or safety reasons does not mean there is not a sense of loss for the client. Clinicians need to be aware of local sentiment in the community concerning those who immigrate and be prepared to address biases that may arise in treatment settings.

Immigration, Acculturation, and Discrimination Stressors

One source of grief experienced by immigrants is associated with leaving their home country (Casado et al., 2010). Not only is immigration a stressful life event, but there is evidence this process creates mental health problems. Losses include both material losses (e.g., homes) and the loss of the familiar, including language, cultural values, and social connections. For the immigrant, these losses may be disenfranchised by the new country, where the focus may be on the positive aspects of their new country with little attention to what has been left behind. "Migratory grief" (Casado et al., 2010, p. 612) is the term applied to this series of losses that occur when leaving one's country. There are also symbolic losses of intangible things, such as loss of status and identity that have psychological and social consequences.

Park et al. (2014) found both acculturation and acculturative stress were predictors of alcohol use in subgroups of Asian immigrants, but these authors also indicated the importance of examining subgroups separately. For example, Vietnamese immigrants demonstrated a significant relationship between alcohol consumption and everyday discrimination and general acculturative stress, whereas Chinese immigrants had a significant relationship between alcohol consumption and family cultural conflict. However, Lo et al. (2014) found recent immigrants had lower levels of heavy drinking than long-term residents, leading to questions about the role of acculturation in establishing drinking patterns versus the role of family support. This further demonstrates the multifactorial nature of substance use behavior among immigrants and their descending generations. Additionally, while research on differences in substance use and problematic gambling behavior between refugees from Southeast Asian countries and other Asian groups are mixed, clinicians may want to be aware of the impact of pre- and post-resettlement experiences of Asians who immigrated to the United States as refugees (Kim & Kim, 2014).

Racial discrimination has shown an indirect relationship with alcohol problems in that discrimination leads to drinking to cope, which in turn leads to alcohol problems (Le & Iwamoto, 2019). In a longitudinal study of Asian American college students, these authors concluded that "experiencing increased racial discrimination was associated with having more alcohol-related problems a year later through drinking to cope" (p. 525). A previous study also found that the presence of an SUD was related to perceived discrimination in three different racial groups (Lo & Cheng, 2012). In particular, the increased rates of SUD were stronger among Asian Americans who were poor, demonstrating the intersectionality of race and poverty.

In extreme cases, prolonged grief disorder can develop for those who witnessed violent deaths of loved ones or experienced multiple deaths, factors that may have prompted immigration; however, there are protective and adaptive factors that can facilitate coping. Belonging to a community, family and community support, supportive relationships, and religious beliefs may facilitate coping (Kokou-Kpolou et al., 2020). One group of potential clients in substance abuse treatment involves those who have been victims of human trafficking (Pascual-Leone et al., 2017). While not all victims of trafficking are immigrants, there are countries that promote sex tourism or fulfill demands for cheap labor in the United States. When the victims are from other countries, their traffickers control them through violence and threats of deportation. Dependency on the traffickers often is facilitated by creating addiction to drugs. Drugs can become a way of coping with the distress and trauma created by being trafficked. Feelings of intense shame and self-blame for falling prey to captors may be experienced, and humiliation over the sexual abuse may complicate feelings of loss. Once freed from captivity, trust will be a major issue in seeking treatment. Support from family may be lacking due to family members who reject those forced into the sex industry, leading to further shame and exclusion from family. If they are in the country by themselves, they would not have direct access to family and community support. Rejection by family may interfere with seeking treatment. Loss of dignity as well as loss of safety and support often are themes that may accompany the recovery process (Pascual-Leone et al., 2017). First-line treatments need to include emotion-focused and emotion regulations strategies, and then move to cognitive restructuring and education about trauma as second-line treatment. These clients may often have to face legal issues related to their status as unlawful immigrants and face the threat of deportation. Hence, counselors may need to assist them to access services that can help them navigate a host of related challenges.

When grief issues are involved in SUD treatment, pressure to express painful feelings may work to the detriment of an Asian client. However, Asian clients may be more receptive of activities related to thoughts and structured activities led by a "wise" expert while working toward empowering them to navigate challenges in a society that prizes self-reliance and upholds values that may seem contrary to theirs. It is also important that cultural practices around grief and loss be valued by the counselor rather than judged according to dominant culture expectations. In areas with large AAPI populations, treatments specifically designed for these groups may create culturally competent approaches that accommodate the values, beliefs, and practices of clients and their families (Kim-Goh et al., 2015). Addressing issues such as the purpose and process of counseling, language match between client and counselor, and openness of discussing cultural issues and culturally congruent intervention can enhance treatment outcomes.

A study of AAPI mental health professionals identified barriers to treatment such as stigma, suppression of emotions, and lack of linguistic congruency (Kim-Goh et al., 2015). The use of culturally compatible approaches, such as cognitive behavioral therapy and more directive, problem-solving approaches, were cited as effective with this population. In addition, mindfulness appeared to mesh well with Asian philosophies. These therapists also emphasized the importance of including family in treatment, which can improve client adherence to the therapeutic process. Rather than an egalitarian relationship, the counselor needs to understand the hierarchical nature of the client-counselor relationship in terms of age, education, and professional status and how this hierarchy will manifest and can be appropriately used to empower when working with the family.

To conclude, we include two case examples to illustrate the complexities clinicians may encounter when providing services to Asian clients who have concerns about substance use and grief and loss. We further include some reflection questions to invite clinicians to apply the concepts discussed in this chapter.

Case 1. A Late-Thirties Female Immigrant From China

Yana came from China to the United States for graduate school 15 years ago. Now in her late thirties, she works as an accountant and is married to a fellow accountant with two young children. Her husband is a biracial American. Yana's days are packed and stressful. To release stress at the end of the day, she would normally have a glass of wine. Mostly, she can keep her drinking to no more than two glasses. Yana's husband shares similar drinking habits. Although excessive use of alcohol and illicit drug use for women in her culture is often frowned upon, Yana feels some shame and prefers not to talk about topics related to drinking because she would find herself drinking more than the usual amount, to the point that she had had to skip work due to a bad hangover when stress levels got very high.

Yana is the only child of her parents who lived in China. Three years ago, Yana's father was diagnosed with cancer. Yana's mother had very poor health, so Yana had been traveling between the two countries to care for her parents. The constant pressure of caring for a terminally ill parent added to Yana's stress physically and emotionally. Before Yana realized it, she turned more and more to drinking for comfort and stress relief. Yana made repeated efforts to stop drinking, but she would relapse when stress built up. This situation became more acute after Yana's father passed away, and she had to take care of the funeral arrangements in China by herself while her husband took care of their children in the States. Grief and shame began to hit her regularly after she returned to the States. Her increased alcohol use has become more problematic than she is willing to admit.

Case 2. A 45-Year-Old South Indian Male

Gaurav is a 45-year-old male who has immigrated from Gujarat, India. He is married to a Gujarati woman and has three children aged 10, 7, and 4. He struggles with alcohol use and complicated grief issues, both of which he denies as problems. Approximately 10 years ago, Gaurav got into a bad car accident at work, and currently, he is on long-term disability. His alcohol use has increased since his accident, which has led to isolation from his family and friends. Gaurav has binge-drinking episodes every weekend, which results in him becoming verbally aggressive to those around him. Often, he has become so intoxicated that his family cannot attend social events, which are important sociocultural systems because there are not many Indian families in the community.

Gaurav lost his father two months before his birth in India. His mother cared for him and his three siblings as a single parent with no money and no steady income due to the cultural expectations at the time. Gaurav grew up in extreme poverty with his family and often witnessed drug use and violence as a child; his mother was too busy trying to provide for the family to give adequate attention to Gaurav or his siblings. When Gaurav stopped working due to his disability, he began presenting with feelings of worthlessness, hopelessness, and overall depression. His mother, who lives with the family, enabled these thoughts and feelings. Both parent and child have not had adequate support to work through the death of the husband/father, which happened 45 years ago. Gaurav refuses to believe that his mental health is affecting his chronic back pain, for which doctors have not been able to identify a medical cause. Gaurav refuses help from a psychologist due to past experiences and prefers only to work with medical doctors.

Reflection Questions

1   Based on the information provided in each of the cases, how might the content in this chapter be helpful for counselors to understand the role of alcohol use/abuse in each of the cases?
2   Should these two individuals seek counseling services, how might culturally informed and responsive services that also honor individual uniqueness for these individuals look like?
3   What may prevent counselors who share similar ethnic backgrounds and cultural experiences with these individuals from effectively serving these individual? Why?

References

Augsberger, A., Hahm, H., Yeung, A., & Dougher, M. (2015). Barriers to substance use and mental health utilization among Asian-American women: Exploring the conflict between emotional distress and cultural stigma. *Addiction Science & Clinical Practice*, *10*(S1), A2–A2. https://doi.org/10.1186/1940-0640-10-S1-A2

Braun, K., & Nichols, R. (1997). Death and dying in four Asian American cultures: A descriptive study. *Death Studies*, *21*(4), 327–359. https://doi.org/10.1080/074811897201877

Bujarski, S., Lau, A., Lee, S., & Ray, L. (2015). Genetic and environmental predictors of alcohol use in Asian American young adults. *Journal of Studies on Alcohol and Drugs*, *76*(5), 690–699. https://doi.org/10.15288/jsad.2015.76.690

Casado, B., Hong, M., & Harrington, D. (2010). Measuring migratory grief and loss associated with the experience of immigration. *Research on Social Work Practice*, *20*(6), 611–620. https://doi.org/10.1177/1049731509360840

Chan, C., Chow, A., Ho, S., Tsui, Y., Tin, A., Koo, B., & Koo, E. (2005). The experience of Chinese bereaved persons: A preliminary study of meaning making and continuing bonds. *Death Studies*, *29*(10), 923–947. https://doi.org/10.1080/07481180500299287

Cook, W., Bond, J., Karriker-Jaffe, K. J., & Zemore, S. (2013). Who's at risk? Ethnic drinking cultures, foreign nativity, and problem drinking among Asian American young adults. *Journal of Studies on Alcohol and Drugs*, *74*(4), 532–541. https://doi.org/10.15288/jsad.2013.74.532

Fang, L., & Schinke, S. (2013). Two-year outcomes of a randomized, family-based substance use prevention trial for Asian American adolescent girls. *Psychology of Addictive Behaviors*, *27*(3), 788–798. https://doi.org/10.1037/a0030925

Garrison, Y., Sahker, E., Yeung, C., Park, S., & Arndt, S. (2019). Asian American and Pacific Islander substance use treatment completion. *Psychological Services, 16*(4), 636–646. https://doi.org/10.1037/ser0000274

Godinet, M. T., McGlinn, L., Nelson, D., & Vakalahi, H. O. (2020). Factors contributing to substance misuse treatment completion among Native Hawaiians, Other Pacific Islanders, and Asian Americans. *Substance Use and Misuse, 55*(1), 133–146. https://doi.org/10.1080/10826084.2019.1657896

Han, Y., Lin, V., Wu, F., & Hser, Y. (2016). Gender comparisons among Asian American and Pacific Islander patients in drug dependency treatment. *Substance Use & Misuse, 51*(6), 752–762. https://doi.org/10.3109/10826084.2016.1155604

Iwamoto, D., Kaya, A., Grivel, M., & Clinton, L. (2016). Under-researched demographics: Heavy episodic drinking and alcohol-related problems among Asian Americans. *Alcohol Research: Current Reviews, 38*(1), 17–25.

Iwamoto, D., Lejuez, C., Hamilton, E., & Grivel, M. (2014). Model minority stereotype, psychological distress, substance use among Asian-American young adults. *Drug and Alcohol Dependence, 146*, e146—e146. https://doi.org/10.1016/j.drugalcdep.2014.09.315

Iwamoto, D., Liao, L., & Liu, W. (2010). Masculine norms, avoidant coping, Asian values, and depression among Asian American men. *Psychology of Men & Masculinity, 11*(1), 15–24. https://doi.org/10.1037/a0017874

Kim, B., Atkinson, D., & Umemoto, D. (2001). Asian cultural values and the counseling process: Current knowledge and directions for future research. *Counseling Psychologist, 29*(4), 570–603. https://doi.org/10.1177/0011000001294006

Kim, B., Atkinson, D., & Yang, P. (1999). The Asian values scale: Development, factor analysis, validation, and reliability. *Journal of Counseling Psychology, 46*(3), 342–352. https://doi.org/10.1037//0022-0167.46.3.342

Kim, B., Yang, P., Atkinson, D., Wolfe, M., & Hong, S. (2001). Cultural value similarities and differences among Asian American ethnic groups. *Cultural Diversity & Ethnic Minority Psychology, 7*(4), 343–361. https://doi.org/10.1037/1099-9809.7.4.343

Kim, I., & Kim, W. (2014). Post-resettlement challenges and mental health of Southeast Asian refugees in the United States. *Best Practices in Mental Health, 10*(2), 63–77.

Kim-Goh, M., Choi, H., & Yoon, M. (2015). Culturally responsive counseling for Asian Americans: Clinician perspectives. *International Journal for the Advancement of Counselling, 37*(1), 63–76. https://doi.org/10.1007/s10447-014-9226-z

Kokou-Kpolou, C., Moukouta, C., Masson, J., Bernoussi, A., Cénat, J., & Bacqué, M. (2020). Correlates of grief-related disorders and mental health outcomes among adult refugees exposed to trauma and bereavement: A systematic review and future research directions. *Journal of Affective Disorders, 267*, 171–184. https://doi.org/10.1016/j.jad.2020.02.026

Le, T., & Iwamoto, D. (2019). A longitudinal investigation of racial discrimination, drinking to cope, and alcohol-related problems among underage Asian American college students. *Psychology of Addictive Behaviors, 33*(6), 520–528. https://doi.org/10.1037/adb0000501

Lei, N., & Pellitteri, J. (2017). Help-seeking and coping behaviors among Asian Americans: The roles of Asian values, emotional intelligence, and optimism. *Asian American Journal of Psychology, 8*(3), 224–234. https://doi.org/10.1037/aap0000086

Li, D., Li, D., Zhao, H., Zhao, H., Gelernter, J., & Gelernter, J. (2012). Strong protective effect of the aldehyde dehydrogenase gene (ALDH2) 504lys (2) allele against alcoholism and alcohol-induced medical diseases in Asians. *Human Genetics*, *131*(5), 725–737. https://doi.org/10.1007/s00439-011-1116-4

Liu, W., & Iwamoto, D. (2007). Conformity to masculine norms, Asian values, coping strategies, peer group influences and substance use among Asian American men. *Psychology of Men & Masculinity*, *8*(1), 25–39. https://doi.org/10.1037/1524-9220.8.1.25

Lo, C., & Cheng, T. (2012). Discrimination's role in minority groups' rates of substance-use disorder. *American Journal on Addictions*, *21*(2), 150–156. https://doi.org/10.1111/j.1521-0391.2011.00205.x

Lo, C., Cheng, T., & Howell, R. (2014). The role of immigration status in heavy drinking among Asian Americans. *Substance Use & Misuse*, *49*(8), 932–940. https://doi.org/10.3109/10826084.2013.852578

Lum, C., Corliss, H. L., Mays, V. M., Cochran, S. D., & Lui, C. K. (2009). Differences in the drinking behaviors of Chinese, Filipino, Korean, and Vietnamese college students. *Journal of Studies on Alcohol and Drugs*, *70*(4), 568–574. https://doi.org/10.15288/jsad.2009.70.568

Masson, C., Shopshire, M., Sen, S., Hoffman, K., Hengl, N., Bartolome, J., McCarty, D., Sorensen, J., & Iguchi, M. (2013). Possible barriers to enrollment in substance abuse treatment among a diverse sample of Asian Americans and Pacific Islanders: Opinions of treatment clients. *Journal of Substance Abuse Treatment*, *44*(3), 309–315. https://doi.org/10.1016/j.jsat.2012.08.005

Matsushita, S., & Higuchi, S. (2017). Review: Use of Asian samples in genetic research of alcohol use disorders: Genetic variation of alcohol metabolizing enzymes and the effects of acetaldehyde. *American Journal on Addictions*, *26*(5), 469–476. https://doi.org/10.1111/ajad.12477

Mercado, M. (2000). The invisible family: Counseling Asian American substance abusers and their families. *Family Journal*, *8*(3), 267–272. https://doi.org/10.1177/1066480700083008

Mericle, A., Ta Park, V., Holck, P., & Arria, A. (2012). Prevalence, patterns, and correlates of co-occurring substance use and mental disorders in the United States: Variations by race/ethnicity. *Comprehensive Psychiatry*, *53*(6), 657–665. https://doi.org/10.1016/j.comppsych.2011.10.002

Museus, S. D., & Kiang, P. N. (2009). Deconstructing the model minority myth and how it contributes to the invisible minority reality in higher education research. *New Directions for Institutional Research*, *142*, 5–15. https://doi.org/10.1002/ir.292

Niv, N., Wong, E., & Hser, Y. (2007). Asian Americans in community-based substance abuse treatment: Service needs, utilization, and outcomes. *Journal of Substance Abuse Treatment*, *33*(3), 313–319. https://doi.org/10.1016/j.jsat.2006.12.012

Park, S., Anastas, J., Shibusawa, T., & Nguyen, D. (2014). The impact of acculturation and acculturative stress on alcohol use across Asian immigrant subgroups. *Substance Use & Misuse*, *49*(8), 922–931. https://doi.org/10.3109/10826084.2013.855232

Pascual-Leone, A., Pascual-Leone, A., Kim, J., Kim, J., Morrison, O., & Morrison, O. (2017). Working with victims of human trafficking. *Journal of Contemporary Psychotherapy*, *47*(1), 51–59. https://doi.org/10.1007/s10879-016-9338-3

Pew Research Center. (2015). *Modern immigrant wave brings 59 million to U.S., driving population growth and change through 2065: Views of immigrations' impact on U.S. society mixed.* Author.

Rastogi, M., & Wadhwa, S. (2006). Substance abuse among Asian Indians in the United States: A consideration of cultural factors in etiology and treatment. *Substance Use & Misuse*, *41*(9), 1239–1249. https://doi.org/10.1080/10826080600754470

Sahker, Y., Yeung, C., Loh, Y., Park, S., & Arndt, S. (2017). Asian American and Pacific Islander substance use treatment admission trends. *Drug and Alcohol Dependence*, *171*, 1–8. https://doi.org/10.1016/j.drugalcdep.2016.11.022

SAMHSA. (2017). Advancing best practices in behavioral health for Asian American, Native Hawaiian, and Pacific Islander boys and men. HHS Publication N. (SMA) 17–5032

Singh, S., McBride, K., & Kak, V. (2015). Role of social support in examining acculturative stress and psychological distress among Asian American immigrants and three sub-groups: Results from NLAAS. *Journal of Immigrant and Minority Health*, *17*(6), 1597–1606. https://doi.org/10.1007/s10903-015-0213-1

Sodowsky, G. R., Kwan, K.-L. K., & Pannu, R. (1995). *Ethnic identity of Asians in the United States*. In J. G. Ponterotto, J. M. Casas, L. A. Suzuki, & C. M. Alexander (Eds.), *Handbook of multicultural counseling* (pp. 123–154). Sage.

U.S. Census Bureau: The Asian Population: 2010. www.census.gov/prod/cen2010/briefs/c2010br-11.pdf

Watkins, W. C., & Ford, J. A. (2011). Prescription drug misuse among Asian-American adults: Results from a national survey. *Substance Use & Misuse*, *46*(13), 1700–1708. https://doi.org/10.3109/10826084.2011.605415

Wong, F., & Halgin, R. (2006). The "model minority": Bane or blessing for Asian Americans? *Journal of Multicultural Counseling and Development*, *34*(1), 38–49. https://doi.org/10.1002/j.2161-1912.2006.tb00025.x

Wu, L., & Blazer, D. (2015). Substance use disorders and co-morbidities among Asian Americans and Native Hawaiians/Pacific Islanders. *Psychological Medicine*, *45*(3), 481–494. https://doi.org/10.1017/S0033291714001330

Yu, J., Clark, L., Chandra, L., Dias, A., & Lai, T.-F. (2009). Reducing cultural barriers to substance abuse treatment among Asian Americans: A case study in New York City. *Journal of Substance Abuse Treatment*, *37*(4), 398–408. https://doi.org/10.1016/j.jsat.2009.05.006

10 Addiction and Grief in the Native American Community

Kathleen Brown-Rice and Vanessa Iverson

My people are few. They resemble the scattering trees of a storm-swept plain. . . . There was a time when our people covered the land as the waves of a wind-ruffled sea cover its shell-paved floor, but that time long since passed away with the greatness of tribes that are now but a mournful memory.
—Chief Seattle, The Chief Seattle's Speech

The American Indian/Native American (AI/NA) community has been subjected to decades of atrocities that have resulted in unimaginable loss of people, land, family, and culture (i.e., *historical losses*; Brave Heart & DeBruyn, 1998; Brown-Rice, 2013; Garrett & Pichette, 2000; Whitbeck et al., 2004). The theory of historical trauma was developed by Brave Heart and DeBruyn (1998) to understand how the past and current struggles in many AI/NA communities are a consequence of "a legacy of chronic trauma and unresolved grief across generations" perpetrated on them by the European dominant culture (p. 60). In that, *historical loss symptoms* (e.g., substance abuse, depression, dysfunctional parenting, obesity, diabetes, uncmployment) are a result of the cross-generational transmission of cultural traumas from *historical losses* (Brown-Rice, 2013; Whitbeck et al., 2004), as seen in Figure 10.1. The impact of the spread of these cultural traumas has and continues to impact AI/NA individuals, families, and communities (Evans-Campbell, 2008) by generating a pathway positioning the present generation at bigger risk of mental and physical suffering, including substance abuse (Big Foot & Funderburk, 2011).

Disintegration of a Culture

From 1492 to 1776, the population of AI/NAs in North American declined by 95% (Plous, 2003) due to the intentional killing of AI/NAs and the exposure of AI/NAs to European illnesses (Trusty et al., 2002). While some exposure to these diseases was unintended on the part of the Europeans, the intentional introduction of disease has been documented. In 1763, Lord Jeffrey Amherst ordered that blankets with smallpox be given to AI/NAs (Plous, 2003). The agenda of U.S. government agencies, churches, and other organizations was

DOI: 10.4324/9781003106906-10

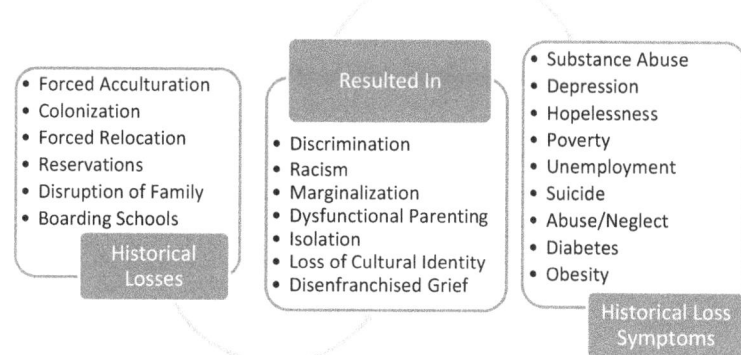

Figure 10.1 Cycle of Historical Trauma

to intrude on the AI/NA population and lands, which led to a disruption to AI/NA culture (Brave Heart & DeBruyn, 1998; Garrett & Pichette, 2000). In that, the goal was to force AI/NAs to completely assimilate to the dominant White culture and fully abandon their own culture (Brown-Rice, 2013).

From the time the United States was formed in 1776 and into the 19th century, the key agenda for most U.S. government officials was to acquire AI/NA lands (e.g., Indian Removal Act of 1830; Duran, 2006; Plous, 2003). By 1876, the majority of AI/NA lands had been confiscated by the U.S. government, and the AI/NA people were forced to either live on reservations or relocate to urban areas (Brave Heart & DeBruyn, 1998; Trusty et al., 2002). Today, approximately 70% of AI/NAs live in urban areas (IHS, 2020) and not on their traditional lands or government-established reservations. Leaving their traditional lands led to a sharp decline in socioeconomic status for AI/NAs, and families became reliant on commodities provided by the U.S. government (Brave Heart & DeBruyn, 1998). "These relocations resulted in the death of thousands of [AI/NAs] and the disruption of families" (Brown-Rice, 2013, p. 119). The loss of life further affected the AI/NA community due to the inability of its members to mourn these lost ones. In 1883, a federal law was passed that forbid AI/NAs from practicing indigenous ceremonies (Brave Heart et al., 2011), which led to disenfranchised grief for many AI/NAs (Brave Heart et al., 2011; Sotero, 2006). It was not until 1978, when the American Indian Religious Freedom Act was passed into law, that AI/NAs could once again engage in traditional mourning practices. However, decades of AI/NAs not being allowed to grieve has left generations with feelings of powerlessness, shame, and subordination to the dominant White culture (Brave Heart & DeBruyn, 1998).

In 1871, Congress passed legislation that declared AI/NAs wards of the U.S. government with the intent to civilize AI/NAs and *Americanize* them to the dominant White European culture (Trusty et al., 2002). In 1892, Captain Richard H. Pratt delivered a speech at the Nineteenth Annual Conference of Charities and Correction regarding how to reeducate AI/NAs, where he proclaimed the only course was to "*Kill the Indian, and Save the Man*" (George Washington University, n.d.). The concepts from this speech were used to set up government- and church-run boarding schools. Four- and five-year-old AI/NA children were taken from their families and relocated to these boarding schools for a minimum of eight years (Brave Heart & DeBruyn, 1998; Garrett & Pichette, 2000). While in the boarding schools, AI/NA children were forced to wear European American clothing, have their hair cut, and were forbidden from speaking their indigenous languages, engaging in traditional practices, or keeping sacred items (Brave Heart & DeBruyn, 1998; Garrett & Pichette, 2000). Sadly, many children were physically and sexually abused, which resulted in them developing dysfunctional coping strategies (e.g., alcohol and drug use, learned helplessness, scapegoating other AI/NA children; Brave Heart & DeBruyn, 1998; Garrett & Pichette, 2000).

Not being allowed to engage in traditional practices led to a loss of cultural identity for many AI/NAs (Garrett & Pichette, 2000). Additionally, for many there has become a clouded perspective from AI/NA to AI/NA regarding what it is to be a *traditional Indian*. In that, it is almost weaponized among the AI/NA to determine if someone is *Indian enough*, which divides the AI/NA people and further complicates recovery from historical trauma. Due to the disintegration of the AI/NA culture and the unresolved grief related to this loss, the perspective of many AI/NAs' racial identity has become a stoic persona. The belief developed that illness must be tolerated (Moss, 2005) along with the belief their substance use would negatively affect the family/community (Gallant et al., 2010). The view evolved that AI/NA individuals need to be strong and not show weakness; as a result, the suffering of the people continues. This inability to process the historical losses because the grief is too complex and multifaceted results in generational and present-day issues. In particular, the use and abuse of substances to numb the pain and grief is the answer for many in this population.

Substance Use and AI/NAs

AI/NA communities had little experience with alcohol and other drugs until Europeans introduced them by trading distilled substances for animal pelts and weapons (Mukosi, 2020). Some substances (e.g., tobacco, peyote) were used by AI/NA tribes for ceremonial purposes; however, these substances were strictly used for ceremonial purposes by indigenous healers (Beauvais, 1998). Recreational use and abuse of substances was not prevalent in indigenous communities. In modern times, the rates of substance abuse for AI/NAs are commonly reported as much higher than those of the general U.S. population (National Institute on Drug Abuse, 2018). However, research has also found similar rates of alcohol use between AI/NAs and Whites (Cunningham et al., 2016; Whitesell et al., 2012). The differences in these findings might be related to where AI/NA participants were located. Studies have found the lifetime prevalence of alcohol use disorder was connected to tribal affiliation: 51%–83% in a Southwestern American Indian tribe, 50%–70% in a Southwest California Indian tribe, and 40%–70% in a Plains American Indian tribe; Ehlers et al., 2004; Enoch & Albaugh, 2017). With 574 federally recognized tribes in 37 states (IHS, 2020), this population is extremely diverse in cultural characteristics. Thus, it is important for researchers and practitioners not to make overreaching assumptions regarding substance use and AI/NA individuals.

While there might be a discrepancy regarding whether the highest rates of alcohol abuse are found in AI/NA individuals, there is research supporting that the results of alcohol abuse and use of illicit drugs are much more problematic for individuals who identify as AI/NA. AI/NAs have been found to have the highest amount of alcohol-induced deaths compared to persons of other racial/ethnic groups (Spillane et al., 2020). Binge drinking and hard drug use are more common in AI/NAs compared to any other racial/ethnic groups (Akins et al., 2013). A study of urban residing AI/NAs in the Midwest found methamphetamines and marijuana were reported as the most used substances (Guenzel & Struwe, 2020). A nationwide investigation found individuals who identified as AI/NA female used at rates identical to or greater than rates of use by those who identified as AI/NA male when assessing alcohol and other drug use across the lifetime and 30-day use of alcohol, methamphetamine, marijuana, and inhalants (Miller et al., 2012). Further, differences in substance use related to sexual orientation and gender identity have been found in this population. Balsam et al. (2004) compared substance use of AI/NAs who identified as heterosexual and AI/NAs who identified as gay, lesbian, bisexual, or transgender (collectively referred to as two-spirit) and found the two-spirit participants reported higher use of illicit drugs other than marijuana.

Allelic Variations

Researchers have studied if AI/NAs have a genetic predisposition for addiction to alcohol and nicotine (Ehlers & Wilhelmsen, 2005; Gizer et al., 2011; Mulligan et al., 2003). Consistently, these studies investigated the alcohol dehydrogenase (ADH) and aldehyde dehydrogenase (ALDH) family of genes and the correlation with difficulty in metabolizing alcohol in AI/NA individuals. Mulligan et al. (2003) identified through their results some significant differences in these genetic alleles, which often lead to higher rates of alcoholism and the risk to develop alcoholism. However, Ehlers and Wilhelmsen (2005) completed an extensive literature review on allelic variations and the increased risk of alcohol addiction. They concluded there were fewer protective factors through these genetic differences but no direct evidence of allelic factors increasing the likelihood of alcohol use disorder. ADH and ALDH gene expression is correlated with a predisposition to develop an alcohol use problem but is not the cause of developing an addiction.

It is important to remember variations of ADH (i.e., ADH4, ADH1B) have been correlated with alcohol abuse not only in AI/NA populations but also their African, Asian, and Caucasian counterparts (Gizer et al., 2011). These finding seem to dispel "the common belief that Native Americans may be more genetically susceptible to developing alcohol dependence owing to unique differences in the metabolism of alcohol" (Gizer et al., 2011, p. 2015). However, differences have been found related to gender. Enoch and colleagues (2006) investigated AI/NA participants diagnosed with a history of alcohol and nicotine use and found significant differences between AI/NA women and men. In particular, they concluded the Val158 allele (linked with having low dopamine levels) was found to be associated with an increase in women's use of tobacco and alcoholism. It was also found Val158 was more frequent in those who used both substances than those that used only one.

Relationship Between Substance Use and Historical Trauma

We might connect the use and/or abuse of substances in this population to the theory of self-medicating; however, this directs our focus on a personal pathology and denies the social and historical influences (Myhra, 2011). Drug use and abuse should be viewed as historical loss symptoms related to the historical losses perpetrated on the AI/NA people. Specifically, substance use "is predicted by pervasive and enduring disadvantage rather than intrinsic ethnic characteristics" (Akins et al., 2013, p. 510). Research with AI/NA participants has supported this hypothesis. It has been found that thoughts about historical losses are associated with substance abuse (Ehlers et al., 2013; Pokhrel & Herzog, 2014), and historical trauma loss symptoms are significantly correlated with past month alcohol use and lifetime use of non-marijuana illicit drugs (Wiechelt et al., 2012).

Disparity in Health and Behavioral Care

The Indian Health Services (IHS) was established and funded by the U.S. government in 1955 to uphold treaty obligations to provide health care services to members of federally recognized AI/NA tribes (Jones, 2006). There are three branches of IHS: (a) an independent, federally operated direct care system, (b) tribal operated health care services, and (c) urban Indian health care services (Sequist et al., 2011). Sixty percent of AI/NAs receive behavioral and medical health services from Indian Health Services (IHS, 2020). IHS (2020) reported that $4,078 was spent per IHS recipient (in comparison to $9,726 for the general population) with less than 10% of these funds being used for behavioral health and substance abuse treatment. This inequality in services might be a reason why consequences of substance abuse are higher for many AI/NA individuals.

Disruption of Family

The removal of children to boarding schools is believed to be "one of the most devastating traumas that occurred to the Native American people because it resulted in the disruption of the family structure, forced assimilation of children, and a disruption in the Native American community" (Brown-Rice, 2013, p. 119), in that the fear of abandonment wound runs so deep in AI/NA country. Research has found insecure or poor attachment can result in an individual engaging in risky substance use (Cassidy et al., 2018). Thus, the consequences of forcibly placing AI/NA children in boarding schools relates to past and current substance abuse for many in this population.

Zephier Olson and Dombrowski (2020) completed a Preferred Reporting Items for Systematic Reviews and Meta-Analyses (PRISMA)-style literature review to investigate substance abuse studies that concentrated on AI/NA populations and experiences at White-run boarding schools. It was found that AI/NA individuals who attended these boarding schools had substantial family discord that was correlated with substance use. In a qualitative study, Myhra (2011) found participants believed historical losses due to cultural traumas were instrumental to their elders' problematic substance abuse and the pattern in some AI/NA families of abusing substances. Cross-generational use of alcohol and other drugs with AI/NA individuals using substances with their children and/or grandchildren has been reported (Guenzel & Struwe, 2020). A national longitudinal research project investigated adverse childhood experiences (ACEs) among persons identifying as Native American, Hispanic, Black, Asian, and White. The project found AI/NAs had the highest average number and variety of ACEs than individuals from any other racial/ethnic group (Richards et al., 2021). In particular, it was found the most reported incidents of parental substance use were reported by both AI/NA females and males.

Continual Grief

The suffering, including substance abuse, that impacts many AI/NA people is a sign and a symptom of a communal grief reaction to generations of persecution, discrimination, and oppression (Brown-Rice, 2013). In traditional AI/NA culture, if a relative or loved one is lost, then a person is told not to be happy for a year (e.g., not attend pow wows, not engage in ceremonies). For many AI/NA people, attending pow wows and community events lifts them up, and positive events give them hope. However, due to so many losses, it could be years before they are able to attend. Failure to comply with the traditional one-year mourning period would result in shame or judgment being brought to the individual and their family. With so much loss in the community, the grief becomes continual in the community.

Dealing With the Past in the Present

There has been a correlation found between AI/NA clients underutilizing medical and behavioral health services and experiencing discrimination (Burgess et al., 2008). Additionally, when a provider's attitude or behavior is perceived as discriminatory, that perception directly affects AI/NA clients' compliance with treatment (Gonzales et al., 2014). Therefore, substance abuse interventions should be designed to reflect the cultural uniqueness of AI/NA people (Gone & Alcántara, 2007), include collaboration with local tribal leaders and members (Lane & Simmons, 2011), acknowledge the cultural traumas inflicted on AI/NA people (Brown-Rice, 2013), and recognize their resilience and strength.

Respect of Cultural Uniqueness

Researchers have theorized that AI/NA cultural identity is a protective factor in treating substance abuse (Barlow et al., 2010; Dickerson & Johnson, 2012). However, it has also been found that utilizing traditional practices was not related to change in behavior of abusing substances (Kropp et al., 2013). These discrepancies could be due to the researchers' lack of acknowledgment of participants' cultural uniqueness. Clinicians "must not make assumptions about a client's cultural identification" and should "assess which cultural contexts are relevant for the client" (Weaver & Brave Heart, 1999, p. 29).

Another rationale for these unexpected results concerns internalized discrimination. Due to forced colonization processes on AI/NAs, there can be a self-perception of shame attached to their cultural identity (Dell & Hopkins, 2011). Such shame can result in the client's belief that he/she is inferior and can potentially trigger initial or continual substance use. Thus, "decolonization must then play a significant role in the planned intervention so that the client can connect to their cultural identity in a positive manner and see their identity as a source of strength" (Dell & Hopkins, 2011, p. 111).

Inclusion of Cultural Collaboration

Culturally appropriate treatment is best achieved by a collective approach (Goodkind et al., 2012; Walters & Simoni, 2009) using traditional culture keepers (e.g., tribal elders, healers; Hartmann & Gone, 2012). Collaborative endeavors should comprise a commitment to long-term, meaningful relationships with members of the AI/NA community, cultural considerations, shared respect and trust, and mutual goals (Rajaram et al., 2014). Evidence-based counseling therapies (i.e., cognitive-behavioral therapy, dialectical behavior therapy) that combine AI/NA tribal-specific strategies have been found to be effective (Beckstead et al., 2015; Novins et al., 2012; Patchell et al., 2015). A study of AI/NA youth found a treatment group that integrated specific tribal ceremonial practices showed significantly declined substance use from baseline after 12 months compared to a group that utilized standard cognitive behavioral therapy (Lowe et al., 2016). Baldwin et al. (2020) found that tailoring interventions to tribal communities was effective in AI/NA adolescent substance use treatment. This included translating materials written in English to specific tribal language and integrating tribal cultural practices and customs. In a qualitative study of AI/NA and non-AI/NA pregnant women, it was found culture was especially relevant to the recovery of AI/NA women (McCarron et al., 2018). However, how they used culture as support in recovery manifested in different ways.

Gone (2013) interviewed 19 staff and clients in a Native American healing lodge regarding the therapeutic approach used to address the legacy of Native American historical trauma. On the basis of thematic content analysis of interviews, four components of healing discourse emerged. First, clients were understood by their counselors to carry pain, leading to adult dysfunction, including substance abuse. Second, counselors believed such pain must be confessed in order to purge its deleterious influence. Third, the cathartic expression of such pain was said by counselors to inaugurate lifelong habits of introspection and self-improvement. Finally, this healing journey entailed a reclamation of indigenous heritage, identity, and spirituality that program staff thought would neutralize the pathogenic effects of colonization. Consideration of this healing discourse suggested that one important way for psychologists to bridge evidence-based and culturally sensitive treatment paradigms was to partner with indigenous programs in the exploration of locally determined therapeutic outcomes for existing culturally sensitive interventions that are maximally responsive to community needs and interests.

Validation of Cultural Traumas

Skewes and Blume (2019) completed a qualitative study to understand substance use disparities in AI/NA communities. AI/NA participants reported substance use and abuse was a direct result of race-based stress due to historical trauma. One participant provided, "Oppression is the overarching umbrella for all sickness with drugs and alcohol" (Skewes & Blume, 2019, p. 94). Counselors need to validate not only the initial historical losses but the continued oppression and discrimination that have deeply affected the AI/NA people (Brave Heart et al., 2011). Healing change will be difficult for AI/NA clients without acknowledgment of not only the past cruelties that occurred to AI/NA communities but validation of the current discriminatory environment (Brown-Rice, 2013). Counselors can utilize different interventions to bring historical losses into session and to assist clients in managing their historical loss symptoms.

Genogram

To understand the cross-generational cycle of substance use, counselors can utilize a version of the genogram with AI/NA clients. Given that AI/NA clients' supports might not come from what is considered a European traditional family, it is suggested that counselors follow these steps with this intervention:

1. Provide the client with a blank sheet of paper and markers, colored pencils, or crayons.
2. Ask the client to write the names of the people who are important to them on the paper.

3. Ask to pick a color for a drug (e.g., alcohol, marijuana, tobacco) and shade over the name of the person they know who uses that substance.
4. The counselor and client then process the genogram in a nonjudgmental and supportive manner.

Medicine Wheel

Historical trauma can permeate all domains of a person's existence (e.g., personal and cultural identity, relationships, memory, spirit, and worldviews; Weisband, 2009). Therefore, healing from these cultural traumas and the related complex grief should connect the client's spiritual, physical, emotional, and mental functioning. To accomplish this, counselors can utilize the Medicine Wheel Model of Wellness, Balance, and Healing (the Medicine Wheel). The Medicine Wheel has numerous variations—as many as 20,000 (Gilgun, 2002). There are four quadrants in the Medicine Wheel, which represent the north, south, east, and west.

The Medicine Wheel has been found to be an effective intervention with AI/NA clients (Gray & Rose, 2012). It has also been found effective in increasing the validity of mainstream counseling interventions with AI/NA population (Big Foot & Schmidt, 2010). Figure 10.2 is an example of a Medicine Wheel that the first author created for her work with AI/NA clients.

Cultural Appropriate Assessments

Unfortunately, there are few assessments that have been developed specifically for AI/NA clients. Garrett and Pichette (2000) developed the Native America Acculturation Scale, which contains 20 self-report items to assist counselors in understanding who clients identify themselves as related to their AI/NA heritage. To assess a client's level of historical trauma, Whitbeck et al. (2004) developed the Historical Loss Scale and the Historical Loss Associated Symptoms Scale. This scale contains 12 self-report items (e.g., distrust of the intentions of the White culture, thoughts about the loss of culture and traditional language, thoughts about the impact of alcoholism on their community).

Respecting Cultural Resiliency

While it might be easy to focus on the pathology that exists in the statistics and data related to this population, it is crucial for practitioners to remember the strength and resilience of members of the AI/NA community. Given the genocide of the AI/NA people from 1492 to 1776 (Plous, 2003), the fact the remaining 5% of original indigenous people have survived and in many cases thrived (e.g., the authors of this chapter) should not be discounted. Counselors need to acknowledge and highlight areas of strengths and resiliency with AI/NA clients (Brave Heart et al., 2011). Assisting clients in this population to

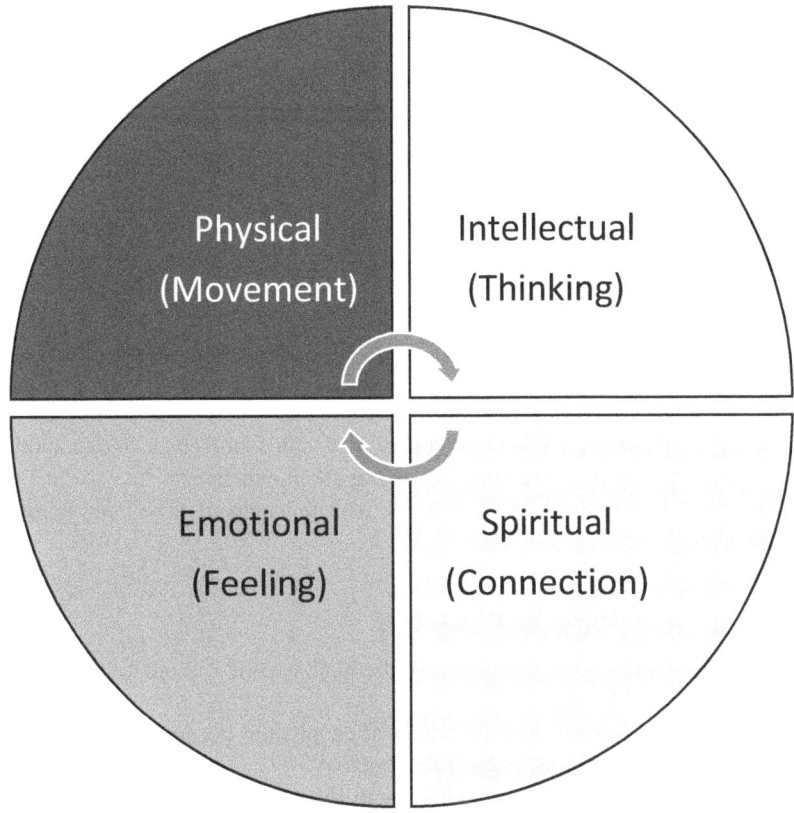

Figure 10.2 The Medicine Wheel of Wellness, Balance, and Healing

understand that while their heritage contains historical and cultural traumas and a history of discrimination and racism that continues today, it also contains a rich history that is admirable. AI/NA research participants have reported how much they respect and admire their elders for their strength and resiliency (Myhra, 2011).

Walking the Red Road

Past cultural traumas have created an unnatural drug-burdened environment in many AI/NA communities. To counteract this, AI/NA individuals struggling with substance abuse are encouraged to *Walk the Red Road* to rediscover their true cultural heritage and heal their body and soul (Thin Elk, 1993). To take this journey, clients engage in the 12 Steps to Wellbriety (White Bison, 2006).

12 Steps to Wellbriety

Finding the Creator

Step 1: Honesty—We admit we are powerless over alcohol and have lost control of our lives.

Step 2: Hope—We come to believe that something greater than ourselves can help us regain control.

Step 3: Faith—We made the decision to ask for help from a higher power and others that understand.

Finding Yourself

Step 4: Courage—We stopped and thought about ourselves, our strengths, and struggles.

Step 5: Integrity—We admitted to the great spirit, ourselves, and to another person the things we think are wrong about ourselves.

Step 6: Willingness—We are ready with the help of the Great Spirit to change.

Finding Your Relationship With Others

Step 7: Humility—We humbly ask the higher spirit and our friends/family to help us change.

Step 8: Forgiveness—We made a lot of people hurt because of our drinking and we want to make up for that hurt.

Step 9: Justice—We are making up to those people as often as we can, except when it would cause them additional hurt.

The Wisdom of Elders

Step 10: Perseverance—We continue to think about our strengths and struggles and when we are wrong, we say so.

Step 11: Spiritual Awakening—We pray and think about ourselves, praying only for the strength to do what is right.

Step 12: Service—We try to help other alcoholics and to practice those principles in all things I do.

Those with higher AI/NA identity may struggle to discuss their experiences of psychological concerns and/or substance use with practitioners (Bird & Parslow, 2002; Fiske et al., 2009). This is due to the shame they believe this disclosure will bring upon their family and community and the disappointment that might fall upon their people for them not walking the Red Road. It is important for counselors to understand that Walking the Red Road relates to no alcohol or other drug use; moderation or harm reduction is never discussed as it relates to the Red Road.

Conclusion

Understanding the historical losses of cultural traumas and how they relate to AI/NA substance abuse is vital for clinicians. Failure to (a) engage in culturally competent strategies, (b) validate the atrocities of the past, and (c) honor the resiliency of the people will continue the cycle of historical trauma. It is important to understand that historical trauma is not an AI/NA issue but a concern for all to acknowledge and be a part of solving. "If you come to help me, you can go home again. But if you see my struggles as part of your own survival, then perhaps we can work together" (Watson, 1985).

References

Akins, S., Lanfear, C., Cline, S., & Mosher, C. (2013). Patterns and correlates of adult American Indian substance use. *Journal of Drug Issues, 43*(4), 497–516.

Baldwin, J. A., Lowe, J., Brooks, J., Charbonneau-Dahlen, B. K., Lawrence, G., Johnson-Jennings, M., . . . Camplain, C. (2020). Formative research and cultural tailoring of a substance abuse prevention program for American Indian youth: Findings from the Intertribal Talking Circle Intervention. *Health Promotion Practice*, 1524839920918551. https://doi.org/10.1177/1524839920918551

Balsam, K. F., Huang, B., Fieland, K. C., Simoni, J. M., & Walters, K. L. (2004). Culture, trauma, and wellness: A comparison of heterosexual and lesbian, gay, bisexual, and two-spirit Native Americans. *Cultural Diversity and Ethnic Minority Psychology, 10*(3), 287–301. https://doi.org/10.1037/1099-9809.10.3.287

Barlow, A., Mullany, B. C., Neault, N., Davis, Y., Billy, T., Hastings, R., et al. (2010). Examining correlates of methamphetamine and other drug use in pregnant American Indian adolescents. *American Indian and Alaska Native Mental Health Research: The Journal of The National Center, 17*(1), 1–24.

Beauvais, F. (1998). American Indians and alcohol. *Health & Research World Journal, 22*, 254–281.

Beckstead, D. J., Lambert, M. J., DuBose, A. P., & Linehan, M. (2015). Dialectical behavior therapy with American Indian/Alaska Native adolescents diagnosed with substance use disorders: Combining an evidence-based treatment with cultural, traditional, and spiritual beliefs. *Addictive Behaviors, 51*, 84–87. https://doi.org/10.1016/j.addbeh.2015.07.018

Big Foot, D. S., & Funderburk, B. W. (2011). Honoring children, making relatives: The cultural translation of parent-child interaction therapy for American Indian and Alaska Native families. *Journal of Psychoactive Drugs, 43*(4), 309–318.

Big Foot, D. S., & Schmidt, S. R. (2010). Honoring children, mending the circle: Cultural adaptation of trauma-focused cognitive-behavioral therapy for American Indian and Alaska Native children. *Journal of Clinical Psychology, 66*(8), 847–856.

Bird, M., & Parslow, R. (2002). Potential for community programs to prevent depression in older people. *Medical Journal of Australia, 177*, S107–S110.

Brave Heart, M. Y. H., Chase, J., Elkins, J., & Altschul, D. B. (2011). Historical trauma among indigenous peoples of the Americas: Concepts, research, and clinical considerations. *Journal of Psychoactive Drugs, 43*(4), 282–290. https://doi.org/10.1080/0 2791072.2011.628913

Brave Heart, M. Y. H., & DeBruyn, L. M. (1998). The American Indian holocaust: Healing historical unresolved grief. *American Indian and Alaska Native Mental Health Research, 8*(2), 60–82.

Brown-Rice, K. (2013). Examining the theoretical underpinnings of historical traumas among Native American. *Professional Counselor: Research and Practice, 3*(3), 117–130.

Burgess, D. J., Ding, Y., Hargreaves, M., van Ryn, M., & Phelan, S. (2008). The association between perceived discrimination and underutilization of needed medical and mental health care in a multi-ethnic community sample. *Journal of Health Care for the Poor & Underserved, 19*(3), 894–911. https://doi.org/10.1353/hpu.0.0063

Cassidy, J., Stern, J. A., Mikulincer, M., Martin, D. R., & Shaver, P. R. (2018). Influences on care for others: Attachment security, personal suffering, and similarity between helper and care recipient. *Personality & Social Psychology Bulletin, 44*(4), 574–588. https://doi.org/10.1177/0146167217746150

Chief Seattle. *The Chief Seattle's speech.* https://suquamish.nsn.us/home/about-us/chief-seattle%20speech/#:~:text=Yonder%20sky%20that%20has%20wept,may%20be%20overcast%20with%20clouds

Cunningham, J. K., Solomon, T. A., & Muramoto, M. L. (2016). Alcohol use among Native Americans compared to whites: Examining the veracity of the "Native American elevated alcohol consumption" belief. *Drug and Alcohol Dependence, 160,* 65–75. https://doi.org/org.ezproxy.shsu.edu/10.1016/j.drugalcdep.2015.12.015

Dell, D., & Hopkins, C. (2011). Residential volatile substance misuse treatment for Indigenous youth in Canada. *Substance Use & Misuse, 46,* 107–113.

Dickerson, D. L., & Johnson, C. L. (2012). Mental health and substance abuse characteristics among a clinical sample of urban American Indian/Alaska Native youths in a large California Metropolitan area: A descriptive study. *Community Mental Health Journal, 48*(1), 56–62. https://doi.org/10.1007/s10597-010-9368-3

Duran, E. (2006). *Healing the soul wound: Counseling with American Indians and other Native peoples.* Teachers College Press.

Ehlers, C. L., Gilder, D. A., Wall, T. L., Phillips, E., Feiler, H., & Wilhelmsen, K. C. (2004). Genomic screen for loci associated with alcohol dependence in Mission Indians. *American Journal of Medical Genetics, 129B,* 110–115.

Ehlers, C. L., Gizer, I. R., Gilder, D. A., Ellingson, J. M., & Yehuda, R. (2013). Measuring historical trauma in an American Indian community sample: Contributions of substance dependence, affective disorder, conduct disorder and PTSD. *Drug & Alcohol Dependence, 133*(1), 180–187. https://doi.org/10.1016/j.drugalcdep.2013.05.011

Ehlers, C. L., & Wilhelmsen, K. C. (2005). Genomic scan for alcohol craving in Mission Indians. *Psychiatric Genetics, 15,* 71–75.

Enoch, M. A., & Albaugh, B. J. (2017). Review: Genetic and environmental risk factors for alcohol use disorders in American Indians and Alaskan Natives. *American Journal on Addictions, 26*(5), 461–468. https://doi.org/org.ezproxy.shsu.edu/10.1111/ajad.12420

Enoch, M. A., Waheed, J. F., Harris, C. R., Albaugh, B., & Goldman, D. (2006). Sex differences in the influence of COMT Val158Met on alcoholism and smoking in plains American Indians. *Alcoholism: Clinical & Experimental Research, 30*(3), 399–406. https://doi.org/10.1111/j.1530-0277.2006.00045.x

Evans-Campbell, T. (2008). Historical trauma in American Indian/Native Alaska communities: A multilevel framework for exploring impacts on individuals, families, and communities. *Journal of Interpersonal Violence, 23*(3), 316–338. https://doi.org/10.1177/0886260507312290

Fiske, A., Wetherell, J., & Gatz, M. (2009). Depression in older adults. *Annual Review of Clinical Psychology, 5,* 363–389.

Gallant, M. P., Spitze, G., & Grove, J. G. (2010). Chronic illness self-care and the family lives of older adults: A synthetic review across four ethnic groups. *Journal of Cross-Cultural Gerontology, 25*(1), 21–43.

Garrett, M. T., & Pichette, E. F. (2000). Red as an apple: Native American acculturation and counseling with or without reservation. *Journal of Counseling & Development, 78*(1), 3–13. https://doi.org/10.1002/j.1556-6676.2000.tb02554x

George Washington University. (n.d.). *"Kill the Indian, and save the man": Capt. Richard H. Pratt on the education of native Americans*. http://historymatters.gmu.edu/d/4929

Gilgun, J. F. (2002). Completing the circle: American Indian medicine wheels and the promotion of resilience of children and youth in care. *Journal of Human Behavior in the Social Environment, 6*(2), 65. https://doi.org/10.1300/J137v06n02_05

Gizer, I. R., Edenberg, H. J., Gilder, D. A., Wilhelmsen, K. C., & Ehlers, C. L. (2011). Association of alcohol dehydrogenase genes with alcohol-related phenotypes in a Native American community sample. *Alcoholism, Clinical and Experimental Research, 35*(11), 2008–2018. https://doi.org/10.1111/j.1530-0277.2011.01552.x

Gone, J. P. (2013). A community-based treatment for native American historical trauma: Prospects for evidence-based practice. *Spirituality in Clinical Practice, 1*(S), 78–94. https://doi.org/10.1037/2326-4500.1.S.78

Gone, J. P., & Alcántara, C. (2007). Identifying effective mental health interventions for American Indians and Alaska natives: A review of the literature. *Cultural Diversity and Ethnic Minority Psychology, 13*(4), 356–363. https://doi.org/10.1037/1099-9809.13.4.356

Gonzales, K. L., Lambert, W. E., Fu, R., Jacob, M., & Harding, A. K. (2014). Perceived racial discrimination in health care, completion of standard diabetes services, and diabetes control among a sample of American Indian women. *Diabetes Educator, 40*(6), 747–755. https://doi.org/10.1177/0145721714551422

Goodkind, J., LaNoue, M., Lee, C., Freeland, L., & Freund, R. (2012). Feasibility, acceptability, and initial findings from a community-based cultural mental health intervention for American Indian youth and their families. *Journal of Community Psychology, 40*(4), 381–405.

Gray, J. S., & Rose, W. J. (2012). Cultural adaptation for therapy with American Indians and Alaska natives. *Journal of Multicultural Counseling and Development, 40*(2), 82–92. https://doi.org/10.1002/j.2161-1912.2012.00008.x

Guenzel, N., & Struwe, L. (2020). Historical trauma, ethnic experience, and mental health in a sample of urban American Indians. *Journal of the American Psychiatric Nurses Association, 26*(2), 145–156. https://doi.org/10.1177/1078390319888266

Hartmann, W. E., & Gone, J. P. (2012). Incorporating traditional healing into an urban American Indian health organization: A case study of community member perspectives. *Journal of Counseling Psychology, 59*(4), 542–554. https://doi.org/10.1037/a0029067

Indian Health Service (IHS). (2020). *IHS profile*. www.ihs.gov/newsroom/factsheets/ihsprofile/

Jones, D. S. (2006). The persistence of American Indian health disparities. *American Journal of Public Health, 96*(12), 2122–2134. https://doi.org/10.2105/AJPH.2004.054262

Kropp, F., Somoza, E., Lilleskov, M., Moccasin, M. G., Moore, M., Lewis, D., . . . Winhusen, T. (2013). Characteristics of Northern Plains American Indians seeking substance abuse treatment in an urban, non-tribal clinic: A descriptive study. *Community Mental Health Journal, 49*(6), 714–721. https://doi.org/10.1007/s10597-012-9537-7

Lane, D. C., & Simmons, J. (2011). American Indian youth substance abuse: Community-driven interventions. *Mount Sinai Journal of Medicine, 78*(3), 362–372. https://doi.org/10.1002/msj.20262

Lowe, J., Liang, H., Henson, J., & Riggs, C. (2016). Preventing substance use among Native American early adolescents. *Journal of Community Psychology, 44*(8), 997–1010. https://doi.org/10.1002/jcop.21823

McCarron, H., Griese, E. R., Dippel, E., & McMahon, T. R. (2018). Cultural and social predictors of substance abuse recovery among American Indian and Non-American Indian pregnant and parenting women. *Journal of Psychoactive Drugs, 50*(4), 322–330. https://doi.org/10.1080/02791072.2018.1481546

Miller, K. A., Stanley, L. R., & Beauvais, F. (2012). Regional differences in drug use rates among American Indian youth. *Drug & Alcohol Dependence, 126*(1/2), 35–41. https://doi.org/10.1016/j.drugalcdep.2012.04.010

Moss, M. (2005). Tolerated illness concept and theory for chronically ill and elderly patients as exemplified in American Indians. *Journal of Cancer Education, 20*(1), 17–22.

Mukosi, L. (2020). Odawa cultural practices to treat substance addictions a tour of the healing to wellness court. *Fourth World Journal, 20*(1), 41–49.

Mulligan, C. J., Robin, R. W., Osier, M. V., Sambuughin, N., Goldfarb, L. G., Kittles, R. A., . . . Long, J. C. (2003). Allelic variation at alcohol metabolism genes (ADH1B, ADH1C, ALDH2) and alcohol dependence in an American Indian population. *Human Genetics, 113*(4), 325–336. https://doi.org/10.1007/s00439-003-0971-z

Myhra, L. L. (2011). "It runs in the family": Intergenerational transmission of historical trauma among urban American Indians and Alaska Natives in culturally specific sobriety maintenance programs. *American Indian and Alaska Native Mental Health Research: The Journal of the National Center, 18*(2), 17–40.

National Institute of Drug Abuse. (2018). *Higher rate of substance use among Native American youth on reservations.* www.drugabuse.gov/news-events/news-releases/2018/05/higher-rate-of-substance-use-among-native-american-youth-on-reservations

Novins, D. K., Boyd, M. L., Brotherton, D. T., Fickenscher, A., Moore, L., & Spicer, P. (2012). Walking on: Celebrating the journeys of Native American adolescents with substance use problems on the winding road to healing. *Journal of Psychoactive Drugs, 44*(2), 153–159. https://doi.org/10.1080/02791072.2012.684628

Patchell, B. A., Robbins, L. K., Lowe, J. A., & Hoke, M. M. (2015). The effect of a culturally tailored substance abuse prevention intervention with Plains Indian adolescents. *Journal of Cultural Diversity, 22*(1), 3–8.

Plous, S. (2003). *Understanding prejudice and discrimination.* McGraw-Hill.

Pokhrel, P., & Herzog, T. A. (2014). Historical trauma and substance use among Native Hawaiian college students. *American Journal of Health Behavior, 38*(3), 420–429, 10p. https://doi.org/10.5993/AJHB.38.3.11

Rajaram, S. S., Grimm, B., Giroux, J., Peck, M., & Ramos, A. (2014). Partnering with American Indian communities in health using methods of strategic collaboration. *Progress in Community Health Partnerships: Research, Education, and Action, 8*(3), 387–395. https://doi.org/10.1353/cpr.2014.0036

Richards, T. N., Schwartz, J. A., & Wright, E. (2021). Examining adverse childhood experiences among Native American persons in a nationally representative sample:

Differences among racial/ethnic groups and race/ethnicity-sex dyads. *Child Abuse & Neglect, 111.* https://doi.org/10.1016/j.chiabu.2020.104812

Sequist, T. D., Cullen, T., & Acton, K. J. (2011). Indian health service innovations have helped reduce health disparities affecting American Indian and Alaska Native people. *Health Affairs, 30*(10), 1965–1973. https://doi.org/10.1377/hlthaff.2011.0630

Skewes, M. C., & Blume, A. W. (2019). Understanding the link between racial trauma and substance use among American Indians. *American Psychologist, 74*(1), 88–100. https://doi.org/10.1037/amp0000331

Sotero, M. M. (2006). A conceptual model of historical trauma: Implications for public health practice and research. *Journal of Health Disparities Research and Practice, 1*(1), 93–108.

Spillane, S., Shiels, M. S., Best, A. F., Haozous, E. A., Withrow, D. R., Chen, Y., . . . Freedman, N. D. (2020). Trends in alcohol-induced deaths in the United States, 2000–2016. *JAMA Network Open, 3*(2), e1921451. https://doi.org/org.ezproxy.shsu.edu/10.1001/jamanetworkopen.2019.21451

Thin Elk, G. (1993). Walking in balance on the Red Road. *Journal of Emotional and Behavioral Problems, 2*(3), 54–57.

Trusty, J., Looby, E. J., & Sandhu, D. S. (2002). *Multicultural counseling: Context, theory and practice, and competence.* Nova Science.

Walters, K. L., & Simoni, J. M. (2009). Decolonizing strategies for mentoring American Indians and Alaska Natives in HIV and mental health research. *American Journal of Public Health, 99*(S1), S71–S76. https://doi.org/10.2105/AJPH.2008.136127

Watson, L. (1985, July 15–26). *Decade for women.* United Nations Conference, Nairobi, Kenya.

Weaver, H. N., & Brave Heart, Y. H. (1999). Examining two facets of American Indian identity exposure to other cultures and the influences of historical trauma. *Journal of Human Behavior in the Social Environment, 2,* 19–33.

Weisband, E. (2009). On the aporetic borderlines of forgiveness: Bereavement as a political form. *Alternatives, 34*(4), 359–381.

Whitbeck, L. B., Adams, G. W., Hoyt, D. R., & Chen, X. (2004). Conceptualizing and measuring historical trauma among American Indian people. *American Journal of Community Psychology, 33*(3–4), 119–130. https://doi.org/10.1023/B:AJCP.0000027000.77357.31

White Bison, Inc. (2006). *The red road to wellbriety: In the Native American way.* Cohyhis.

Whitesell, N. R., Beals, J., Crow, C. B., Mitchell, C. M., & Novins, D. K. (2012). Epidemiology and etiology of substance use among American Indians and Alaska Natives: Risk, protection, and implications for prevention. *American Journal of Drug & Alcohol Abuse, 38*(5), 376–382. https://doi.org/10.3109/00952990.2012.694527

Wiechelt, S. A., Gryczynski, J., Johnson, J. L., & Caldwell, D. (2012). Historical trauma among urban American Indians: Impact on substance abuse and family cohesion. *Journal of Loss & Trauma, 17*(4), 319–336. https://doi.org/10.1080/15325024.2011.616837

Zephier Olson, M. D., & Dombrowski, K. (2020). A systematic review of Indian boarding schools and attachment in the context of substance use studies of Native Americans. *Journal of Racial and Ethnic Health Disparities, 7*(1), 62–71. https://doi.org/10.1007/s40615-019-00634-4

11 Addiction and Grief in the LGBTQ+ Community

Pamela S. Lassiter, Michael S. Spivey, and Derrick Johnson

Lesbian, gay, bisexual, transgender, queer/questioning, plus (LGBTQ+) individuals have a greater likelihood of having a substance use disorder than non-LGBTQ+ individuals. In addition to experiencing substance use disorders at higher rates than their nonminority counterparts experience them, they are also more likely to have comorbid disorders, such as depression, generalized anxiety disorder, or suicidality, and may engage in self-harm. These rates also vary among individuals who belong to the LGBTQ+ community and are even higher for transgender and nonbinary individuals. As members of a minority community, LGBTQ+ individuals experience discrimination and oppression at high rates. This discrimination and oppression often translate into a number of losses that occur throughout the development life cycle. Many of these losses are invisible to the broader, majority community. Because of this invisibility, their losses are often disenfranchised in that others view the loss as not worthy of grieving. To cope with these losses, many members of the LGBTQ+ community may resort to avoidant strategies such as alcohol and other substances.

The impact of oppression, discrimination, and stigma associated with identity weaves throughout the life span of LGBTQ+ individuals. Members of this group historically have been marginalized, as they often do not conform to the traditional gender roles and other heterosexual societal expectations. One commonality that exists for all LGBTQ+ individuals is they are a group of "others" (Institute of Medicine [IOM], 2011). "This 'otherness' is the basis for stigma and its attendant prejudice, discrimination, and violence, which underlie society's general lack of attention to their health needs" (IOM, 2011, p. 13). The intersectionality of their "otherness" is further complicated by the "additional dimensions of inequality such as race, ethnicity, and socioeconomic status, resulting in stigma at multiple levels" (IOM, 2011, p. 13).

As individuals move through the life span from childhood to older adulthood, there are many barriers and losses they may experience along the way. These losses are especially significant for LGBTQ+ persons. Many individuals experience legal discrimination and oppression when it comes to housing, employment, marriage, adoption, retirement benefits, and health insurance. For others, it is a lack of social programs and support in their communities. LGBTQ+ persons often experience a shortage of health care providers who

DOI: 10.4324/9781003106906-11

possess the cultural competency needed to support their mental and health care needs (Office of Disease Prevention and Health Promotion [ODPHP], 2020).

From a very young age, LGBTQ+ individuals begin to experience various types of discrimination and oppression. For example, children and adolescents often experience a lack of support from family and friends, especially as they begin to explore their sexual orientation and gender identity (IOM, 2011; Centers for Disease Control and Prevention [CDC], 2016). This lack of support often overlaps with a feeling of being unsafe in school environments. Students who report experiencing harassment, violence, bullying and victimization often indicate they lack support from faculty, staff, and administrators when they report these aggressions. This lack of support by adults in their lives often results in lower grades than their non-LGBTQ+ peers. As these children grow into adolescents, many turn to alcohol, tobacco, and illegal drugs to cope with the many stressors they face day to day (CDC, 2016; IOM, 2011). There is also research to support that higher rates of childhood abuse exists among LGBTQ+ youth than their non-LGTBQ+ peers (IOM, 2011). The lack of support from family and friends often results in higher rates of homelessness among LGB adolescents, and these rates are even higher among the transgender and nonbinary populations (IOM, 2011; The Trevor Project, 2020). Additional factors can contribute to the reasons why LGBTQ+ youth and young adults (ages 13–24) often do not seek mental health care. Many report that in addition to an inability to find affordable health and mental health care, they have fears of being outed by a health care professional. Other factors that contribute to not seeking out health care is many often lack transportation options to get to appointments, may have had a negative previous experience with a health care provider, and worry about having to get parental or caregiver permission to be seen in a health care setting (The Trevor Project, 2020).

As LGBTQ+ individuals move into early, middle, and older adulthood, discrimination and oppression are still very much a part of daily life. The forms of the discrimination and oppression continue to evolve. For example, as individuals begin to enter the workforce, their sexual and gender minority status tends to lead to an increase in discriminatory and oppression actions toward them. Their sexual and gender minority status often affects their ability to obtain and maintain employment, including positions that offer health insurance benefits, and their ability to advance in certain careers (CDC, 2016). In addition to these workplace stressors, LGBTQ+ individuals often experience stress when it comes to their romantic and sexual relationships. For many sexual and gender minorities, their inability to maintain long-term same-sex relationships not only affects their mental health but may also affect their physical health. By not forming long-lasting sexual relationships, LGBTQ+ persons are at greater risk of contracting HIV or sexually transmitted infections and/or diseases (CDC, 2016).

As LGBTQ+ individuals move into older adulthood, discrimination often manifests itself in the form of new challenges in health care, housing, and finding retirement communities where they feel safe and supported (IOM, 2011).

Many older LGBTQ+ persons have experienced higher rates of a lifetime of violence and substance use and may have been less likely to seek assistance for their health care needs. In cases where they did not establish long-term romantic or sexual relationships, they may find themselves feeling alone and isolated as they age (IOM, 2011). All of these factors contribute to a lifetime of stress and loss.

For transgender and nonbinary individuals, many of them experience the same stressors and losses as other sexual minorities. However, when they do experience the same forms of discrimination and oppression, they often do so at a much higher level (IOM, 2011; Korell & Lorah, 2013). For example, many lack support systems—family, friends, and culturally competent mental health and medical providers—just as their other sexual minority counterparts.

Many of the additional stressors they experience are a direct result of trying to navigate the health care profession (Korell & Lorah, 2013). Often times, this population will encounter health care providers who make certain assumptions about treatment. For instance, not all transgender individuals want gender affirming surgery, nor do they all want hormone treatments. Because some health care providers make such assumptions combined with the high cost of many treatments, this population often feels multiple layers of oppression and discrimination (Korell & Lorah, 2013). Other stressors this population experiences center on proper pronoun use or the lack thereof. The importance of proper pronoun usage is an essential part of their gender identification and can affect their mental health (The Trevor Project, 2020).

When looking at the many barriers and stressors LGBTQ+ individuals encounter, yet another aspect to be considered is that of their spirituality. Barret and Logan (2002) argued it is important to consider the "wounds from religious rejection" when considering stressors LGBTQ+ persons may face (p. 158). Many LGBTQ+ individuals struggle with their spirituality, and this struggle can take on many forms. Individuals may find they are questioning their own religious beliefs and how they align with a religious belief system they were exposed to during their formative years (Barret & Logan, 2002). This crisis of spirituality can be transformational and at the same time a very painful life experience, as LGBTQ+ individuals often feel separated from their religious community.

No matter at what point in the life span an LGBTQ+ individual comes out, there is always the risk of exposing oneself to a negative coming out experience due to the lack of support of family, friends, and community (CDC, 2016; National Alliance on Mental Illness [NAMI], n.d.; Substance Abuse and Mental Health Services Administration [SAMHSA], 2018). The rejection by family and friends and possible harassment and assault in the school or work environment are often unbearable for many. The trauma from bullying and the constant negative messaging and stigma associated with being a sexual or gender minority often leads to internalized shame. This internal shame or internalized homophobia may lead to self-destructive behaviors in order to cope (CDC, 2016; NAMI, n.d.; SAMHSA, 2018).

For many LGBTQ+ individuals, dealing with the stresses of discrimination and oppression may be overwhelming and exhausting and often leads to feelings of grief and loss. This grieving process often takes place in isolation, compounded by the fact this loss is often invisible to non-LGBTQ+ persons. Searching for a way to cope with these losses may lead to avoidant strategies such as substance use, self-harm, or even suicidal ideation. The intersectionality of race and ethnicity combined with being a member of the LGBTQ+ community only compounds the losses and creates multiple layers of stressors (IOM, 2011; Meyer, 2003, 2013; Weber & Dodge, 2017). The isolation, hiding, anger, internalized homophobia, and fear lead to substance use as a means to cope with the ongoing daily stresses and losses (Capuzzi & Stauffer, 2016; Meyer, 2003, 2013; ODPHP, 2020; Weber & Dodge, 2017).

LGB individuals are twice as likely as heterosexual adults to have a substance use disorder, and transgender and nonbinary individuals are four times more likely than cisgender adults to have a substance use disorder. Illicit drug use is also significantly higher in high school–aged LGB youth (NAMI, n.d.). According to SAMHSA (2020), 3 in 5 LGB adults with a substance use disorder struggled with alcohol use, 1 in 2 struggled with illicit drugs, and 1 in 6 struggled with illicit drugs and alcohol.

Substance Use (Using Within the Previous 12 Months)	Sexual Minority (LGB) Aged 18 and Older	National Average
Illicit drug use	40.3%	18%
Marijuana	31.1%	13.8%
Misuse of prescription pain reliever	10.5%	4.5%
Heroin	0.9%	0.4%
Alcohol	64.2%	55.5%
Binge drinking	36.2%	26.5%
Heavy alcohol use	34.5%	31.9%

Source: SAMHSA (2018, November 21).

In addition to experiencing higher rates of substance use, LGBTQ+ individuals are also more likely to have comorbid disorders, such as depression, generalized anxiety disorder, suicidality, and self-harm (CDC, 2016; IOM, 2011; NAMI, n.d.). LGB adults are twice as likely as non-LGBTQ+ individuals to experience a mental health condition (NAMI, n.d.; SAMHSA, 2020). The findings from the most recent National Survey on Drug Use and Health indicate LGB persons (ages 18–25 and 26–49) who suffer from serious mental illness have increased significantly since the 2016 study (SAMHSA, 2020). Additional findings indicated that 2 out of 5 (38.2%, or 2.6 million) LGB adults had a serious mental illness compared to 14.1% (1.5 million) in 2016 (SAMHSA, 2020).

Mental Health (Within the Previous 12 Months)	Sexual Minority (LGB) Aged 18 and Older	National Average
Any mental illness	39.9%	18.1%
Serious mental illness	14.1%	4.1%
Mental health treatment or counseling	27.2%	14.3%

Source: SAMHSA (2018, November 21).

When faced with anti-LGBTQ+ sentiment at every turn, these feelings often become internalized. The internalized stigma can become layered in with the multitude of other stressors, which may lead LGBTQ+ persons to engage in self-harm or suicidal thoughts and behaviors (Hatzenbuehler & Pachankis, 2016; NAMI, n.d.; ODPHP, 2020). It is often difficult to arrive at accurate death rates by suicide for LGBTQ+ persons because government fatal injury reports and death records do not capture sexual orientation or gender identity (ODPHP, 2020). However, as more data becomes available through self-report surveys, the rates of suicidal behavior among LGBTQ+ persons are also higher than the national average (NAMI, n.d.; ODPHP, 2020). When compared to the overall population, LGB adults are twice as likely to attempt suicide than the general population, and for gay and bisexual men, the risk is four times greater over a lifetime to attempt suicide than the general population (King et al., 2008). The most significant risk of suicidal behavior is among LGBTQ+ youth (ages 13–24). According to a 2020 survey of 40,000 LGBTQ+ youth from across the United States, 40% of LGB youth considered attempting suicide in the past 12 months, and more than 50% of transgender and nonbinary youth seriously considered suicide in the last 12 months (The Trevor Project, 2020).

Homelessness is another stressor and often begins early in the life of LGBTQ+ individuals. Among LGBTQ+ individuals ages 13–24, 29% experience some form of housing instability (either they were kicked out of their homes or they ran away) that results in homelessness (The Trevor Project, 2020). LGBTQ+ youth and young adults are reported to have a 120% higher risk of experiencing homelessness than their nonminority peers (NAMI, n.d.; Roberts et al., 2012). Homelessness brings additional forms of discrimination for LGBTQ+ youth. Many homeless shelters are not welcoming or do not accommodate LGBTQ+ youth. LGBTQ+ individuals also experience increased instances of harassment and abuse in shelters due to their sexual orientation and gender identity (NAMI, n.d.).

Finally, throughout the life span, LGBTQ+ individuals are at a greater risk for violence both intimate partner and sexual assault. This violence is attributed to homophobia, harassment, and violent acts directed toward sexual minorities (D'Inverno et al., 2019; Walters et al., 2013). The lifetime prevalence of intimate partner violence among LGBTQ+ persons is higher than the general population of the United States; LGB persons experience violence at rates equal to or higher than heterosexuals (Walters et al., 2013). These violent acts can be classified as intimate partner violence, sexual violence, and stalking (D'Inverno et al., 2019; Walters et al., 2013). Bisexual women experience intimate partner violence and sexual violence at significantly higher rates over their lifetimes than lesbian and heterosexual women (Walters et al., 2013). Nearly 1 out of 3 bisexual women (37%) and 1 out of 7 heterosexual women (16%) were injured as a result of rape, physical violence, and/or stalking by an intimate partner (Walters et al., 2013).

Lifetime Prevalence of Rape, Physical Violence, and/or Stalking by Intimate Partner

Women		Men	
Lesbian	44%	Gay	26%
Bisexual	61%	Bisexual	37%
Heterosexual	35%	Heterosexual	29%

Source: CDC (2011).

LGBTQ+ Grief and Loss

In Western culture, school plays, proms, and "finding that special one" is part of a societal narrative that is strongly influenced by societal norms and expectations. In most cases, these are rituals one looks forward to and represent an understood rite of passage. Normally these milestones entail implicit support from family, friends, places of work and worship, and the community at large; however, among sexual minorities this same sense of belonging is met with rejection, stigmatization, and discrimination (Herek et al., 2013).

D'Augelli et al. (2002) identified 15% to 51% of LGBTQ+ individuals do not experience acceptance but rather live with negativity and rejections, making them vulnerable to negative emotional and physical pathologies and ongoing issues surrounding belonging. Compared to heterosexual counterparts, LGBTQ+ individuals are at a higher risk of experiencing psychopathology, including substance abuse, suicidal ideation, suicidal attempts, depression, and anxiety (Case et al., 2004). These stressors suggest LGBTQ+ individuals face a wide range of challenges that affect physical and emotional health and leave them with unique lifelong grief and loss issues (Berg et al., 2015) that in many cases are disenfranchised or rather losses people respond to with less compassion or see as insignificant.

Of profound significance is the experience of coming out. For the LGBTQ+ individual, coming out is an integral part of LGBTQ+ identity formation. In other words, knowing, acknowledging, and accepting a nonheterosexual identity is a profound marker that validates sexual identity and creates congruence between many aspects of one's life (Ben-Ari et al., 1995). For the LGBTQ+ person, family acceptance is critical to self-acceptance and validation

(Shilo et al., 2011) and decreases the risk of experiencing depression, suicidal ideation, suicide attempts, and substance abuse (Padilla et al., 2010). Disclosure is a time of immense stress for the individual coming out because of concern of negative reactions, something particularly relevant when coming out to one's family (Ben-Ari et al., 1995). For many, these negative reactions culminate in family, work, and peer rejection, an ongoing loss that is grieved and is related to increased heterosexism (Pachankis et al., 2008). Central to family rejection is how the rejection becomes the lived experience of what is portrayed and perceived. Carastathis et al. (2017) purported some rejections as subtle and some blatant, which included verbal abuse, physical abuse, disownment, and punishment. However, overt expression of disgust was most oppressive, and these blatant forms of rejection were associated with internalization of negative thoughts, which contribute to engaging in self-harming behaviors and substance abuse.

Regardless of the rejection experience, many LGBT people continue the maintenance of some sense of family relationships; however, for many, being gay, lesbian, bisexual, and/or transgender violates the perception of familial love, which comes with the condition of being heterosexual (Carastathis et al., 2017). This is important because it highlights yet another loss for LGBTQ+ people: acceptance and parity recognition of same sex relationships. From the onset, same-gender couples are aware of stigma consciousness or rather are keenly aware of their differences from the heteronormative couple and therefore are expectant of critical judgment and discrimination (Pinel, 1999).

Marriage in the United States carries potent symbolic power and prestige (Ocobock, 2013). Moreover, for Americans, marriage defines family and assigns family status (Powell et al., 2010). Arguments against same-sex marriage are abundant, and critics render marriage between one man and one woman and adhere to strict boundaries regarding marriage legitimacy. These same censors "normalize being married as healthy and moral and unmarried as abnormal, unhealthy, and deviant" (Green, 2010, p. 406). Without legal marriage, same-sex couples forgo rituals and status, something that leads to a keener sense of belonging in heterosexual couples. In one 2010 study conducted among gay men in Iowa, men specifically cited they felt "they needed marriage so others would view their relationship as a serious one" (Ocobock, 2013, p. 195). This same study found same-sex couples felt differently after being married. Specifically, the participants stated they felt more legitimate, real, and solid. This highlights marginalization that same sex couples feel without the same civil privileges extended to their heterosexual counterparts. This lack of recognition contributes to higher incidences of lower self-esteem and negatively impacts emotional and physical well-being. Unfortunately, as the LGBTQ+ person ages and moves into later life years, the sense of accomplishment and belonging experienced by heterosexual couples can be experienced as one of oppression and despair by members of the LGBTQ+ community.

Implications for Counseling

It is important for counselors to examine their own biases about the LGBTQ+ community, including those internalized societal biases and assumptions we have all internalized to greater or lesser degrees. This is important because trust, safety, and affirmation are particularly crucial to this population given the history of oppression and the need to come out to the counselor. Some guiding questions for the counselor in beginning this process might include the following:

- What was the first reference to gays or lesbians you ever remember hearing?
- What do you remember about the first person you ever saw or met who you identified as gay or lesbian?
- What did your parents teach you about people who are gay and lesbian?
- Do you currently have friends or acquaintances who you know to be gay or lesbian? If not, why do you think this is so?

Exploring these questions may reveal an internalized and unconscious bias that could surface in the counseling relationship. Beginning this personal exploration of potential internalized bias can help the counselor become more effective and aware as they build relationships with LGBTQ+ clients.

Because one must come out as LGBTQ+, it is also important for counselors to use language that signifies this is a safe person. Using language such as "gay lifestyle" or "sexual preference" implies the counselor believes the client's sexual identity is a choice and therefore can be unchosen. This strategy is typical of reparative therapy and conservative religious groups who attempt to "pray the gay away" or to change the person. Conversely, a counselor who uses terms such as "sexual identity" or "orientation," does not use heterosexist terminology or assumptions, and uses the preferred labels of the client demonstrates this may be a safe place. Additionally, understanding the history of oppression for LGBTQ+ people, having knowledge of sexual identity development and transgender identity development models, and understanding the kitchen table or everyday issues for this population are all important to providing culturally competent counseling services. Understanding the impact of intersectional identities is also important to working effectively with this population, especially in terms of grief issues, because of deeply rooted cultural traditions and beliefs related to loss and grieving.

Additionally, it is crucial for counselors to set a tone of affirmation with this population and not tolerance or acceptance. Because of bias, LGBTQ+ people wish for acceptance from family, friends, and society at large; however, the counseling relationship is one where clients need to be affirmed for who they are and not merely tolerated. Establishing strong rapport is the key to any counseling relationship and for this population, being affirmed for one's identity is at the core of that healing relationship.

Counselors should be particularly attuned to suicidal ideation and substance use disorders in the LGBTQ+ client population because prevalence rates are higher than their heterosexual, cisgendered counterparts. Being prepared to assess risk and to intervene as needed is vital to the overall health and wellness of clients. Assessment procedures with people who abuse substances typically involve clinical interviews with the client and with people who may be in their family of origin or members of their support group in combination with objective assessment instruments. Potential barriers to a strong therapeutic alliance include interviews that assume heterosexuality and assessment tools laden with heterosexist or gender binary bias. Counselors should ask about family and other relationships in a manner that communicates acceptance to people of all sexual identities. Each client, regardless of cultural context, should be asked about sexual orientation in a relaxed way, as a normal part of the assessment procedure. Additionally, inclusion of partners in the assessment process is crucial. A client who is struggling with addiction may face bias in the treatment environment as well. If inpatient treatment is needed, the housing environment may present obstacles for LGBTQ+ individuals due to binary gender constructions around housing and restrooms. Counselors should prepare clients for situations like these, including potential bias in 12-step support communities and in group therapy, a common modality in addiction treatment. Clients struggling with addiction and grief and loss issues while managing coming out issues in a heteronormative environment can be overwhelmed, which may lead to higher dropout rates for treatment.

Assisting LGBTQ+ clients with the coming out process is an important role for the counselor. Clients with addiction issues may not be out to family, friends, or in the workplace. Recovery often leads to wanting to live a more authentic life, so it is not uncommon for LGBTQ+ people in early recovery to feel the need to disclose to significant others and sponsors in 12-step programs. The following should guide the counseling process regarding coming out by exploring the associated *who, what, why, where,* and *when* questions. First, help clients determine *why* they are planning on coming out. Help them explore the ramifications, potential outcomes, and pitfalls. Help clients decide *what* to say when they come out. For example, prepare a written statement or role-play various scenarios. Prepare your clients for potential questions they might be asked such as, *Are you sure you're gay, trans, bisexual? How long have you been gay, bisexual or trans? Have you tried to change? Have you tried to be involved with a person of the opposite sex?* Help your clients decide *where* they will disclose, whether it is in a letter, over the phone, or, preferably, in a quiet, private place. Finally, help clients to determine *when* they will come out. Encourage your clients not to disclose during an event or holiday. It is an important occasion, so let it have the full attention it deserves. Also, prepare clients for the reactions of others, which may be similar to the grief process. Significant others may experience phases of an acceptance process such as shock, denial, guilt, anger or hostility, coping, and then acceptance. The following is offered as a guide to working with LGBTQ+ clients in counseling:

1 Counselors should first help clients process the recognition of being or feeling different.
2 Counselors should be able to assist the client in management of their sexual or gender identity across contexts and intersectional identities.
3 Counselors should help clients identify impact of internalized homonegativity. This is important in moving toward greater self-acceptance.
4 Counselors should assist clients in the management of oppression and stigma.

Regardless of the complexity of issues, abstinence and sobriety should be a priority in assisting the LGBTQ+ client. Establishing a safe, affirmative counseling environment will help in developing a strong therapeutic alliance. Co-occurring issues may include losses such as alienation from family, trauma history, HIV/AIDS, suicide potential, domestic violence, and family formation issues. Alienation from family and friends due to a combination of social damage from addictive behavior and sexual orientation or transgender stigma creates complex barriers for the LGBTQ+ client to overcome. Culturally competent treatment strategies provide the best opportunity for sexual minority clients to benefit from treatment and lead healthy lives.

References

Barret, B., & Logan, C. (2002). *Counseling gay men and lesbians*. Brooks/Cole.

Ben-Ari, A. (1995). The discovery that an offspring is gay: Parents', gay men's, and lesbian perspectives. *Journal of Homosexuality, 30*(1), 89–112. https://doi.org/10.1300/J082v30n01_05

Berg, R., Weatherburn, P., Ross, M., & Schmidt, A. (2015). The relationship of internalized homonegativity to sexual health and well-being among men in 38 European countries who have sex with men. *Journal of Gay & Lesbian Mental Health, 19*(3), 285–302. https://doi.org/10.1080/19359705.2015.1024375

Capuzzi, D., & Stauffer, M. D. (2016). *Foundations of addictions counseling* (3rd ed.). Pearson.

Carastathis, G., Cohen, L., Kaczmarek, E., & Chang, P. (2017). Rejected by family for being gay or lesbian: Portrayals, perceptions, and resilience. *Journal of Homosexuality, 64*(3), 289–320. https://doi.org/10.1080/00918369.2016.1179035

Case, P., Austin, S., Hunter, D., Manson, J., Malspeis, S., Willett, W., & Spiegelman, D. (2004). Sexual orientation, health risk factors, and physical functioning in the Nurses' Health Study II. *Journal of Women's Health (Larchmont, N.Y. 2002), 13*(9), 1033–1047. https://doi.org/10.1089/jwh.2004.13.1033

CDC (Centers for Disease Control and Prevention). (2011). *NISVS: An overview of 2010 findings on victimization by sexual orientation.* www.cdc.gov/violenceprevention/pdf/cdc_nisvs_victimization_final-a.pdf

CDC (Centers for Disease Control and Prevention). (2016, February). *Stigma and discrimination.* www.cdc.gov/msmhealth/stigma-and-discrimination.htm

D'Augelli, A. R. (2002). Mental health problems among lesbian, gay, and bisexual youths ages 14–21. *Clinical Child Psychology and Psychiatry, 7,* 433–456. https://doi.org/10.1177/1359104502007003010

D'Inverno, A. S., Smith, S. G., Zhang, X., & Chen, J. (2019). *The impact of intimate partner violence: A 2015 NISVS research-in-brief.* Centers for Disease Control and Prevention. www.cdc.gov/violenceprevention/pdf/nisvs/nisvs-impactbrief-508.pdf

Green, A. I. (2010). Queer unions: Same-sex spouses marrying tradition and innovation. *Canadian Journal of Sociology, 35,* 399–436.

Hatzenbuehler, M. L., & Pachankis, J. E. (2016). Stigma and minority stress as social determinants of health among lesbian, gay, bisexual, and transgender youth: Research evidence and clinical implications. *Pediatric Clinics of North America, 63*(6), 985–999. https://doi.org/10.1016/j.pcl.2016.07.003

Herek, G. M., & McLemore, K. A. (2013). Sexual prejudice. *Annual Review of Psychology, 64*(1), 309–333. https://doi.org/10.1146/annurev-psych-113011-143826

IOM (Institute of Medicine). (2011). *The health of lesbian, gay, bisexual, and transgender people: Building a foundation for better understanding.* National Academies Press. https://doi.org/10.17226/13128

King, M., Semlyen, J., Tai, S. S., Killaspy, H., Osborn, D., Popelyuk, D., & Nazareth, I. (2008). A systematic review of mental disorder, suicide, and deliberate self-harm in lesbian, gay and bisexual people. *BMC Psychiatry, 8*(1), 70. https://doi.org/10.1186/1471-244X-8-70

Korell, S. C., & Lorah, P. (2013). An overview of affirmative psychotherapy and counseling with transgender clients. In K. Bieschke, R. M. Perez, & K. A. DeBord (Eds.), *Handbook of counseling and psychotherapy with lesbian, gay, bisexual, and transgender clients* (pp. 271–288). American Psychological Association.

Meyer, I. H. (2003). Prejudice, social stress, and mental health in lesbian, gay, and bisexual populations: Conceptual issues and research evidence. *Psychological Bulletin, 129*(5), 674–697. https://doi.org/10.1037/0033-2909.129.5.674

Meyer, I. H. (2013). Prejudice, social stress, and mental health in lesbian, gay, and bisexual populations: Conceptual issues and research evidence. *Psychology of Sexual Orientation and Gender Diversity, 1*(S), 3–26. https://doi.org/10.1037/2329-0382.1.S.3

NAMI (National Alliance on Mental Illness). (n.d.). *LGBTQI.* www.nami.org/Your-Journey/Identity-and-Cultural-Dimensions/LGBTQI

Ocobock, A. (2013). The power and limits of marriage: Married gay men's family relationships. *Journal of Marriage and Family, 75,* 191–205. https://doi.org/10.1111/j.1741-3737.2012.01032.x

ODPHP (Office of Disease Prevention and Health Promotion). (2020, October 8). Lesbian, gay, bisexual, transgender health. *HealthyPeople.* www.healthypeople.gov/2020/topics-objectives/topic/lesbian-gay-bisexual-and-transgender-health

Pachankis, J. E., Goldfried, M. R., & Ramrattan, M. E. (2008). Extension of rejection sensitivity construct to the interpersonal functioning of gay men. *Journal of Counseling and Clinical Psychology, 76,* 306–317. https://doi.org/101037/0022-006X.76.2.306

Padilla, Y. C., Crisp, C., & Rew, D. L. (2010). Parental acceptance and illegal drugs use among gay, lesbian, and bisexual adolescents: Results from a national survey. *Social Work, 55,* 265–275. https://doi.org/10.1093/sw/55.3.265

Pinel, E. C. (1999). Stigma consciousness: The psychological legacy of social stereotypes. *Journal of Personality and Social Psychology, 76,* 114–128.

Powell, B., Bolzendahl, C., Geist, C., & Carr Streelman, L. (2010). *Counted out: Same sex relations and Americans' definitions of Family.* Russell Sage Foundation.

Roberts, A. L., Rosario, M., Corliss, H. L., Koenen, K. C., & Bryan Austin, S. (2012). Elevated risk of posttraumatic stress in sexual minority youths: Mediation by childhood abuse and gender nonconformity. *American Journal of Public Health (1971), 102*(8), 1587–1593. https://doi.org/10.2105/AJPH.2011.300530

SAMHSA (Substance Abuse and Mental Health Services Administration). (2018, November 21). *2015–2016 NSDUH: Sexual orientation summary sheets.* SAMHSA. www.samhsa.gov/data/report/2015-2016-nsduh-sexual-orientation-summary-sheets

SAMHSA (Substance Abuse and Mental Health Services Administration). (2020, November 18). *2019 National survey on drug use and health: Lesbian, gay, & bisexual (LGB) adults.* SAMHSA. www.samhsa.gov/data/report/2019-nsduh-lesbian-gay-bisexual-lgb-adults

Shilo, G., & Savaya, R. (2011). Effects of family and friend support on LGB youths' mental health and sexual orientations milestones. *Family Relations, 60,* 318–330. https://doi.org/10/1111/j.741-3729.2011.00648.x

The Trevor Project. (2020). *2020 National survey on LGBTQ youth mental health.* www.thetrevorproject.org/survey-2020/

Walters, M. L., Chen, J., & Breiding, M. J. (2013). *The national intimate partner and sexual violence survey (NISVS): 2010 findings on victimization by sexual orientation.* Centers for Disease Control and Prevention. www.cdc.gov/violenceprevention/pdf/nisvs_sofindings.pdf

Weber, G., & Dodge, A. (2017). Substance use among gender and sexual minority youth and adults. In K. B. Smalley, J. C. Warren, & K. N. Barefoot (Eds.), *LGBT health: Meeting the needs of gender and sexual minorities* (pp. 199–214). Springer.

12 Addiction and Grief in the Military

Henry L. Harris and Lyndon P. Abrams

The U.S. military represents a unique cultural group where individuals form strong bonds at times, under stressful situations that may directly change one's life forever. Numerous deployments, separation from family, physical injuries, and stressful combat situations are some of the critical experiences active duty service members (ADSMs) have encountered. For example, deployed service members, particularly those in combat, have encountered stressors that include receiving enemy artillery attacks, suicide bombers, blasts from improvised explosive devices (IEDs), witnessing injury, deaths of others, exposure to decomposed bodies, and being wounded or taken as a prisoner of war (Bøg et al., 2018).

While the military projects an aura of strength and confidence, service members do indeed encounter concerns related to substance abuse and grief, similar to civilian populations. For example, from 2003 to 2013, service members experienced multiple combat deployments in Iraq and Afghanistan; thousands were injured and many gave the ultimate sacrifice (Leskin, 2015). A larger number of them suffered from physical injuries and various other mental health challenges. Post-traumatic stress disorder (PTSD), depression, and generalized anxiety disorder were reported by nearly 18% of ADSMs, and nearly 10% met the criteria for two or more of these disorders (Meadows et al., 2018).

For some service members, grief and loss is another area that has not been examined extensively within the confines of the U.S. military (Delaney et al., 2017), yet it has impacted substance use. In one of the earliest studies that followed the loss of 248 soldiers in an accidental plane crash, the survivors who used persistent avoidance in addressing the tragedy demonstrated the most dysfunction, which included heavy drinking. Many at certain stages of their grief resorted to using tranquilizers and alcohol to help with impaired sleeping and relieve tension (Bartone & Wright, 1990). Regardless of contributing factors impacting substance abuse, ADSMs could be criminally charged or face a dishonorable discharge if they are caught using illegal drugs or fail a drug test.

Military Demographic Profile

The U.S. military reflects an all-volunteer force that has decreased in size over the past few decades. For example, in 1990 during the time period of

DOI: 10.4324/9781003106906-12

the Persian Gulf War, there were more than two million active duty service members (ADSMs); yet even during conflicts with Iraq and Afghanistan that began in 2010, the number of ADSMs decreased to 1.46 million (Pew Research Center, 2019). In 2019, there were 1,326,200 ADSMs, and 82% (n =1,087,484) were enlisted, with an average age of approximately 27 years. Eighteen percent (n = 238,716) were officers, with an average age of 34 years. The Army represents the largest branch of the U.S. Armed Forces at 36% (n = 479,785), followed by the Navy with 25% (n = 332,528), the Air Force at 25.5% (n = 327,878), and the Marine Corps with 14% (n = 186,009). The majority (87%) were stationed in the United States or U.S. territories followed by East Asia (6.5%) and Europe (5%). It also important to note that while the Navy increased mildly in numbers from 2010–2019, the Air Force, Army, and Marine Corps suffered decreases (U.S. Department of Defense, 2019).

In 2019, nearly 51% (n = 676,362) of ADSMs were married, 80% (n = 869,984) of enlisted ADSMs held a high school diploma, and almost 9% (n = 97,873) had a bachelor's or advanced degree. In contrast, nearly 86% (n = 205,295) of officers held similar degrees. From a gender perspective, males represented 83% (n = 1,101,440) of the ADSMs, and females accounted for the remaining 17% (n = 224,760). In addition, 31% (n = 413,764) of the ADSMs were from racial minority groups that included African Americans, American Indian or Alaska Native, Asian, Native Hawaiian or Other Pacific Islander, multiracial, or other/unknown. Hispanics or Latinos represented the largest minority group at nearly 17% (n = 70,339; U.S. Department of Defense, 2019).

Selected Reserve Force

In addition to the active duty force, members serving in the Selected Reserve Force (SRF) are worthy of recognition because of their integral role supporting the mission of the U.S. Armed Forces. The SRF members generally serve on a part-time basis that typically calls for training one weekend per month and two weeks annually. However, they may be called to serve active duty when the president issues a mobilization order during war or national emergency (Congressional Research Service, 2020; SAMHSA, 2010). The SRF comprises 807,602 members from seven different organizations: (a) Coast Guard Reserve (6,277); (b) Marine Corps Reserve (38,389); (c) Navy Reserve (59,658); (d) Air Force Reserve (69,389); (e) Air National Guard (107,197); (f) Army Reserve (190,719); and (g) Army National Guard (335,973; U.S. Department of Defense, 2019). Military service members are well trained and must be ready to respond to conflicts and or natural disasters anywhere in the world.

Veterans

A military veteran is a man or woman who has served on active duty in the U.S. Armed Forces. According to Vespa (2020), data from the 2018 American

Community Survey indicated there were approximately 18 million veterans in the United States, a decline from 26 million in 2000. Males accounted for 91% of the population; however, by 2040, the number of female veterans is expected to increase to 17%. In 2018, the largest group of veterans (6.4 million) served during the Vietnam War (1964–1975), and the median age of this group is 71 years. Veterans from the post-9/11 era have a median age of 37. Veterans have made numerous sacrifices and as a result of their military service have unique health concerns. When compared to the civilians who have never served, veterans are more likely to suffer from mental health disorders, trauma-connected injuries, and substance use (Olenick et al., 2015).

Military Culture

Mental health providers are expected to provide culturally competent services to individuals from different cultural backgrounds in a highly effective manner. In order to meet this challenge most effectively with military personnel, it is essential that providers understand the culture of the military (Meyer, 2015). The military is a unique cultural organization characterized by a different set of values, laws, customs, expectations, language, traditions, and courtesies that impacts every aspects of the lives of service members. They relinquish certain levels of personal freedom and privacy and are made aware of this commitment from basic training throughout their career that these sacrifices are needed in order to ensure military mission success (Meyer, 2015).

Structure

The military environment has been characterized as a fortress reflected by a firm authoritarian structure where rules and regulations must be followed. Rank and order are highly valued, and questioning authority is most often not tolerated by military service members (Wertsch, 1991). Following the chain of command is an essential element of military culture and solely based on the rank of the individual. There is typically one person in charge of the unit who assumes all responsibility. When individuals meet certain benchmarks, they are promoted up the chain of command that also includes additional responsibilities and pay. All service members have a specific person who addresses specific problems or concerns, and when the chain of command is not followed, this could cause informal or formal disciplinary actions. The chain of command is further reflected in officer and enlisted ranks. Officers typically have more postsecondary educational degrees than enlisted members. In addition, they have more power, a different rank system, higher pay scale, separate living quarters, and limited socialization with enlisted members outside of work. Wertsch (1991) contended supporting the mission and giving the ultimate sacrifice on the battlefield is the sole equality between officers and enlisted service members. Hall further noted (2011) that it is a universal belief that a rigid hierarchical system characterized by subordination and dominance is required for the military to function most effectively.

Understanding generic military language and the uniqueness of each military branch is another cultural characteristic that must be taken into consideration. For example, some of the Air Force values include *excellence in all we do* and *integrity*; the Army conveys *integrity first, duty, honor*, and *loyalty*; the Coast Guard values *devotion to duty, honor*, and *respect*; and the Navy and Marines promote *honor, courage*, and *commitment*. Regardless of the branch, military service members are taught the significance of understanding custom and courtesies; how to listen, stay focused, maintain self-discipline, and display emotional self-control at all times are essential characteristics of service members (SAMHSA, 2010).

Substance Use

Persons in the military are conditioned to conduct themselves in a manner that requires discipline and self-control at all times. ADSMs must be ready at any given moment to perform their duties at a high level, and being under the influence of drugs negatively impacts their ability to maintain mission readiness. It is not uncommon for service members to participate in random urine testing, and they must comply because substance use in the military is not tolerated. A positive test may also be accompanied with severe consequences because military persons are governed by a different set of laws known as the Uniform Code of Military Justice (UCMJ). These laws forbid the possession and use of controlled substances, which is reflective of the zero-tolerance policy supported by all branches of the Armed Forces (Drug Crimes, 2019). ADSMs and selected reserve members (SRMs) could also face military punishment for other drug-related matters, such as refusing to provide a requested urine sample, being in possession of certain drugs, tampering with a drug test, testing positive for an illegal substance, being in possession of banned drug paraphernalia, and distributing drugs either by growing, trafficking, or selling. If an ADSM or SRM is charged and convicted of a drug offense, severe punishment can be expected under the UCMJ guidelines. Penalties may range from reduction in rank, dishonorable discharge from the military, and even incarceration (Drug Crimes, 2019).

Alcohol

Alcohol is a legal substance; however, the abuse of alcohol is a significant issue that impacts military personnel and their families. Service members have been known to use alcohol recreationally (i.e., holidays, sporting events, and base celebrations), to relax and reward themselves for a hard day's work, and to build comradery with other service members. Alcohol is easily attainable, inexpensive, and readily available for purchase on most military bases. Some of the known negative effects of alcohol abuse include unintentional injury, cancers, cardiovascular disease, and liver damage (Room et al., 2005). According to Waller et al. (2015), the misuse of alcohol significantly impacts service members' health and other behavioral and performance concerns, such as driving while intoxicated and failing to be promoted (Mattiko et al., 2011). In addition, results from a 2015 Health Related Behaviors Survey (HRBS) of ADSMs found that 35% consumed alcohol at such a level that would categorize them as hazardous drinkers, as measured by the Alcohol Use Disorders Identification Test (AUDIT). Another 30% of the ADSMs were considered binge drinkers, nearly 70% regarded the military environment supportive of drinking, and 42% stated their supervisor did not discourage the use of alcohol. The last two viewpoints were more commonly held by younger enlisted service members. Finally, slightly over 8% of members experienced serious consequences after excessive drinking (Meadows et al., 2018).

The Selective Reserve Force and veterans are not immune from alcohol-related issues. For example, in one study of Ohio Army National Guard soldiers ($n = 671$), alcohol use was the highest reported substance use disorder, at 44% (Fink et al., 2016). In a 2018 National Survey on Drug Use and Health, nearly four million veterans with a mental health and/or substance use issue struggled the most with alcohol use (SAMHSA, 2018). Alcohol abuse is more common among male veterans than female veterans. Further, veterans exposed to higher levels of combat are also at a greater risk to engage in binge drinking and drink more heavily when compare to other military veterans (Teeters et al., 2017).

Illicit Drug Use

Illicit drugs include a wide variety of substances such as marijuana, opium, heroin, cocaine, and the nonmedical use of prescription drugs. In 2015, only 0.7% of ADSMs reported using any illicit drugs, such as synthetic cannabis or marijuana. This level of use is much lower than the general U.S. population and further reflects how illicit drug use has decreased over the years and was impacted by earlier wars and conflicts. For example, during the Vietnam War, 45% of Army soldiers reported using narcotics, and 80% used marijuana (Robins, 1993). In part due to the widespread drug use of the Vietnam era, the Department of Defense adopted the "zero tolerance" drug policy, which further initiated mandatory urine testing of service members for illegal substances (Bachman et al., 1999). Even with this zero tolerance policy, in 2017–2018 the Army reported an 18% increase in the number of positive drug tests for THC (tetrahydrocannabinol in cannabis) for soldiers in states where marijuana was legalized (Szoldra, 2019).

In a survey exploring illicit drug use among veterans, 11% reported using marijuana, 1% used cocaine, 0.8% used hallucinogens, and 0.9% used methamphetamines, inhalants, and/or heroin (SAMHSA, 2018). Regarding use of marijuana or cannabis, there have been some efforts to increase veterans' access to medical cannabis. In a recent study of 93 military veterans who were given the opportunity, the majority of them reported using cannabinoids as a substitute for either prescription medications, tobacco, alcohol, or illicit substances. Additional results further indicated they used cannabis as a primary source to self-treat their mental health conditions and physical health issues as well. The findings suggest more guidance on using medical cannabis with veterans is warranted because of the potential helpful and harmful outcomes (Loflin et al., 2019).

Prescription Medications

There are numerous types of prescription medications, and some of the most used are opioids. Opioids are medications designed with the intended purpose of relieving severe pain and are most often prescribed for individuals suffering from chronic pain and recovering surgery or an injury. In 2015, slightly over 6% of ADSMs indicated using opioid pain medication, a decrease of 4% compared to 2011. Four percent of ADSMs reported misusing one or more prescription drugs over the past year, and pain relievers and sedatives were the drugs most often used. Additionally, the majority of ADSMs obtained their prescription drugs from a military treatment facility (Meadows et al., 2018). Veterans have also been affected by the misuse of prescription drugs. In 2018, 2.7% of veterans (562,000) reported misuse of prescription pain relievers, including hydrocodone, oxycodone, and fentanyl. These numbers are much lower than the general population and further represent a significant decrease in prescription drug misuse for veterans between 2015 and 2018 (SAMHSA, 2018). Even so, abuse of prescription medication remains an area of concern because in a study of 124,000 veterans, when compared to individuals receiving the lowest doses of opioid pain relievers, those who received the highest doses were more than twice as likely to end their lives by suicide (Ilgen et al., 2016).

Grief and Military

Grief is a normal response to loss. Whether the loss involves death, physical injury, or other incapacity, grief is a waypoint on the route toward resolution and recovery (Humphrey, 2009). For those engaged in military service, several factors may preclude the grieving process. When the grief process is thwarted, the normal resolution of grief is disrupted. In this context, three common factors may play a role in disrupting the normal grief process: (a) delay in the process grief, (b) disenfranchisement from the grieving experience, and (c) traumatic loss. While these factors are considerations in any grief context, they are of particular concern for armed services personnel (Delaney et al., 2017). Significant losses that occur in the military theater may be sudden and occur at a time and place that do not readily facilitate the grieving process. Consider a loss that occurs during an active military conflict where intense attention needs to be focused on the ongoing dangers. That situation allows little time or space for acknowledging and dealing with loss (Simon et al., 2020).

Disenfranchised grief may be the result of a service person's attempts to avoid the grief process because the military or personal cultural context does not condone open recognition of loss (Smith, 1999). In a situation where there is a need to see oneself as invulnerable, delving into loss may challenge military self-efficacy, which was created by the invulnerability cloak necessary for normal functioning in a highly dangerous situation. In active military conflicts, the chances of traumatic loss are great; still, the shock associated with the death or dismemberment of one's colleagues or significant personal injury may result in a stress-related response (i.e., PTSD). The mitigation of these factors will impact the way the grief one experiences is worked through effectively or is complicated.

Complicated grief generally occurs after significant losses in about 7% of the general population (Shear, 2012). The prevalence of complicated grief among members of the military is unknown, but in one study, active-duty personnel and retirees seeking mental health services were screened for complicated grief using the Inventory of Complicated Grief. These researchers found that 46.1% were screened as positive for complicated grief, with 43.5% of the same sample population indicating they had experienced a loss that continues to impact them (Delaney et al., 2017). While we do not know the exact percentage of service personnel and veterans positive for complicated grief, we can say with a measure of confidence that it is higher than the percentage in the general population. Shear (2012) has compared complicated grief to an infection that interrupts the healing process, which if left unresolved will ultimately destroy. Sometimes infection resolves itself, but the better course is to treat the infection directly.

Stigma and Military Grief

The literature points to several barriers military service members may encounter as they attempt to work through traumatic loss. The following quote illustrates broadly the complexity of grief for military service members:

> Death is a fact of life in the military culture given the potential lethal nature of the profession of arms. The military as a whole is not psychologically prepared to deal with death and grief. Military leaders and soldiers have learned from society that it is not okay to openly express their grief, which has a profound impact on morale in the Army.
>
> (Smith, 1999, p. iii)

The American Psychiatric Association (2021) defines psychological stigma as prejudice and discrimination against people with people with mental illness. This prejudice can be directed at others, self, or institutions. The preceding quote suggests that the culture of the military, in all branches, places service persons at risk of being bound by stigma with peers, self, and within the military institutions. This creates a conundrum for individuals who find themselves in need of support in the aftermath of some grief-evoking event. In the state of needing help but resisting it because of stigma, the individuals find themselves facing additional psychological challenges such as reduced self-confidence, reduced self-efficacy, challenges to interpersonal relationships, and difficulty in duty assignment and daily living (Smith, 1999).

With the recognition of the danger of stigma, efforts have been made to increase psychological help seeking among service personnel. Miggantz (2014) identified recent strategies to reduce stigma. Some have included (a) utilizing military peers to share success stories of working through mental health challenges, (b) creating a duty readiness continuum that allows mental health to factor into a service person's readiness for duty, (c) embedding of mental health professionals into military units, and (d) integrating psychological services into primary medical care military settings. While all are well-intentioned, these interventions have not been fully embraced by service personnel.

In a review of the literature, we found researchers have studied the impact of grief and loss on the families of military service members much more than grief's impact on the service members themselves. The military's cultural notion of pushing through the personal in effort to meet the aims of the mission has facilitated neglect of the needs of the service personnel. Prior to 2008, the suicide rate of the general public was greater than that of the U.S. military population (Nock et al., 2013). However, in 2019 the U.S. Department of Defense (2019) reported the suicide rate for veterans was 1.5 times greater than that of nonmilitary adults. The links between military service, complicated grief, and suicide are easily established and have been understood from studying veterans and serving military personnel from the Vietnam conflict forward (Currier & Holland, 2012). Arguably the problems have been in existence for much longer, but myriad factors have obscured our recognition of these issues.

Substance Abuse and Grief

The literature appears to be devoid of information with a focus on grief and addiction in the military. This is significant, because grief and addiction are often so deeply connected that working through grief is an essential part of recovering from substance use (Hairston, 2021). The military reflects a segment of society, and service members and veterans are not immune to grief and substance abuse issues. Research has indicated that some types of grief, such as bereavement, may increase risks of developing an alcohol-related substance use disorder (Stahl & Schulz, 2014). In addition, individuals suffering from complicated grief appear to be more prone to develop an addiction in their attempt to deal with their mourning. Additional research on the effect of grief on brain function discovered that complicated grief activated a part of the brain's reward center that impacted addiction-related behaviors (O'Connor et al., 2008).

Regardless of the event that caused the grief, it is important to keep in mind that some military personnel may use substances as a way to numb feelings of pain, shock, loss, anger, resentment, and helplessness. Use of substances could eventually make things more difficult because when the grieving ends, the substance abuse could be even more pronounced and uncontrolled.

Mental Health Implications

Working with military personnel has challenges that may not be covered in human services preparation programs. Developing competency to work effectively with this unique population requires self-awareness along with an empathic understanding on the need to apply military-sensitive interventions. The following are suggestions that some mental health providers may find useful. However, please keep in mind that each military branch provides specific mental health treatment and support to its service members. For the veteran population, the Veterans Administration offers various types of mental health and addiction treatment programs. Organizations such as Veterans and Family Care, Fisher House, Warrior Care Network, and Veterans Wellness Alliance also have provided valuable support.

Military Cultural Awareness

Initially, it is important for the clinician to convene all services with an appreciation of military culture (Hall, 2011; Meyer, 2015). Just as cultural competency regarding issues such as race, ethnicity, national origin, religion, and so forth is essential, the practitioner must be (a) aware of their attitudes and biases toward military personnel, (b) knowledgeable of the cultural frame of the military and its various branches, and (c) skilled in applying interventions that fit into that framework. McGuire (2013) suggested that "veterans need to know that clinicians are aware that veterans are trained warriors; they need to know that clinicians value their service and recognize that freedom is not free" (p. 182). With that understanding, the clinician is positioned to embody and transmit a sense of respect and appreciation of the personhood and purpose of the service person (Meyer, 2015).

Additionally, the counselor needs to be aware of supports and services afforded to military personnel and veterans, as they are complex and layered. Add to that knowledge of the nature of governmental bureaucracies that often make help seeking difficult on individual service members. It is important to note that supports may vary according to various factors such as military branch, rank, and status (i.e., active duty, reservist, retired). This information needs to be known and understood by the helper and must be communicated to the service member or veteran.

Mental health providers should also be mindful of the stigma ADSMs and veterans may encounter when they seek mental health services. Historically, the military has attempted to create a culture with minimum tolerance for moral, physical, or mental weakness. As a result of this environment, mental health issues have often been associated with personal weakness, which may cause some to refrain from seeking counseling (Nash et al., 2009). Some do not trust the system and (a) may not be ready to discuss their problems, (b) believe they can solve it themselves, (c) believe the problem will simply "go away," and (d) fear negative consequences. There are also some career-related matters involving seeking treatment that include commanders having access to their mental health records, being rated or perceived as unfit for duty, and not being able to attain high-level security clearance (Gibbons et al., 2014). It is essential to point out that the military has taken appropriate steps to portray mental health and substance treatment more positively over the past three decades. It is not uncommon to see posters with slogans reading "Comprehensive Soldier & Family Fitness: Strong Minds*Strong Bodies" or "Warriors Don't Fight Alone: Knowing When to Get Help Takes Strength." Additionally, the military branches have adopted specific ways to destigmatize mental health and substance abuse treatment.

Rituals

Built into military culture are myriad rituals. Ceremonies are held for induction into and upon completion of basic training, and often graduation ceremonies are held to signify the establishment of the end of recruit status and the commencement of full-fledged service. Days begin with reveille and the close of the day is signaled by the playing of taps. This is often done audibly with the expectation that all attired personnel will be attentive and respectful of the reverence of all these events. Ritual is an integral part of military life. Even in death, personnel who have honorably served are entitled to a military funeral as a final salute to the individual for their service.

McGuire (2013) has suggested that the use of ritual can be especially meaningful and helpful to the service person working through unresolved grief. McGuire described a therapeutic intervention with a group of veterans at an Ohio State Veterans Home. The ceremony was created and led by clinicians working with a chaplain. The group gathered in a large room as patriotic music was played. Participants were instructed to think of a comrade they had lost. The room's lighting was dimmed. As the veterans entered, they were offered small rocks intended to represent fallen comrades. A chaplain opened the ceremony with prayer and another clinician led the group through a guided imagery activity. The veterans were given prompts to address unfinished business that might have previously gone unaddressed. One by one, the service members delivered their rocks to a table designated as a sacred space where the rocks would be collected before being transported to a permanent reflection space (i.e., garden or park) that the veterans had ready access to and could visit later. McGuire reported that some group members requested additional rocks to represent additional losses.

McGuire (2013) identified Byock's (1997) five stages of ritual as the theoretical underpinning of the ritual just presented. Imbedded in the ritual were

Byrock's five tasks for closure: (a) asking for forgiveness, (b) extending forgiveness to others, (c) expressing thanks, (d) expressing love, and (e) saying goodbye. The tasks were all addressed during the ritual, with many being addressed during the guided imagery activity.

Equine-Facilitated Therapy

Equine-assisted therapy is a mode of animal-assisted therapy that has been employed with increasing frequency in recent years. It is an experiential mode of therapy that pairs equine-related activities with more traditional talk therapy. Marchand et al. (2021) reported that the number of accredited Professional Association of Therapeutic Horsemanship International (PATH) of equine therapy programs that provided services for veterans grew from 89 to 335 between 2009 and 2016. Much of the research on equine-assisted therapy with veterans has focused on PTSD, individuals with traumatic brain injuries, substance abuse, depression, and anxiety. Symington (2012) specifically advocated for the use of equine-assisted therapy with clients working through grief-related issues. While there has been increasing interest in this kind of program and this approach appears to be well received, Kinney et al. (2019) encouraged further study before declaring this an evidence-based methodology.

Family Systems

Given the transitory nature of military assignments, often military families operate with limited extended family or community support. While military communities often are positioned to offer support to individuals impacted by grief, it is important to note the needs of the family system when working through issues of grief with a service person. Lester and Flake (2013) argued there is much we do not know about the impact of military service on families, as much research has been flawed by design. It then seems incumbent on the clinician to consider the systemic impact of any intervention applied to any aspect of a military family system. Some service members might also benefit from participating in support groups. For example, Military Support Groups of America is a federation of respected organizations that were created to support, protect, and enhance the lives of ADSMs and veterans.

Complicated Grief Therapy

Complicated grief therapy is a relatively new approach (Loebach-Wetherell, 2012) that blends traditional cognitive behavior therapy with attachment theory and interpersonal theory. Participants of this approach work through a highly structured 16-session protocol that relies on repeatedly telling the story of the loss paired with in vivo exposure activities. In a randomized controlled study, Loebach-Wetherell (2012) reported faster recovery for participants assigned to the treatment group where complicated grief theory was utilized.

Bibliotherapy

Briggs and Pehrsson (2008) suggested that bibliotherapy can be readily used with traditional talk therapy in grief counseling. Bibliotherapy can be used as a stand-alone resource for individuals experiencing mild symptoms and an additional support for those engaged in more extensive therapeutic treatment modes (U.S. Department of Veterans Affairs, n.d.). Care should be exercised to ensure that materials are carefully selected with a number of factors, such as developmental level, appropriateness of language, and reading capacity of the client considered. Clients should be carefully guided through the materials (Briggs & Pehrsson, 2008). The U.S. Department of Veterans Affairs (n.d.) has identified a number of bibliotherapy resources suitable for active-duty personnel and veterans.

Conclusion

ADSMs, National Guard and Reservists, and veterans represent a unique collection of individuals who have made sacrifices to support the mission of the U.S. Armed Forces. Supporting this mission has helped make possible the liberty and freedom we experience today. It is not uncommon for some ADSMs, National Guard and Reservists, and veterans to have experienced a physical injury, witnessed death, experienced combat, participated in multiple deployments, or have other underlying mental health concerns; these events could also make them more susceptible to a substance abuse disorder. Because of the uniqueness of their assigned duties and responsibilities, it is imperative for society and the military to continue to seek ways to decrease the stigma for being treated and for those in need of treatment. Recovering from addiction is a lifelong process and while the rate of addiction for ADSMs, National Guard and Reservists, and veterans is lower than the civilian population, there are levels of substance abuse that warrant attention. Mental health professionals must continue to respond with empathy, compassion, and understanding in a manner that will help past, present, and future military personnel confront any substance abuse issue they may encounter.

References

American Psychiatric Association. (2021). Stigma, prejudice and discrimination against people with mental illness. www.psychiatry.org/patients-families/stigma-and-discrimination

Bachman, J. G., Freedman-Doan, P., O'Malley, P. M., Johnston, L. D., & Segal, D. R. (1999). Changing patterns of drug use among US military recruits before and after enlistment. *American Journal of Public Health*, 89, 672–677. https://doi.org/10.2105/ajph.89.5.672

Bartone, P. T., Wright, K. M. (1990). Grief and group recovery following a military air disaster. *Journal of Trauma Stress*, 3(4), 523–539. https://doi.org/10.1007/BF02039586

Bøg, M., Filges, T., & Jørgensen, A. M. K. (2018). *Deployment of personnel to military operations: Impact on mental health and social functioning.* Campbell Systematic Reviews. https://doi.org/10.4073/csr.2018.6

Briggs, C., & Pehrsson, D. (2008). Use of bibliotherapy in the treatment of grief and loss: A guide to current counseling practices. *Adultspan Journal, 7*(1), 32–42. https://doi.org/10.1002/j.2161-0029.2008.tb00041.x

Byock, I. (1997). *Dying well: Peace and possibilities at end of life.* Riverhead Books.

Congressional Research Service. (2020). *Reserve component personnel issues: Questions and answers.* https://fas.org/sgp/crs/natsec/RL30802.pdf

Currier, J. M., & Holland, J. M. (2012). Examining the role of combat loss among Vietnam War veterans. *Journal of Traumatic Stress, 25*, 102–105. https://doi.org/10.1002/jts.21655

Delaney, E. M., Holloway, K. J., Miletich, D. M., Webb-Murphy, J. A., & Lanouette, N. M. (2017). Screening for complicated grief in a military mental health clinic. *Military Medicine, 182*(9), 1751–1756. https://doi.org/10.7205/MILMED-D-17-00003

Drug Crimes. (2019). *Consequences of drug use in the military.* https://armycourtmartialdefense.info/2019/11/consequences-of-drug-use-in-the-military/

Fink, D. S., Gallaway, M. S., Tamburrino, M. B., Liberzon, I., Chan, P., Cohen, G. H., . . . Galea, S. (2016). Onset of alcohol use disorders and comorbid psychiatric disorders in a military cohort: Are there critical periods for prevention of alcohol use disorders? *Prevention Science, 17*, 347–356.

Gibbons, S. W., Migliore, M., Convoy, S. P., Greiner, S., & DeLeon, P. H. (2014). Military mental health stigma challenges: Policy and practice considerations. *Journal for Nurse Practitioners, 10*(6). Elsevier. https://doi.org/10.1016/j.nurpra.2014.03.021

Hairston, S. (2021). *Grief and substance abuse.* The Recovery Village. www.therecoveryvillage.com/mental-health/grief/substance-abuse/

Hall, L. K. (2011). The importance of understanding military culture. *Social Work in Health Care, 50*, 4–18. https://doi.org/10.1080/00981389.2010.513914

Humphrey, K. M. (2009). *Counseling strategies for grief and loss.* American Counseling Association.

Ilgen, M. A., Bohnert, A. S. B., Ganoczy, D., Blair, M. D., McCarthy, J. F., & Blow, F. C. (2016). Opioid dose and risk of suicide. *Pain, 157*(5).

Kinney, A. R., Eakman, A. M., Lassell, R., & Wood, W. (2019). Equine-assisted interventions for veterans with service-related health conditions: A systematic mapping review. *Military Medical Research, 6*, 1–15, 28. https://doi.org/10.1186/s40779-019-0217-6

Leskin, G. (2015). Preventing substance abuse in military members and their families. *Prevention Tactics, 9*(14). www.ca-cpi.org/publication/preventing—substance-abuse-in-military-members-and-their-families/

Lester, P., & Flake, L. C. E. (U.S. Air Force). (2013). How wartime military service affects children and families. *Future of Children, 23*(2), 121–141. https://doi.org/10.1353/foc.2013.0015

Loebach-Wetherell, J. (2012). Complicated grief therapy as a new treatment approach. *Dialogues in Clinical Neuroscience, 14*(2), 159–166.

Loflin, M., Babson, K., Sottile, J., Norman, S., Gruber, S., & Bonn-Miller, M. (2019). A cross-sectional examination of choice and behavior of veterans with access to free medicinal cannabis. *American Journal of Drug and Alcohol Abuse, 45*(5), 506–513. https://doi.org/10.1080/00952990.2019.1604722

Marchand, W., Andersen, S., Smith, J., Hoopes, K., & Carlson, J. (2021). Equine-assisted activities and therapies for veterans with posttraumatic stress disorder: Current state, challenges and future directions. *Chronic Stress, 5,* 1–11. https://doi.org/10.1177/2470547021991556

Mattiko, M. J., Olmsted, K. L., Brown, J. M., & Bray, R. M. (2011). Alcohol use and negative consequences among active duty military personnel. *Addictive Behaviors, 36*(6), 608–614. https://doi.org/10.1016/j.addbeh.2011.01.023

McGuire, P. (2013). Serving the bereavement needs of veterans and their families. In K. J. Doka & A. S. Tucci (Eds.), *Improving care for veterans facing illness and death.* Hospice Foundation of America.

Meadows, S. O., Engel, C. C., Collins, R. L., Beckman, R. L., Cefalu, M., Hawes-Dawson, J., . . . Williams, K. M. (2018). 2015 Department of Defense health related behaviors survey (HRBS). *Rand Health Quarterly, 8*(2), 5. www.ncbi.nlm.nih.gov/pmc/articles/PMC6183770/

Meyer, E. G. (2015). The importance of understanding military culture. *Academic Psychiatry, 39,* 416–418. https://doi.org/10.1007/s40596-015-0285-1

Miggantz, E. L. (2014). *Stigma of mental health care in the military.* www.med.navy.mil/sites/nmcsd/nccosc/healthProfessionalsV2/reports/Documents/Stigma%20White%20Paper.pdf

Nash, W. P., Silva, C., & Litz, B. (2009). The historic origins of military and veteran mental health stigma and the stress injury model as a means to reduce it. *Psychiatric Annals, 39*(8), 789–794. https://doi.org/10.3928/00485713-20090728-05

Nock, M. K., Deming, C. A., Fullerton, C. S., Gilman, S. E., Goldenberg, M., Kessler, R. C., . . . Schoenbaum, M. (2013). Suicide among soldiers: A review of psychosocial risk and protective factors. *Psychiatry, 76*(2), 97–125. https://doi.org/10.1521/psyc.2013.76.2.97.

O'Connor, M. F., Wellisch, D. K., Stanton, A. L., Eisenberger, N. I., Irwin, M. R., & Lieberman, M. D. (2008). Craving love? Enduring grief activates brain's reward center. *Neuroimage, 42*(2), 969–972. https://doi.org/10.1016/j.neuroimage.2008.04.256

Olenick, M., Flowers, M., & Diaz, V. J. (2015). U.S. veterans and their unique issues: Enhancing health care professional awareness. *Advances in Medical Education and Practice, 6,* 635–639. https://doi.org/10.2147/AMEP.S89479

Pew Research Center (2019). *The changing profile of the U.S. military: Smaller in size, more diverse, more women in leadership.* www.pewresearch.org/fact-tank/2019/09/10/the-changing-profile-of-the-u-s-military/

Robins, L. N. (1993). Vietnam veterans' rapid recovery from heroin addiction: A fluke or normal expectation? *Addiction, 88,* 1041–1054.

Room, R., Babor, T., & Rehm, J. (2005). Alcohol and public health. *Lancet, 365,* 519 530. https://doi.org/10.1016/S0140-6736(05)17870-2

SAMHSA. (2010). *Understanding the military: The institution, the culture, and the people.* Department of Health and Human Services. www.samhsa.gov/sites/default/files/military_white_paper_final.pdf

SAMHSA. (2018). *National survey on drug use and health: Veterans.* Department of Health and Human Services. www.samhsa.gov/data/sites/default/files/reports / rpt23251/6_Veteran_2020_01_14_508.pdf

Shear, M. (2012). Grief and mourning gone awry: Pathway and course of complicated grief. *Dialogues in Clinical Neuroscience, 14*(2), 119–128. https://doi.org/10.31887%2FDCNS.2012.14.2%2Fmshear

Simon, N., Hoeppner, S., Lubin, R., Robinaugh, D., Malgaroli, M., Norman, S., . . . Rauch, S. (2020). Understanding the impact of complicated grief on combat related posttraumatic stress disorder, guilt, suicide, and functional impairment in a clinical trial of post-9/11 service members and veterans. *Depression and Anxiety, 37*(1), 63–72. https://doi.org/10.1002/da.22911

Smith, A. L. (1999). *Coping with death and grief: A strategy for army leadership.* DTIC Technical Reports.

Stahl, S. T., & Schulz, R. (2014). Changes in routine health behaviors following late-life bereavement: A systematic review. *Journal of Behavioral Medicine, 37*(4), 736–755. https://doi.org/10.1007/s10865-013-9524-7

Symington, A. (2012). Grief and horses: Putting the pieces together. *Journal of Creativity in Mental Health, 7*(2), 165–174. https://doi.org/10.1080/15401383.2012.685017

Szoldra, P. (2019). Soldiers are smoking a whole lot more weed in states where it's legalized. *Task & Purpose.* https://taskandpurpose.com/news/army-marijuana-legalization/

Teeters, J. B., Lancaster, C. L., Brown, D. G., & Back, S. E. (2017). Substance use disorders in military veterans: Prevalence and treatment challenges. *Substance Abuse and Rehabilitation, 8*, 69–77. https://doi.org/10.2147/SAR.S116720

U.S. Department of Defense. (2019). 2019 *Demographics profile of the military community.* www.militaryonesource.mil/data-research-and-statistics/military-community-demographics/

United States Department of Veterans Affairs. (n.d.). *Department of Veterans Affairs bibliotherapy resource guide. Mental illness research, education and clinical centers.* Office of Mental Health Services, VA Central Office.

Vespa, J. E. (2020). *Those who served: America's veterans from World War II to the war on terror.* United States Census Bureau. www.census.gov/library/publications/2020/demo/acs-43.html

Waller, M., McGuire, A. C., & Dobson, A. J. (2015). Alcohol use in the military: Associations with health and wellbeing. *Substance Abuse Treatment Prevention Policy, 10*, 27. https://doi.org/10.1186/s13011-015-0023-4

Wertsch, M. E. (1991). *Military brats: Legacies of childhood inside the fortress.* Harmony Books; currently published by Brightwell.

13 Addiction and Grief in Older Adults

Christine Chasek

Substance use among older adults is often a hidden problem. Some researchers have gone so far as to characterize substance misuse among the elderly as an invisible epidemic (Levin & Kruger, 2000) due to stereotyping and ageism. Ageism, as coined by Butler in 1975, refers to the systemic stereotyping of older generations across many areas of life. The social and professional ageism toward older people fosters the belief that the elderly will not be harmed by substance use and that they deserve to be happy with the time they have left (Culberson, 2006). Many people, including health care providers, avoid talking about substance use among older adults for these reasons. These factors contribute to a substance misuse problem that will only grow as the baby boom generation enters older adulthood.

The leading edge of the baby boom cohort, referring to persons born in the United States after World War II between 1946 and 1964, has begun to enter into the older adult population. By 2030, it is expected that there will be 72.1 million adults living in the United States who are over the age of 65, doubling the current number of older adults (Administration on Aging, 2011). The aging of the baby boom generation will greatly influence many segments of society including the economy, social programs, and the health care system. This is especially true for the mental health and substance use health care system, as baby boomers come into older age having used more alcohol and drugs than previous generations (Agency for Healthcare Research and Quality, 2010; Benshoff et al., 2003). In fact, researchers estimate that the number of older adults who will need substance use treatment will increase from 1.7 million to 4.4 million by 2030 (Chhatre et al., 2017). Admissions for substance use treatment for older adults have already increased from 3.4% in 2000 to 7.0% in 2012. This creates a demand for specialty substance use treatment and providers who understand the unique issues and concerns the older population brings into treatment (Kuerbis, 2019; Substance Abuse and Mental Health Services Administration [SAMHSA], 2019). These unique issues include the prevailing cultural norms surrounding substance misuse; risk factors for substance use in older adults; the intersection of grief, loss, and addiction in the older population; and the need for evidence-based strategies and treatment techniques for older adults.

DOI: 10.4324/9781003106906-13

Cultural Norms and Prevalence of Substance Use in Older Adults

The older adult population includes two distinct categories defined by age: (a) adults from ages 50 to 63 (older adults) and (b) adults ages 65 and over (elderly). Examining the substance use trends across both categories of the older adult population reveals some alarming statistics. Overall, alcohol is the most frequently reported substance for persons over the age of 50, followed by misuse of prescription drugs and illicit drugs (Bogunovic, 2012; Kuerbis, 2019). Results from the 2018 National Survey on Drug Use and Health (SAMHSA, 2019) found the following rates of binge alcohol use, prescription drug misuse, and illegal substance use in adults age 50 or older:

- Among adults 50 and older, 47% reported lifetime use of illicit drugs, with 12% reporting use in the past year and 7.6% reporting use in the past month. Marijuana was the most frequently used illicit drug at 43.7% over the lifetime, 9.5% in the past year, and 6.5% in the past month.
- Prescription drug misuse was reported at 34% lifetime use, with 2.3% reporting misuse in the past year but less than 1% reporting misuse in the past month. The 50 and older age group, however, reported the highest rate of misuse out of all age groups.
- Binge alcohol use, defined as drinking more than five drinks for males and four drinks for females in a single session, was reported at 49.2% over the lifetime, with 17.1% reporting binge drinking in the past year and 4.5% in the past month.

These reports are even more disturbing given the lowered national guidelines for alcohol and substance use consumption for older adults. Three nationally recognized organizations, the American Geriatrics Society, the National Institute of Alcohol Abuse and Alcoholism (NIAAA), and the National Institute on Aging have modified and defined the alcohol use limits for older adults based on their decreased ability to metabolize alcohol and other drugs as a result of the aging process. The American Geriatrics Society guidelines indicate that two or more drinks a day within the past 30 days is considered at-risk drinking for older adults. The National Institute on Aging and the NIAAA further define at-risk drinking for those aged 65 and older as more than one drink a day and no more than seven standard drinks per week (American Geriatrics Society, 2003; National Institute on Aging, 2013; National Institute of Alcohol Abuse and Alcoholism, 2013). It is clear from the National Survey on Drug Use and Health (NSDUH) data on binge drinking rates that most older adults are drinking more than the recommended amount of alcohol.

In addition to the concerns related to alcohol use, prescription drug misuse is increasing in the older population. The 2018 NSDUH indicated the older adult population constitutes the largest group of adults misusing prescription medication. This is likely a result of the large number of medications that older adults are prescribed due to health concerns; three-quarters of those aged 50–64 use prescription drugs, while 91% of those aged 80 and older are prescribed medications (Health Policy Institute, 2021). Older adults are often given multiple prescriptions based on legitimate needs; however, this can lead to unintentional misuse and worsening of existing mental health issues. Schepis et al. (2019) found that 25% of patients who misused prescription opioids or benzodiazepines expressed suicidal ideation compared to 2% who did not use them. Older adults are also at risk for opioid use disorder as a result of prescribed pain medications. Huhn et al. (2018) reported that the number of older adults using heroin more than doubled between 2013 and 2015, in part due to the need to switch from more expensive prescription pain medication to cheaper and more readily available illicit substances.

Data from the 2018 NSDUH relating to marijuana highlights an emerging trend of increased cannabis use in the older adult population. This is backed up by Han et al. (2016), who found that past-year cannabis use among adults aged 50 increased significantly from 2006 to 2013, with a 57.8% increase for adults aged 50–64 and a 250% increase for those aged 65 and older. This dramatic increase could be due to the fact that medical marijuana is more often prescribed to older adults. In another study conducted by Han and Palamar (2018), close to 25% of cannabis users aged 65 and older reported that a doctor had recommended using marijuana to them in the past year. While there has been emerging research to suggest that medical marijuana may relieve some health symptoms, the potential benefits must be weighed against the risks, especially for older adults who have substance use problems or take other prescribed medications (Abuhasira et al., 2019). The physiological effects of cannabis may lead to poorer outcomes for older adults who are at increased risk of cardiovascular disease, poorer cognitive functioning, and increased risk of falls and chronic health conditions.

Risk Factors for Substance Misuse in Older Adults

There are several risk factors associated with substance misuse among older adults. Due to the aging process, the brain changes in a variety of ways that are developmentally determined. Older adults metabolize substances more slowly and their brains are more sensitive to the effects of drugs (Benshoff et al., 2003; Colliver et al., 2006). Due to the age-related changes in the neurotransmitter system that mediate the effects of substances in the brain, even moderate amounts of substance use can present greater risks for older adults (Benyon, 2009; Brown University, 2008; Colliver et al., 2006; Wu & Blazer, 2011).

Physical changes in the aging body also play a large role in the risk factors of substance misuse and abuse in older adults. Changes in body composition and decreased liver and digestive functions result in more damage to the central nervous system and vital organs when older adults misuse alcohol (Barry & Blow, 2016; Caputo et al., 2012; Kuerbis, 2019). Decreased kidney functioning and reductions in body mass and water content increase the amount of drug serum in older adults who misuse prescription and illicit drugs. This can cause significant effects from even a small amount of drug use in older adults (Benyon, 2009; Kuerbis, 2019; Wang & Andrade, 2013), as substances remain in the body for longer amounts of time at higher concentration levels. From these physiological effects, it is easy to see why guidelines for alcohol and substance use are much lower for older adults and must be taken into consideration when working with an older adult population.

In addition to the effects of substances on the aging body, it is also important to note the risk factors associated with mental health concerns and substance use in older adults. Depressive disorders are more common among the elderly than in younger people, and substance use often co-occurs with depression (Kuerbis, 2019; Morin et al., 2013; Schladitz et al., 2021; Wang & Andrade, 2013). This sets up a vicious cycle of substance misuse exacerbating mental health symptoms, which leads to coping with more substance use (Carr, 2020). Among adults older than 65, those with alcohol use disorders are approximately three times more likely to exhibit a major depressive disorder than those without an alcohol use disorder (Simoni-Wastila & Yang, 2006). Wilson et al. (2014) found that symptoms of depression were the leading factors in identifying older adults as risky and hazardous drinkers; therefore, it is imperative that mental health symptoms are addressed and understood when treating older adults.

Intersection of Grief, Addiction, and Older Adults

Depression is a commonly reported mental health issue in later life (Buchtemann et al., 2012; Maust et al., 2015; Salmon & Forester, 2012), and studies consistently connect depression with use of substances (Choi et al., 2015; Chorlton & Smith, 2016; Green et al., 2015; Kuerbis, 2019; Satre, 2015; Schonfeld et al., 2010; Simoni-Wastila & Yang, 2006; Wang & Andrade, 2013). A common risk factor that connects substance misuse and depression among older adults is grief. Furthermore, previous research has established that grief and loss are connected to substance use disorders (Beechem et al., 1996; Blankfield, 1982; Chambers & Wallingford, 2017; Furr et al., 2015; Parisi et al., 2019). Grief can be found at all stages of substance use: prior to substance use, during initiation of misuse, throughout substance abuse, and during recovery. There are special considerations, however, when it comes to older adults, grief, and substance use.

Life transitions that are connected to grief and loss are common in the older adult population. Bereavement due to death of a partner, significant other, or friends, loneliness, poor health, caring for ill loved ones, and loss of position in society all impact older adults and can influence substance misuse, contributing to depression symptoms (Kuerbis, 2019). Loneliness is a significant risk factor for depression (Schladitz et al., 2021) and is often triggered by loss, especially emotionally significant losses, such as the loss of loved ones or loss of health. These losses are frequent for older adults and have many implications for their mental well-being. When an older person loses a loved one, they also lose social relationships, social structure, and often income. As these losses culminate, the impacts can be extremely distressing. In some older adults, grief can increase the risk of and contribute to depression symptoms (Kuerbis, 2019) and substance misuse, especially alcohol and tobacco use. Grieving older adults may misuse substances as a way of coping with their loss. If this is their main method of coping, it can be a barrier to entering treatment, as they likely will not want to quit. Masferrer et al. (2017) found that the presence of complicated grief, defined as intense grief experience in either time or degree, contributed to substance use disorder vulnerability in those who were experiencing complicated grief.

There are other losses that are unique to older adults outside of losing significant others and mortality issues. Retirement, described as a transition process rather than an event, is often experienced as an ongoing loss and has a significant impact on substance misuse as found by Kuerbis and Sacco (2012). Retirement is not a one-time event; it is on ongoing process with a long adjustment phase that has implications for life satisfaction. Those who were very satisfied with work prior to retirement experience significant loss when retiring, leading to an increased risk of substance use to cope with the loss. Conversely those who were very stressed and using substances to cope while working carried that stress and substance use over into retirement. Finally, involuntary retirement also increases the likelihood of older adults misusing substances into retirement as they are often dissatisfied with their new life status and feel pushed out of the workforce (Kuerbis & Sacco, 2012).

Grief and loss are not only risk factors for substance misuse; they are also a result of substance misuse. Bergstrom (2017) conducted a study with people aged 55–69 who struggled with ongoing long-term alcohol problems. Participants shared how they conceptualized the past, present, and future in an attempt to understand how substance use had impacted their lives. Grief, loss, and loneliness were highlighted as themes in the study. Participants shared they had a great deal of resentment over the losses their drinking caused, such as loss of jobs, loss of relationships, and loss of enjoyable recreation. Gratitude for the past, however, also emerged as a theme and as a resource for possible future recovery. The authors concluded that this hope can be strengthened by increasing social support and decreasing isolation to improve the odds of recovery.

Evidence-Based Strategies and Techniques for Older Adults

According to SAMHSA (2020) and the Center for Substance Abuse Treatment (2005), brief motivational approaches, cognitive behavioral therapy approaches, and specialized care options such group-based approaches, individual counseling, medical and psychiatric approaches, family therapy, case management, and community-based services are recommended for older adults. The challenge, however, is getting the older adult into substance use treatment. Due to ageism, lack of resources, lack of attention from the field, misdiagnosis, and the belief that older individuals will "age out of" substance use (Benshoff et al., 2003; Quinn & Mowbray, 2018), very few older adults make it into treatment services and far fewer acknowledge the need for treatment. Bartels et al. (2004), however, found that older adults were more open to substance use treatment and mental health care when it was included as part of their primary care. If screening for substance misuse can be integrated into primary care, a larger portion of the older adult population will have access to care as substance use treatment.

For the older adult population, an integrated care model of brief intervention followed by intervention strategies using motivational interviewing has been recommended by several researchers and has been adopted by the SAMHSA as an evidence-based practice (Chang et al., 2015; Chhatre et al., 2017; Mowbray & Quinn, 2016; Quinn & Mowbray, 2018; SAMHSA, 2020; Schonfeld et al., 2010). When combined with brief motivational intervention approaches, services that takes place in primary care settings offer the best evidence for effective treatment among substance using older adults (Quinn & Mowbray, 2018). Furthermore, Quinn and Mowbray (2018) found that physicians who delivered brief motivational-enhancement interventions were the most effective for reducing substance use among the baby boomer population. Brief interventions are also a good fit for other settings that focus on older adult care, such as social service agencies, outpatient clinics, and other emergency room settings. They are cost-effective, low intensity, and efficient.

For older adults who need further services beyond screening and brief intervention, cognitive behavioral–based treatments are recommended (Chhatre et al., 2017; Quinn & Mowbray, 2018; SAMHSA, 2020). Group therapy using cognitive behavioral techniques is also very effective for older adults (CSAT, 2005; Quinn & Mowbray, 2018; SAMHSA, 2020; Schonfeld et al., 2010). Experts recommend that these services take into account the issues related to older adults including the unique physical, psychological, social, and vocational changes that occur in later life. They should focus on the developmental needs of older adults including grief, loss, loneliness, and medical issues (Bogunovic, 2012; Quinn & Mowbray, 2018; SAMHSA, 2020). Treatment plans must include age-specific goals and objectives and be tailored to the older adults' level of cognitive functioning. The intervention strategies should be nonconfrontational and supportive. Research with older adults has found they prefer programs that are led by warm, caring, nonconfrontational therapists and those that include their family and friends in an individualized manner (Holland et al., 2016; Kuerbis, 2019; SAMHSA, 2020).

Beyond formalized treatment, participation in self-help and support groups such as Alcoholics Anonymous or Smart Recovery can be very beneficial for older adults, especially taking into consideration the grief, loss, and loneliness that often accompany substance misuse. Age-matched support groups can provide essential peer bonding that help alleviate social isolation and loneliness and other triggers for relapse (Bogunovic, 2012). Just as loneliness, grief, loss, and other developmental challenges that come with aging can contribute to substance misuse, connection, meaningful relationships, and purpose can be protective factors against substance abuse and relapse.

Counselors, physicians, and other behavioral health providers can engage older adults in a variety of ways to address substance misuse concerns. It is important to remember to take into account the unique needs of older adults ensuring that services are tailored to their needs and developmental concerns. Combating ageism and providing evidence-based services will go a long way to ensure the older years can be good years.

References

Abuhasira, R., Ron, A., Sikorin, I., & Noack, V. (2019). Medical cannabis for older patients: Treatment protocol and initial results. *Journal of Clinical Medicine, 8*(11), 1819. https://doi.org/10.3390/jcm8111819

Administration on Aging. (2011). *A profile of older Americans: 2011*. U.S. Department of Health and Human Services.

Agency for Healthcare Research and Quality. (2010). *Hospitalizations for medication and illicit drug-related conditions on the rise among Americans ages 45 and older*. AHRQ.

American Geriatrics Society. (2003). *Clinical guidelines for alcohol use disorder in older adults*. www.americangeriatrics.org/products/positionpapers/alcohol.shtml

Barry, K. L., & Blow, F. C. (2016). Drinking over the lifespan: Focus on older adults. *Alcohol Research & Health, 38*(4), 115–120.

Bartels, S. J., Coakley, E. H., Zubritsky, C., Ware, J. H., Miles, K. M., Arean, P. A., & Levkoff, S. E. (2004). Improving access to geriatric mental health services: A randomized trial comparing treatment engagement with integrated versus enhanced referral care for depression anxiety, and at-risk alcohol use. *American Journal of Psychiatry, 161*(8), 1455–1462.

Benshoff, J. J., Harrawood, L. K., & Koch, D. (2003). Substance abuse and the elderly: Unique issues and concerns. *Journal of Rehabilitation, 69*(2), 43–48.

Benyon, C. (2009). Drug use and ageing: Older people do take drugs. *Age and Ageing, 38*, 8–10.

Bergstrom, M. (2017). "I could've had a better life": Reflective life reviews told by late-middle-aged and older women and men with ongoing long-term alcohol problems. *Nordic Studies on Alcohol and Drugs, 34*(1), 6–17. https://doi.org/10.1177/1455072516682436

Blankfield, A. (1982). Grief and alcohol. *American Journal of Drug and Alcohol Abuse, 9*(4), 435–446.

Bogunovic, O. (2012, August). Substance abuse in aging and elderly adults. *Psychiatric Times*, 39–40.

Brown University. (2008, April). Substance use and the aging brain: Screening, diagnosis, and treatment. *Brown University Geriatric Psychopharmacology Update, 12*(4), 1–6.

Buchtemann, D., Luppa, M., Bramesfeld, A., & Riedel-Heller, S. (2012). Incidence of late-life depression: A systematic review. *Journal of Affective Disorders, 142*(1–3), 172–179.

Butler, R. (1975). *Why survive? Being old in America*. Harper & Row.

Caputo, F., Vignoli, T., Leggio, L., Addolorato, G., Zoli, G., & Bernardi, M. (2012). Alcohol use disorders in the elderly: A brief overview from epidemiology to treatment options. *Experimental Gerontology*, *47*, 411–416.

Carr, D. (2020). Mental health of older widows and widowers: Which coping strategies are most protective? *Aging & Mental Health*, *24*(2), 291–299.

Center for Substance Abuse Treatment. (2005). *Substance abuse relapse prevention: A group treatment approach for older adults*. Substance Abuse and Mental Health Services Administration.

Chambers, A. R., & Wallingford, S. C. (2017). On mourning and recovery: Integrating stages of grief and change toward a neuroscience-based model of attachment adaptation in addiction treatment. *Psychodynamic Psychiatry*, *45*(4), 451–474. https://doi.org.unk.idm.oclc.org/10.1521/pdps.2017.45.4.451

Chang, Y., Compton, P., Almeter, P., & Fox, C. H. (2015). The effect of motivational interviewing on prescription opioid adherence among older adults with chronic pain. *Perspectives in Psychiatric Care*, *51*, 211–291. https://doi.org/10.1111/ppc.12082

Chhatre, S., Cook, R., Maliik, E., & Jayadevappa, R. (2017). Trends in substance use admission among older adults. *BMC Health Services Research*, *17*, 1–8. https://doi.org/10.1186/s12913-017-2538-z

Choi, N. G., DiNitto, D. M., & Marti, C. N. (2015). Alcohol and other substance use, mental health treatment use, and perceived unmet treatment need: Comparison between baby boomers and older adults. *American Journal on Addictions*, *24*(4), 299–307.

Chorlton, E., & Smith, I. C. (2016). Understanding how people with mental health difficulties experience substance use. *Substance Use and Misuse*, *51*(3), 318–329.

Colliver, J. D., Compton, W. M., Gfroerer, J. C., & Condon, T. (2006). Projecting drug use among aging baby boomers in 2020. *Annals of Epidemiology*, *16*(4), 257–265.

Culberson, J. (2006). Alcohol use in the elderly: Beyond the CAGE. *Geriatrics*, *61*(10), 23–27.

Furr, S., Johnson, W. D., & Goodall, C. S. (2015). Grief and recovery: The prevalence of grief and loss in substance abuse treatment. *Journal of Addictions & Offender Counseling*, *36*, 43–56. https://doi.org/10.1002/j.2161-1874.2015.00034.x

Green, C. A., Yarborough, M. T., Polen, M. R., Janoff, S. L., & Yarborough, B. J. H. (2015). Dual recovery among people with serious mental illnesses and substance use problems: A qualitative analysis. *Journal of Dual Diagnosis*, *11*(1), 33–41.

Han, B. H., & Palamar, J. J. (2018). Marijuana use by middle-aged and older adults in the United States, 2015–2016. *Drug and Alcohol Dependence*, *191*, 374–381. www.ncbi.nlm.nih.gov/pubmed/30197051

Han, B. H., Sherman, S., Mauro, P. M., Martins, S. S., Rotenberg, J., & Palamar, J. J. (2016). Demographic trends among older cannabis users in the United States, 2006–13. *Addiction*, *112*, 516–525.

Health Policy Institute. (2021). *Prescription drugs*. Georgetown University. https://hpi.georgetown.edu/rxdrugs/#

Holland, J. M., Rozalski, V., Beckman, L., Rakhkovskaya, L. M., Klingspon, K. L., Donohue, B., . . . Gallagher-Thompson, D. (2016). Treatment preference of older adults with substance use problems. *Clinical Gerontologist*, *39*(1), 15–24.

Huhn, A. S., Strain, E. C., Tompkins, D. A., & Dunn, K. E. (2018). A hidden aspect of the U.S. opioid crisis: Rise in first-time treatment admissions for older adults with opioid use disorder. *Drug and Alcohol Dependence, 193*, 142–147. https://doi.org/10.1016/j.drugalcdep.2018

Kuerbis, A. (2019). Substance use among older adults: An update on prevalence, etiology, assessment, and intervention. *Gerontology, 66*, 249–258. https://doi.org/10.1159/000504363

Kuerbis, A., & Sacco, P. (2012). The impact of retirement on the drinking patterns of older adults: A review. *Addictive Behaviors, 37*, 587–595. https://doi.org/10.1016/j.addbeh.2012.01.022

Levin, S. M., & Kruger, J. (Eds.). (2000). *Substance abuse among older adults: A guide for social service providers*. Substance Abuse and Mental Health Services Administration.

Masferrer, L., Garre-Olmo, J., & Caparrós, B. (2017). Is complicated grief a risk factor for substance use? A comparison of substance-users and normative grievers. *Addiction Research and Theory, 25*(5), 361–367. https://doi.org/10.1080/16066359.2017.1285912

Maust, D., Kales, H., & Blow, F. C. (2015). National trends in antidepressant use among Baby Boomers: 1995–2010. *American Journal of Geriatric Psychiatry, 23*(3), S177–S178.

Morin, J., Wiktorsson, S., Marlow, T., Olesen, P. J., Skoog, I., & Waern, M. (2013). Alcohol use disorder in elderly suicide attempters: A comparison study. *American Journal of Geriatric Psychiatry, 21*(2), 196–203. https://doi.org/10.1016/j.jagp.2012.10.020

Mowbray, O., & Quinn, A. (2016). A scoping review of treatment for older adults with substance use problems. *Research on Social Work Practice, 26*(1), 74–87.

National Institute on Aging. (2013). *Facts about aging and alcohol*. www.dietaryguidelines.gov/sites/default/files/2020-12/Dietary_Guidelines_for_Americans_2020-2025.pdf

National Institute on Alcohol Abuse and Alcoholism. (2013). *Drinking guidelines for older adults*. www.niaaa.nih.gov/alcohol-health/special-populations-co-occurring-disorders/older-adults

Parisi, A., Sharma, A., Howard, M. O., & Wilson, A. B. (2019). The relationship between substance misuse and complicated grief: A systematic review. *Journal of Substance Abuse Treatment, 103*, 43–57. https://doi.org.unk.idm.oclc.org/10.1016/j.jsat.2019.05.012

Quinn, A., & Mowbray, O. (2018). Effective treatments for older adult baby boomers with alcohol-use disorders: A literature review. *Journal of Social Work Practice in the Addictions, 18*, 389–410. https://doi.org/10.1080/1533256X.2018.1516987

Salmon, J. M., & Forester, B. (2012). Substance use and co-occurring psychiatric disorders in older adults: A clinical case and review of the relevant literature. *Journal of Dual Diagnosis, 8*(1), 74–84.

Satre, D. D. (2015). Alcohol drug use problems among older adults. *Clinical Psychology: Science and Practice, 22*(3), 238–254.

Schepis, T. S., Simoni-Wastila, L., & McCabe, S. E. (2019). Prescription opioid and benzodiazepine misuse is associated with suicidal ideation in older adults. *International Journal of Geriatric Psychiatry, 34*(1), 122–129. https://doi.org/10.1002/gps.4999

Schladitz, K., Lobner, M., Stein, J., Weyerer, S., Werle, J., Wagner, M., . . . Riedel-Heller, G. (2021). Grief and loss in old age: Exploration of the association between grief and depression. *Journal of Affective Disorders, 283*, 285–292.

Schonfeld, L., King-Kallimanis, B. L., Duchene, D. M., Ethridge, R. L., Herrera, J. R., Barry, K. L., & Lynn, N. (2010). Screening and brief intervention for substance misuse among older adults: The Florida BRITE project. *American Journal of Public Health, 100*(1), 108–114.

Simoni-Wastila, L., & Yang, H. K. (2006). Psychoactive drug abuse in older adults. *American Journal of Geriatric Pharmacotherapy, 4*(4), 380–394.

Substance Abuse and Mental Health Services Administration. (2019). *Results from the 2018 national survey on drug use and health: Detailed tables.* Center for Behavioral Health Statistics and Quality, Substance Abuse and Mental Health Services Administration. www.samhsa.gov/data/report/2019-nsduh-detailed-tables

Substance Abuse and Mental Health Services Administration. (2020). *Treating substance use disorder in older adults.* Treatment Improvement Protocol (TIP) Series No. 26, SAMHSA Publication No. PEP20-02-01-011. Substance Abuse and Mental Health Services Administration.

Wang, Y., & Andrade, L. H. (2013). Epidemiology of alcohol and drug use in the elderly. *Psychiatry, 26,* 343–438.

Wilson, S. R., Knowles, S., Huang, Q., & Fink, A. (2014). The prevalence of harmful and hazardous alcohol consumption in older U.S. adults: Data from the 2005–2008 national health and nutrition examination survey. *Journal of General International Medicine, 29*(2), 312–319. https://doi.org/10.1007/s11606-013-2577-z

Wu, L., & Blazer, D. G. (2011). Illicit and nonmedical drug use among older adults: A review. *Journal of Aging and Health, 23*(3), 481–504. https://doi.org/10.1177/08

14 Grieving Traumatic Experiences and Addiction

An Adolescent Perspective

Regina R. Moro

Adolescence is a developmental period marked by numerous changes for individuals. While the majority of adolescents move through this period without major life challenges, some are not as fortunate. For those who experience trauma in early childhood or experience repetitive traumatic events into their teenage years, they are at an increased risk for using substances and developing addiction. This chapter explores the prevalence of substance use among adolescents and the etiology of addiction, including the influence of trauma and how to approach work with this population from a grief perspective.

Prevalence of Substance Use and Disorders Among Adolescents

Despite positive downward trends over the past two decades, substance use by adolescents and young adults continues to be prevalent in our society. According to the 2019 National Survey on Drug Use and Health (NSDUH) conducted by the Substance Abuse and Mental Health Services Administration (SAMHSA, 2020a) roughly 1 in 10 youths ages 12–17 used alcohol in the past month, with about half of these uses being binge drinking. Additionally, 2.2 million youths aged 12–17 used illicit drugs in the past month, according to the report. While any use of a mood-altering substance by a minor is concerning, this report highlights a trend in which past-month alcohol use and past-month binge use has decreased over a 17-year period. These downward trends are further identified for other substances such as cigarettes, marijuana, and cocaine, although there were no reported changes in hallucinogen use by this age group.

The NSDUH (SAMHSA, 2020a) report highlighted that there is continued use of substances by youth in our country and given the normative process for adolescents to experiment with substances (Hogue et al., 2018) this trend makes sense. However, this experimentation can escalate to problematic use over time. Among youth ages 12–17, approximately 1.1 million report a past-year substance use disorder (alcohol or illicit drugs; SAMHSA, 2020b).

DOI: 10.4324/9781003106906-14

The following are the latest estimated prevalence rates of use disorders reported in the past year by the respective substance for the adolescent population:

- 414,000, alcohol use disorder
- 894,000, illicit drug use disorder
- 699,000, marijuana use disorder
- 5,000, cocaine use disorder
- 19,000, methamphetamine use disorder
- 66,000, prescription stimulant use disorder
- 96,000, prescription tranquilizer or sedative use disorder
- 87,000, prescription pain reliever use disorder. (SAMHSA, 2020b)

Tarter (2002) noted that it is important to consider how survey data results like those above likely do not include a full picture of the true prevalence rates. This is due to the highest risk youth who are more likely to have dropped out of school, be absent on data collection days perhaps because they are receiving treatment services, or in the custody of the juvenile justice system. While the accuracy of these numbers can be debated, it is clear that substance use continues to effect adolescents in our society.

Once an adolescent is identified as needing services, it is crucial to get them into appropriate treatment. This, however, can be a challenge. Despite approximately 1.1 million adolescents meeting the criteria for a substance use disorder (SUD) in 2019, only 93,000 (8.3%) reported receiving any substance use treatment in the past year (SAMHSA, 2020b). This low number is perhaps due to a high percentage (98.5%) of adolescents who perceive they do not need treatment despite being diagnosed with a past-year SUD (SAMHSA, 2020b). While this perception of not needing treatment may account for some of those folks not receiving treatment, another issue is treatment availability. The Center for Substance Abuse Treatment recommends that effective treatment for adolescent SUDs requires separation of adolescent and adult services (Knudsen, 2009). However, a little more than one quarter (3,537) of addiction treatment facilities in the United States offer specific adolescent programs (Alinsky et al., 2020). For counselors working in the addiction treatment arena, it is important to advocate for the separation of services. For counselors who are working in other areas of clinical practice, it is important to recognize these adolescents will likely seek assistance through other means if they are not able to get into treatment facilities. This chapter will lay the groundwork for counselors who find themselves working with one adolescents who has a history of risky use of substances.

Development of Addiction

There are many different factors that contribute to an individual's development of addiction. According to Tarter (2002), these factors can be classified as a configuration of biological, behavioral characteristics, and environment characteristics—more specifically, an individual's biochemistry, physiology, psychopathology, behavior, family, peers, and environment. An individual's unique configuration of characteristics determines their personal risk (Tarter, 2002). One well-known factor leading to addiction is the experience of trauma during childhood.

Childhood Trauma

The National Child Traumatic Stress Network (NCTSN) defines trauma as occurring "when a child feels intensely threatened by an event he or she is involved in or witnesses" (NCTSN, n.d., para. 1). Types of trauma include bullying, natural disaster exposure, witnessing intimate partner violence, medical trauma, physical abuse, sexual abuse, terrorism and violence, and many other forms. In the past couple of decades, more attention has been given to traumatic experiences of youth, and more specifically, what are now known as adverse childhood experiences. The original Adverse Childhood Experiences (ACE) study conducted by Felitti and colleagues (1998) examined youths' adverse experiences categorized as either abuse/neglect (psychological, physical, or sexual) or as household dysfunction (substance abuse/mental illness within the household, mother/stepmother treated violently, and criminal behavior in the household). Further research expanded the categories of ACEs to also include losing a parent/guardian to abandonment/divorce and/or having a family member in jail (Merrick et al., 2018). These authors found that when children do experience these events in childhood, they go on to develop health risk behaviors and diseases as adults (e.g., SUDs, depression, obesity, cancer, lung disease), and the more they experience, the greater their chances for risk and disease later on. In addition, children who are exposed to a greater number of traumatic events, or over a span of time, are at risk for developing complex trauma.

Complex Trauma

The term *complex trauma* is used to refer to severe traumatic events as well as the resulting symptoms experienced following exposure to traumatic events (Kliethermes et al., 2014). A complex traumatic event is one that "is repetitive and occurs over an extended period of time, undermines primary caregiving relationships, and occurs at sensitive times with regard to brain development" (Kliethermes et al., 2014, p. 340). The pattern of symptoms that emerge following a complex traumatic event(s) includes problems with attachment and relationship patterns, emotional and behavioral dysregulation, cognitive and attention deficits, and physical health concerns (Cohen et al., 2012; Kliethermes et al., 2014). One key feature of complex trauma is dissociation, which occurs when an individual is faced with reminders of the trauma and disconnects from physical and psychological awareness (Racco & Vis, 2015). Dissociation is a protective state the individual has adapted to protect themselves (Racco & Vis, 2015).

Prevalence of Childhood Trauma

Accurate prevalence rates of childhood trauma are difficult to estimate due to underreporting, however, it is clear that this is a significant problem in our society (Garner et al., 2014). Continued research from the original ACE study has found that approximately 61% of adults surveyed report experiencing at least one type of ACE as a child, and a little more than 16% report experiencing four or more ACEs (Centers for Disease Control and Prevention, 2020).

As mentioned, prevalence rates are affected by underreporting, which can also impact a counselor's assessment process. Clients who have experienced trauma may not be forthcoming with information due to their own avoidance of trauma stimuli; that is, they avoid talking about the experience as a protective measure for themselves, and/or they also may not trust the counselor due to historical attachment injuries (Cohen et al., 2012). Counselors need to be mindful and sensitive to these issues when working with adolescents.

Connecting Trauma and Addiction

Exposure to trauma in childhood increases the likelihood that individuals will go on to develop any number of concerning behaviors in adolescence (Dube et al., 2006), such as risky substance use and addiction. There are two main theories that provide a framework for understanding how trauma influences an individual's risk for developing an addiction. The first theory is the self-medicating hypothesis, and the second is a neurobiological perspective (Rothman et al., 2010). Each of these theories assists counselors with understanding possible mechanisms that led to their clients' struggle with substances.

Self-Medicating Hypothesis

Khantzian (1997) explained that some adolescents use substances as a way to alleviate their own internal distress. This author suggested individuals with SUDs struggle with self-regulating their emotions, and using substances helped to reduce the painful affects when these individuals experience extreme emotions. The research on the self-medicating hypothesis continues to be inconclusive (Rothman et al., 2010); however, individuals reported that relieving their psychological distress is an important reason for their use (Khantzian, 1997). Also relevant is that this internal drive to reduce psychological discomfort is associated with higher abuse risk, compared to adolescents who use due to external reasons (e.g., peer pressure), which is associated with more experimental use (Newcomb & Bentler, 1989).

Neurobiological Development

The neurobiological explanation suggests childhood trauma affects neurodevelopment (Rothman et al., 2010). According to Dube et al. (2006), the impact of trauma on neurodevelopment can lead to the initiation of using mood-altering substances. For example, children exposed to a traumatic event (or events) show higher levels of stress hormones (i.e., cortisol and norepinephrine), which can lead to physiological changes, such as increased resting heart rates. This theoretical perspective highlights that experiencing these physiological changes may then disrupt an individual's own ability to cope with these feelings. That is, the trauma leads to physical changes in one's body that reduce their own ability to regulate their emotions and behaviors (Dube et al., 2006). This inability to cope with emotional/behavioral regulation then leads individuals to seek out substances to assist with this process. While this sounds similar to the self-medicating hypothesis, this theory suggests that it is ultimately due to the problems with neurodevelopment and physiological experiences that leads to the use of substances, not solely for alleviating distressing emotions.

Treatment Considerations

There is positive news related to childhood trauma and the resulting SUDs despite the negative picture that has been painted thus far. Research shows that adolescents who enter treatment with a history of severe childhood maltreatment have greater reductions in substance use compared to their peers who had low levels or no maltreatment in childhood (Garner et al., 2014). In addition, research has explored how an adolescent's reasons for substance use are connected to treatment outcomes. Dow and Kelly (2013) explored how use, characterized as either positive reinforcement (i.e., "using to enhance a positive state"; p. 6) or negative reinforcement (e.g., school problems, stress/personal problems, family problems) was predictive of treatment outcome. These authors found that adolescents who reported use of the negative reinforcement category were more likely to show a positive treatment response compared to the positive reinforcement adolescents. This is helpful to highlight that although these folks might be using substances to self-medicate their experience of distress, they are an important population that can benefit from treatment access.

There are many reasons adolescents may not seek treatment, such as not believing they need help, not knowing where to go for help, or possibly being concerned about the stigma of mental health and substance use (NCTSN, 2008a). Once teenagers are in front of the counselor, it is crucial to be intentional about engaging them in the process. As anyone who has worked with adolescents is aware, this can be a challenge. The NCTSN (2008a) recommended that establishing rapport, setting clear boundaries, and allowing for autonomy are important for engagement. In addition, it is recommended to explore what the adolescent wants to discuss to allow for meaningful conversations. It is crucial that counselors are intentional with this engagement process to support the rest of the work to come.

The National Child Traumatic Stress Network (2008b) recommended several treatments that address both traumatic stress and substance use issues in an integrated fashion, as well as each as the primary focus. Table 14.1 outlines the recommended treatments.

The list below provides a comprehensive overview of available treatment models for clinicians to use that are grounded in research. The focus of the rest of this chapter involves how counselors can attend to adolescent trauma histories and/or the recovery process from a grief perspective.

Grieving the Traumatic Event(s)

With the vast majority of adolescents who seek SUD treatment having exposure to one or more traumatic events in childhood, it is crucial that counselors

Table 14.1 Recommended Treatments for Traumatic Stress and/or Substance Use Disorders for Adolescents

Focus of Treatment Model	Treatment Model Name	Author(s)
Integrated	Seeking Safety	Najavits (2001) Najavits et al. (2006)
	Risk Reduction Through Family Therapy	Danielson (2006)
	Trauma Systems Therapy for Substance Abuse in Adolescents	Saxe et al. (2006)
Trauma-Focused	Trauma-Focused Cognitive Behavioral Therapy (TF-CBT)	Cohen et al. (2000)
	Cognitive Behavioral Intervention for Trauma in Schools (CBITS)	Stein et al. (2003)
	Trauma Systems Therapy (TST)	Saxe et al. (2005)
Substance-Focused	Cognitive Behavioral Therapy (CBT)	Beck (1993)
	Motivational Interviewing	Miller and Rollnick (1991)
	Motivational Enhancement Therapy and Cognitive Behavioral Therapy for Cannabis Users	Sampl and Kadden (2001)
	Multidimensional Family Therapy (MDFT)	Liddle et al. (2001)
	Brief Strategic Family Therapy for Adolescent Drug Abuse	Robbins et al. (2009)
	Multisystemic Therapy	Henggeler and Borduin (1990)
	Adolescent Community Reinforcement Approach (ARCA)	Godley et al. (2001)

Note: Adapted from National Child Traumatic Stress Network (2008b).

do not ignore this in the treatment process. Counselors can work with clients to grieve the trauma(s) in intentional ways once a collaborative relationship has been established where the clients feel safety and autonomy. It is important that counselors "move at the speed of trust" with their clients, particularly as it relates to exploring trauma (Marcano as cited in Brown, 2017, p. 42). A crucial step in acting from a trauma-informed lens is offering an invitation to the client, not a mandate, to collaborate in the treatment process (SAMHSA, 2014). In addition, counselors need to understand that this is an ongoing process, and the client's trust in the counselor and their ability to engage in the process may change from session to session, or even within one session. Patience and compassion are of the utmost importance for the counselor to embody and convey.

When the client and counselor agree that exploring the trauma history is appropriate, counselors need to identify what the client may need to grieve specifically. This may be personal relationships that were lost or harmed because of trauma, it might be experiences they missed out on, feelings/thoughts they did not get to experience because of the trauma, and any number of other things. Counselors can consider using the following prompts to explore grief foci:

- Counselor: I invite you to think back to that time in your life.
- Who was not around you at that time that you needed/wanted?
- What life events were impacted by your experiences?
- What feelings/thoughts were common for you at that time?
- What feelings/thoughts were you not experiencing at that time?

Counselors may also find it can be helpful to externalize the traumatic event(s), which is a common practice in Narrative Therapy (White & Epston, 1990). For example, clients can be invited to give the trauma(s) a name so the trauma can be referenced by both the client and the counselor. Examples of questions using the externalizing process follow:

- What do you want to say to [name of trauma(s)]?
- If you could tell [name of trauma(s)] anything, what would that be?
- Please describe events you think you missed out on in your life because of [name of trauma(s)]?
- How do you think [name of trauma(s)] is still impacting you today?
- How can we help [name of trauma(s)] stop interfering in your life?

Another useful counseling strategy is the Miracle Question from Solution-Focused Brief Therapy (De Jong & Berg, 2013). The name of this technique implies that it is one singular question; however, this should be thought of more as an intervention. The counselor can prompt the client to think creatively and pretend there is a magical way they are able to go back in time. The counselor can invite the client to consider what if the trauma(s) did not happen to them, and then to explore how they would know it did not happen. This will give the counselor insight into what the client perceives as the ideal life and therefore what was missing from their own life. It is important for counselors to truly spend time here, not rushing to get to an answer, and being sensitive to the fact that the trauma did happen. The counselor's intention is not to minimize or distort the experience but to explore what the client needs to grieve. Below is an example of how a counselor could implement this skill in a session with an adolescent client:

> Pat is a counselor who has been working with Jasmine for four sessions. Jasmine is a 17-year-old cisgender female who has presented to counseling due to difficulty with depression. Throughout their time together, Pat has learned that Jasmine is the youngest of four children, all raised by a single parent due to their mother's incarceration approximately eight years ago. Jasmine experienced physical abuse by her mother from the age of four until eight. Her mother was physically abusive to all four children, and one of her older brothers (age 13) spoke to his school counselor about the abuse, which ultimately led to a child protective investigation and the incarceration of her mother. Jasmine has been in and out of counseling services since the discovery of the abuse. She has displayed risky behaviors such as being caught with alcohol and a vape pen on school property and engaging in sexual behavior with numerous partners since the age of 13. She demonstrates understandable trust issues with adults, and Pat has been mindful of this throughout their work together. Pat is interested in using the miracle question in today's session in order to explore what Jasmine might feel the need to grieve from her childhood.

PAT (COUNSELOR): Thank you for being here today, Jasmine. I appreciate your continued dedication to showing up and working with me in this process. How would you like to spend our time today?

JASMINE (CLIENT): Umm, I don't know.

PAT: Well, in that case, I was wondering if we could do a sort of creative thinking exercise today. How would that be?

JASMINE: Umm, I guess so. You know I'm not very creative though.

PAT: You're wondering if you will be able to do this.

JASMINE: Yeah.

PAT: Well, how about we give it a try, and at any time you want to stop, you just let me know.

JASMINE: Ok, I guess we can try.

PAT: Ok, Jasmine, I'd like you to close your eyes if that is comfortable to you, or perhaps have a soft gaze at the floor. Now, imagine that tonight you go to sleep just like normal. While you are in a deep sleep a little fairy sneaks into your room and sprinkles you with magical dust. This magical dust is actually time-traveling dust and you are taken back to the age of four, before you were harmed by your mother.

JASMINE: But, time traveling dust isn't real.

PAT: You are struggling with the creativity. It's hard to believe in something you know is not real.

JASMINE: Yeah, of course I am.

PAT: I believe you can do this.

JASMINE: Whatever you say.

PAT: We can stop if this does not feel ok.

JASMINE: Nah, it's fine, I'll try again. Ok . . . fairy dust.

PAT: Yes, so you are back at the age of four, and you wake up one morning after having not experienced abuse the night before. What is the first thing you notice that is different?

JASMINE: I want my mom.

PAT: When you wake up you have an urge to go see your mom.

JASMINE: Yeah, I want a hug.

PAT: You notice the desire to feel an embrace.

JASMINE: [Nods head softly.]

PAT: [Uses silence first—long pause.] What else do you notice?

JASMINE: I'm hungry, I used to always like to eat right when I woke up back then. Pancakes, those were my favorite. My mom would put chocolate chips in them sometimes, before the bad stuff started. After, she just poured us cereal, if she even did that.

PAT: So, as you think back then, this magical fairy dust is helping you see that you would notice things are different, that the bad things didn't happen because you are looking for your mom to give her a hug, and you are ready to eat.

JASMINE: Ha, yeah, two things I hate now!

PAT: I wonder if there is anything else you notice that is different because the bad things didn't happen.

JASMINE: Umm, umm, not really.

PAT: Take your time.

JASMINE: Well maybe I see that my older brothers are all around. They kind of disappeared a lot after things started going downhill with mom.

PAT: You are smiling now. It is as if you are feeling joy from being surrounded by your brothers.

JASMINE: Yeah, and I think I'd see my dad there joking around with us, instead of being so serious all of the time.

PAT: So, you're not only surrounded by your siblings, but your dad is there and things are lighthearted. And your mom is cooking for you.

JASMINE: Yeah, wow this would be so great if this was real.

PAT: As you think about this image in comparison to the reality you experienced you are feeling sad this was not your life.

JASMINE: Yeah, of course. I mean pretending is nice, but it doesn't erase what happened.

PAT: It does not. You experienced things that no child should, but they happened. My intention for us was to explore what you feel the abuse stole from your childhood, and it sounds like we got some ideas.

JASMINE: What do you mean, because I wanted chocolate chip pancakes?

PAT: For me, it seems like those chocolate chip pancakes were about feeling sad that the younger you did not get those, that was something that was stolen from you by your mom. Also, you missed out on all those hugs because you were scared to get close to your mom back then.

JASMINE: Yeah, it seems weird that when I was that little I knew to stay clear of mom, but it's like I just avoided her because I didn't want to get hurt.

PAT: You learned how to protect yourself, but that doesn't mean you didn't miss out on something too.

JASMINE: Yeah, it really sucks, even now. I want to be able to hug someone, I just don't even know how to do it.

PAT: It sounds like hugs are something you missed out on back then, but also now.

JASMINE: Yeah, it seems so silly.

Pat and Jasmine go on to process the miracle question activity for the rest of the session. By using this skill, Pat was able to glean important information about what Jasmine might want to grieve, such as the loss of hugs, the loss of nurturance from her mom, and the loss of bonding time with her brothers and her dad. This exchange demonstrates just how important it is to stay focused with the client throughout this process.

Trauma affects children and adolescents in a multitude of ways and can result in the absence of important life events. Counselors can work with their clients to explore what has been lost for them in a caring, compassionate, collaborative, and intentional way. Counselors can then use this information to work with their clients on the grieving process.

Grieving an Addiction

Individuals who have developed an addiction to a substance may experience painful feelings of loss following the removal of that substance from their lives (Jennings, 1991). This is particularly relevant for adolescents who have experienced trauma and have used substances to cope, and/or adolescents whose neurobiology has driven substance use. These individuals often struggle with forming close relationships and secure attachments (Kliethermes et al., 2014). While the substance use is likely causing numerous negative consequences, it is nonetheless always there, when adults and stable attachment figures are not.

Counselors need to honor the relationships adolescents have formed to substances. The externalizing process (White & Epston, 1990) just described for grieving trauma can be used here. Clients can be invited to name their addiction, and once named, the client and the counselor have an agreed-upon way of addressing the addiction. Just as the counselor needs to identify what needs to be grieved due to trauma, the counselor needs to explore what specifically the client needs to grieve in relation to losing their addiction. The following prompts may be useful:

- When you think of not being able to spend time with [Addiction's Name], what comes to your mind?
- What will you miss most about not spending time with [Addiction's Name]?
- What will [Addiction's Name] do without you?
- Who will be there to support you when [Addiction's Name] is not there?
- When will you miss [Addiction's Name] the most?
- How will you cope with not having [Addiction's Name] in your life?
- Where in your body do you feel a sensation when you think about not spending time with [Addiction's Name]?

These questions will provide counselors information to individualize each client's needs in relation to what the focus of the grief work should be.

Grief Interventions for Adolescents

Counselors working with adolescents who have experienced trauma and have developed problematic substance use are in a unique position to work on processing the client's unresolved grief. Slyter (2012) noted that adolescents have a distinctly different grief reaction than adults. This is marked by grieving with more intensity and grief following a lifelong trajectory (Slyter, 2012). The use of creative techniques with grieving adolescents is recommended for the developmental considerations (Edgar-Bailey & Kress, 2010; Slyter, 2012). Creative techniques assist with reorganizing the lower regulatory systems of the brain that were disrupted due to childhood trauma. This reorganizing focuses on key areas such as those responsible for impulsivity, self-regulation and attention (Edgar-Bailey & Kress, 2010).

Writing

The use of the written word is a powerful intervention for clients of all presenting problems, but specifically for addiction and trauma. Edgar-Bailey and Kress (2010) suggested a variety of different writing interventions with clients, such as constructing a trauma narrative. Trauma narratives are a key component of Trauma-Focused Cognitive Behavioral Therapy and involve telling one's life story (TFCBT; Cohen et al., 2012). This story creation attends to the individual's life from birth, and they are encouraged to include as much specificity as they are able, including attention to specific sensations, experiences, thoughts, and emotional responses (Cohen et al., 2012). The construction of this narrative allows adolescents to reprocess the events in a systematic order and in the safety of the relationship with the counselor (Edgar-Bailey & Kress, 2010).

Other writing interventions can build on the externalizing technique from Narrative Therapy (White & Epston, 1990) that counselors may have introduced when exploring the client's presenting grief. In this intervention, clients are invited to write a letter to the trauma(s) and/or to the addiction. The following prompts may be useful:

- Write a letter to your trauma/addiction that covers the following items as you are comfortable:
  - Your earliest memory of the trauma/addiction
  - Describe your relationship with the trauma/addiction and how it evolved over time
  - Describe how the trauma/addiction has been helpful for you
  - Describe how the trauma/addiction has been harmful for you
  - Describe what the trauma/addiction has taken from your life
  - Offer a goodbye to the trauma/addiction, releasing it from controlling your life.

Depending on the nature of trauma in an individual's life, and/or their substances of choice, clients may choose to write numerous letters. The technique of letter writing can offer clients the opportunity to say what they never had the chance to and offer closure in order to reorient to the future (Edgar-Bailey & Kress, 2010). Other writing interventions include poem, song, or epitaph construction (Edgar-Bailey & Kress, 2010). The above prompts could guide the construction of these expressions.

Drama

Drama therapy is a developmentally appropriate intervention for adolescents (Edgar-Bailey & Kress, 2010; Slyter, 2012). Clients can be encouraged to role-play key moments from their lives in relation to either trauma or addiction. For example, clients may role-play the moment they met their substance of choice for the first time. Drama therapy allows adolescents to express the conflicting emotions they may be experiencing (Slyter, 2012). They may feel anger for the presence of the trauma/addiction but fearful of the unknown for what will happen when the trauma/addiction is no longer the dominant story in their lives. In addition, drama therapy helps adolescents learn how to stay grounded in the present experience (Edgar-Bailey & Kress, 2010), which is often difficult due to neurodevelopment disruptions from childhood trauma.

Visual Arts

Adolescents are sometimes lost for words to describe their experiences. In this case, it can be very useful to use art to assist clients with expressing themselves. Counselors could consider using the prompts suggested in the writing section for clients to construct an artistic representation of their experiences.

For example, a client can be encouraged to draw or perhaps create a collage representing the time they first met their addiction and then another one saying goodbye to the addiction.

Music

Counselors can utilize music in the therapeutic process. Clients can be encouraged to bring in songs that represent their experiences at different points in their life. They may choose songs that represent their childhood trauma experience(s), when they first met their substance of choice, a song that represents their relationship with their substance of choice, and a song that represents saying goodbye to their addiction. Integrating music into the counseling process is one way to encourage emotional expression. It is not uncommon for adolescents to feel validated by the lyrics of a song (Slyter, 2012).

There are many creative interventions counselors can use with clients in order to process the grief experience they bring to the counseling relationship. It is important that counselors have appropriate training in the modalities they choose to utilize and seek supervision to enhance their skill development with the techniques. In addition, it is crucial to allow clients' autonomy with this process and for the counselor to spend adequate time processing the experience.

Conclusion

Adolescents in our society often turn to mood-altering substances for a variety of reasons. For many, this is a direct result of experiencing trauma during childhood. Counselors working with traumatized youth who have developed risky relationships with substances are encouraged due to research that support treatment successes for this population. Grief interventions focused on helping clients explore their personal relationship to the trauma and/or addiction are powerful interventions. Counselors are encouraged to consider the use of creative techniques to allow for adolescent expression of the myriad of emotions and cognitions they are experiencing. It is possible for these young folks to honor their experiences and look to the future with optimism.

References

Alinsky, R. H., Hadland, S. E., Matson, P. A., Cerda, M., & Saloner, B. (2020). Adolescent-serving addiction treatment facilities in the United States and availability of medications for opioid use disorder. *Journal of Adolescent Health, 67*, 542–549. https://doi.org/10.1016/j.jadohealth.2020.03.005

Beck, A. T. (1993). Cognitive therapy: Past, present, and future. *Journal of Consulting and Clinical Psychology, 61*(2), 194–198.

Brown, A. M. (2017). *Emergent strategy: Shaping change, changing worlds.* AK Press.

Centers for Disease Control and Prevention. (2020, April 3). *Preventing adverse childhood experiences.* www.cdc.gov/violenceprevention/aces/fastfact.html

Cohen, J. A., Mannarino, A. P., Berliner, L., & Deblinger, E. (2000). Trauma-focused cognitive behavioral therapy for children and adolescents: An empirical update. *Journal of Interpersonal Violence, 15*(11), 1202–1223.10.1177/088626000015 011007

Cohen, J. A., Mannarino, A. P., Kliethermes, M., & Murray, L. A. (2012). Trauma-focused CBT for youth with complex trauma. *Child Abuse & Neglect, 36,* 528–541. https://doi.org/10.1016/j.chiabu.2012.03.007

Danielson, C. (2006). *Risk reduction through family therapy treatment manual.* National Crime Victims Research & Treatment Center.

De Jong, P., & Berg, I. K. (2013). *Interviewing for solutions* (4th ed.). Cengage.

Dow, S. J., & Kelly, J. F. (2013). Listening to youth: Adolescents' reasons for substance use as a unique predictor of treatment response and outcome. *Psychology of Addictive Behaviors, 27*(4), 1122–1131. https://doi.org/10.1037/a0031065

Dube, S. R., Miller, J. W., Brown, D. W., Giles, W. H., Felitti, V. J., Dong, M., & Anda, R. F. (2006). Adverse childhood experiences and the association with ever using alcohol and initiating alcohol use during adolescence. *Journal of Adolescent Health, 38,* 444.e1–444.e10. https://doi.org/10.1016/j.jadohealth.2005.06.006

Edgar-Bailey, M., & Kress, V. E. (2010). Resolving child and adolescent traumatic grief: Creative techniques and interventions. *Journal of Creativity in Mental Health, 5*(2), 158–176. https://doi.org/10.1080/15401383.2010.485090

Felitti, V. J., Anda, R. F., Nordenberg, D., Williamson, D. F., Spitz, A. M., Edwards, V., Koss, M. P., & Marks, J. S. (1998). Relationship of childhood abuse and household dysfunction to many of the leading causes of death in adults: The adverse childhood experiences (ACE) study. *American Journal of Preventive Medicine, 14*(4), 245–258.

Garner, B. R., Hunter, B. D., Smith, D. C., Smith, J. E., & Godley, M. D. (2014). The relationship between child maltreatment and substance abuse treatment outcomes among emerging adults and adolescents. *Child Maltreatment, 19*(3–4), 267–269. https://doi.org/10.1177/1077559514547264

Godley, S. H., Meyers, R. J., Smith, J. E., Karvinen, T., Titus, J. C., Godley, M. D., . . . Kelberg, P. (2001). *The adolescent community reinforcement approach for adolescent cannabis users.* Cannabis Youth Treatment (CYT) Series, Volume 4. DHS Pub. No. 01–3489. Center for Substance Abuse Treatment, Substance Abuse and Mental Health Services Administration.

Henggeler, S. W., & Borduin, C. M. (1990). *Family therapy and beyond: A multisystemic approach to treating the behaviour problem of children and adolescents.* Brooks/Cole.

Hogue, A., Henderson, C. E., Becker, S. J., & Knight, D. K. (2018). Evidence base on outpatient behavioral treatments for adolescent substance use, 2014–2017: Outcomes, treatment delivery, and promising horizons. *Journal of Clinical Child & Adolescent Psychology, 47*(4), 499–526. https://doi.org/10.1080/15374416.2018.1 466307

Jennings, P. S. (1991). To surrender drugs: A grief process in its own right. *Journal of Substance Abuse Treatment, 8*(4), 221–226. https://doi.org/10.1016/0740-5472(91) 90042-9

Khantzian, E. (1997). The self-medication hypothesis of substance use disorders: A reconsideration and recent applications. *Harvard Review of Psychiatry, 4*(5), 231–244. https://doi.org/10.3109/10673229709030550

Kliethermes, M., Schacht, M., & Drewry, K. (2014). Complex trauma. *Child and Adolescent Psychiatric Clinics of North America, 23*(2), 339–361.10.1016/j.chc.2013.12.009

Knudsen, H. K. (2009). Adolescent-only substance abuse treatment: Availability and adoption of components of quality. *Journal of Substance Abuse Treatment, 36*, 195–204. https://doi.org/10.1016/j.jsat.2008.06.002

Liddle, H. A., Dakof, G. A., Parker, K., Diamond, G. S., Barrett, K., & Tejeda, M. (2001). Multidimensional family therapy for adolescent drug abuse: Results of a randomized clinical trial. *American Journal of Drug and Alcohol Abuse, 27*(4), 651–688.

Merrick, M. T., Ford, D. C., Ports, K. A., & Guinn, A. S. (2018). Prevalence of adverse childhood experiences from the 2011–2014 behavioral risk factor surveillance system in 23 states. *Journal of the American Medical Association Pediatrics, 172*(11), 1038–1044. https://doi.org/10.1001/jamapediatrics.2018.2537

Miller, W. R., & Rollnick, S. (1991). *Motivational interviewing: Preparing people to change addictive behavior*. Guilford Press.

Najavits, L. M. (2001). *Seeking safety: A treatment manual for substance abuse*. Guilford Press.

Najavits, L. M., Gallop, R. J., & Weiss, R. D. (2006). Seeking safety therapy for adolescent girls with PTSD and substance use disorder: A randomized controlled trial. *Journal of Behavioral Health Services & Research, 33*(4), 453–463. https://doi.org/10.1007/s11414-006-9034-2

National Child Traumatic Stress Network. (n.d.). *Trauma types*. www.nctsn.org/what-is-child-trauma/trauma-types

National Child Traumatic Stress Network. (2008a). *Engaging adolescents in treatment*. www.nctsn.org/sites/default/files/resources//engaging_adolescents_emotional_substance_use_in_treatment.pdf

National Child Traumatic Stress Network. (2008b). *Understanding the link between adolescent trauma and substance abuse: A toolkit for providers* (2nd ed.). www.nctsn.org/sites/default/files/resources//understanding_the_links_between_adolescent_trauma_and_substance_abuse.pdf

Newcomb, M. D., & Bentler, P. M. (1989). Substance use and abuse among children and teenagers. *American Psychologist, 44*(2), 242–248. https://doi.org/10.1037/0003-066X.44.2.242

Racco, A., & Vis, J. (2015). Evidence based trauma treatment for children and youth. *Child and Adolescent Social Work Journal, 32*, 121–129. https://doi.org/10.1007/s10560-014-0347-3

Robbins, M. S., Szapocznik, J., Horigian, V. E., Feaster, D. J., Puccinelli, M., Jacobs, P., . . . Brigham, G. (2009). Brief strategic family therapy™ for adolescent drug abusers: A multi-site effectiveness study. *Contemporary Clinical Trials, 30*(3), 269–278. https://doi.org/10.1016/j.cct.2009.01.004

Rothman, E. F., Bernstein, J., & Strunin, L. (2010). Why might adverse childhood experiences lead to underage drinking among US youth? Findings from an emergency department-based qualitative pilot study. *Substance Use & Misuse, 45*, 2281–2290. https://doi.org/10.3109/10826084.2010.482369

Sampl, S., & Kadden, R. (2001). *Motivational enhancement therapy and cognitive behavioral therapy for adolescent cannabis users: 5 sessions*. SMA-01–3486. Substance Abuse and Mental Health Services Administration.

Saxe, G., Ellis, B. H., Fogler, J., Hansen, S., & Sorkin, B. (2005). Comprehensive care for traumatized children: An open trial examines treatment using Trauma Systems Therapy. *Psychiatric Annals, 35*(5), 443–448. https://doi.org/10.3928/00485713-20050501-10

Saxe, G., Ellis, B. H., & Kaplow, J. (2006). *Collaborative treatment of traumatized children and teens: The trauma systems therapy approach.* Guilford Press.

Slyter, M. (2012). Creative counseling interventions for grieving adolescents. *Journal of Creativity in Mental Health, 7*(1), 17–34. https://doi.org/10.1080/15401383.2012.657593

Stein, B. D., Jaycox, L. H., Kataoka, S. H., Wong, M., Tu, W., Elliott, M. N., & Fink, A. (2003). A mental health intervention for school children exposed to violence: A randomized controlled trial. *Journal of the American Medical Association, 290*(5), 603–611. https://doi.org/10.1001/jama.290.5.603

Substance Abuse and Mental Health Services Administration. (2014). *Trauma-informed care in behavioral health services.* Treatment Improvement Protocol (TIP) Series 57. HHS Publications No. (SMA) 13–4801. Substance Abuse and Mental Health Services Administration.

Substance Abuse and Mental Health Services Administration. (2020a). Behavioral health barometer: United States, Volume 6: Indicators as measured through the 2019 National Survey on Drug Use and Health and the National Survey of Substance Abuse Treatment Services. HHS Publication N. PEP20-07-02-001. Substance Abuse and Mental Health Services Administration.

Substance Abuse and Mental Health Services Administration. (2020b). *Key substance use and mental health indicators in the United States: Results from the 2019 national survey on drug use and health (HHS Publication No. PEP-20-07-01-001, NSDUH Series H-55).* Center for Behavioral Health Statistics and Quality, Substance Abuse and Mental Health Services Administration.

Tarter, R. E. (2002). Etiology of adolescent substance abuse: A developmental perspective. *American Journal of Addiction, 11*, 171–191. https://doi.org/10.1080/10550490290087965

White, M., & Epston, D. (1990). *Narrative means to therapeutic ends.* W. W. Norton.

15 Addiction and Grief in the Prison Population

Leigh Falls Holman

Despite the dramatic increase in numbers of prisoners with substance use disorders (SUDs) over the past 40 years, few receive competent addiction treatment (Karberg & James, 2005; Mumola & Karberg, 2006). In fact, although approximately half of the 7.1 million adults under supervision in the justice system meet the criteria for diagnosis of an addictive disorder, only about 20% receive treatment, other than psychoeducation (Jensen et al., 2004; Karberg & James, 2005; Mumola & Karberg, 2006; Taxman et al., 2007). These individuals also have significantly higher risks of recidivism post-release. Frequently, they live with the stigma of dual status as an offender and as an addict, which may also affect their support systems and their ability to obtain housing and employment, further increasing their risks of relapse and recidivism (Field, 2004; Shivy et al., 2007). However, a risk factor that many do not discuss is the link between unresolved traumatic grief and higher rates of recidivism (Leach et al., 2008).

Grief and loss are among the emotional challenges that prisoners experience both prior to incarceration and because of incarceration. In most cases, the loss prisoners experience is complicated by the context within which they live. In fact, the tasks of grieving, which one needs to accomplish in order to resolve the mourning process, are often prevented in a prison setting. This results in complicated and unresolved grief. For this reason, there are potential negative consequences for successful reintegration into the community (Hendry, 2008; Worden, 2018).

Correctional Context

Although mental health professionals and many working in the criminal justice system would likely agree that appropriate treatment intervention is important, the debate between criminal justice and counseling approaches to mental health intervention leads us to ask, What is "appropriate" in this environment? Psychological work in prison adds a layer of complexity that counselors must factor into treatment in addition to all the other individual, cultural, and societal factors that affect recovery. For instance, an additional challenge that may lead to relapse and recidivism, which treatment providers must address, is the

DOI: 10.4324/9781003106906-15

need to facilitate the offenders' process of mourning losses they encountered because of their incarceration. For offenders with SUDs, the losses associated with their addictive behaviors are intertwined with losses associated with leaving behind criminal behavior and relationships tied to criminal enterprises, as well (Finlay & Jones, 2000; Harner et al., 2011; Hester & Taylor, 2011; Lansing et al., 2018).

The most obvious of these is their loss of freedom. Additionally, prisoners may experience existential crises, such as how to live with meaning in their lives, even within the prison walls. They may also experience death and dying as existential crises differently than they might have prior to incarceration. Issues facing prisoners are related to death, including their own mortality, the possibility of dying in prison, the death of a significant loved one like a parent or child, or witnessing the long-term illness and death of a fellow inmate. Due to the complex nature of these experiences occurring within a correctional setting, the grief process is often complicated because these settings are not always psychologically safe spaces (Finlay & Jones, 2000; Hester & Taylor, 2011).

What is psychological safety? Basically, in a correctional setting people experience the need to stifle their emotions and stay emotionally isolated, except in rare circumstances. Prisoners use terms like "putting on my game face" or "putting up a wall" as they leave a counseling session to metaphorically express the need to protect themselves from this harsh environment, which lacks empathy or social support. Counselors can use these metaphors to help prisoners transition into and out of individual or group sessions so that they can "do the work" of counseling. The counselor may guide a client or a group through a visualization of taking bricks out of their wall or unplugging a dam and letting the water of emotions flow at the beginning of the group or individual session, and then guide visualization using the same metaphor to contain intense emotion, so that they can reenter the prison unit in a psychologically protected space.

Counselors must acknowledge and respect the reality that this type of vulnerability in prison may in fact result in physical violence, if weakness is sensed by another inmate or even by correctional officers. Ferszt (2002) described an unwritten code of conduct in prison culture that demands toughness, loyalty to other inmates and lack of trust in others, and no allowances for "soft" emotion, which includes anything other than anger and resulting aggression. These cultural norms necessarily impact grief work when counseling inmates. Even within women's units, hegemonic masculinity is predominant in prisons (Sabo et al., 2001; Stohr & Hemmens, 2004). *Hegemonic masculinity* is characterized by distrust in others, which inhibits the social support aspects of grieving and rejection of feminine traits, including "soft" emotions associated with crying or sadness, which is perceived as weak and vulnerable, thus making the inmate a target for violence (Hendry, 2009). However, the inability to publicly express their grief may result in ambiguous loss and subsequent lack of clarity in meaning making following loss, which is important for the inmate's healing

(Gilbert, 2007; Parkes, 1998; Young, 2003). Subsequently, incarcerated individuals are likely to experience a complicated form of disenfranchised grief, which can raise their risks of relapse and recidivism. Therefore, it is important for counselors to address inmates' grief and loss issues.

An example is Ferszt's (2002) work, which found women in prison experienced restrictions in their ability to grieve familial losses because they feared disciplinary action from supervisors if they demonstrated strong emotions associated with grieving. This experience is often consistent with their pre-incarceration lives when many feelings were not "safe" to have, often resulting from living in complicated family systems, unsafe neighborhoods with few community resources, and repeated experiences of trauma, including the trauma of oppression (Afuape, 2020; Root, 2000). Leach et al. (2008) analyzed the literature on grief and loss among prisoners and documented links between these unresolved interpersonal adverse childhood experiences (ACEs) and the development of maladaptive behaviors leading to addictions and criminal behavior. Research further revealed that losses and unresolved grief earlier in life could be further complicated by new losses resulting in grief that was traumatic and subsequently contributed to relapse and recidivism (Leach et al., 2008). *Traumatic grief* "arises as a result of interpersonal trauma experienced as a betrayal of attachment" (Leach et al., 2008, p. 104).

One phenomenological inquiry of prisoners' experiences of traumatic grief described four elements that characterize grieving in prison. The first element is *temporality*, which is described as experiencing grief as if "frozen in time" (p. 458), where prisoners discussed a lack of closure around losses because they felt they were not able to grieve them, so they carried the weight of the loss with them, sometimes for years (Harner et al., 2011). The second element is *spatiality*. Since there is no privacy, prisoners did not have personal space to grieve, and although there were people around, they did not feel like there was empathy for their grieving experiences. For instance, many are told about the death of a child or parent in the presence of others, with little regard for the intensely personal nature of these losses (Harner et al., 2011).

The third element is *corporeality*, which describes the need to quickly block intense emotional responses to loss because there is a risk that vulnerability, associated with expressing emotions, presents in a correctional setting. One concern prisoners discussed was that their expressions of grief would result in correctional officers identifying them for suicidal risk and isolate them from other inmates, who may otherwise provide some emotional support (Harner et al., 2011). Finally, the element of *relationality* is described as being lonely, although never alone, which results in a unique experience of lacking support or empathy to aid their process of grieving, often because once they are part of the correctional system, they are not viewed as human or in need of kindness or care (Harner et al., 2011). Unexpressed emotions, particularly strong feelings of anger, loss, loneliness, or shame, often associated with incarceration, further trigger emotional dysregulation, which is a conditioned cue for many people struggling with addictions and offending behaviors (e.g., interpersonal violence) that "automatically activate the reward/motivation neurocircuitry and can trigger an intense desire to consume drugs (craving)" (Chandler et al., 2008, p. 184).

Common Losses in Prison

Given the significance of disenfranchised traumatic grief that prisoners frequently develop, it is important for counselors to be aware of the various forms of loss typical among this population, in order to intentionally scan for these potential issues when working with inmates. Although some experiences are shared with losses experienced in the outside world, such as the death of a loved one, the ability to grieve within the prison context is much more complicated to navigate.

Loss of Freedom: Ambiguous Loss

The first, and perhaps most obvious, form of loss is the loss of freedom that prisoners experience. This loss of freedom is described by Hendry (2009):

> Prisoners are at the mercy of the system and their lives are determined by the decisions of others in a tightly controlled environment. Daily life is governed by incessant rules, and this, combined with lack of privacy and personal space, interferes with adaptive strategies that people use under stress, such as going for walks, exercise, art, and writing in journals.
>
> (Hendry, 2009, p. 273)

Due to these restrictions, prisoners may experience limitations on their ability to engage in therapeutic activities necessary for healing and growth from previous trauma. Loss of freedom can result in two types of *ambiguous loss*, including

(a) [Perceiving people] as physically present but psychologically absent: addictions, chronic mental illness; [or]
(b) [Perceiving people] as being psychologically present but physically absent: missing people, prisoners. (Leach et al., 2008)

Inmates have different experiences of losing their freedom. For instance, many people who end up in prison felt like prisoners, restricted in their ability to live freely, for much of their lives, due to frequently overlapping traumas. For these inmates, the loss of freedom associated with prison is one more in a sequence of traumatic events.

However, for counselors working in this setting, it is often a very different experience from any they have had previously. Therefore, counselors are also impacted by working in the prison setting (Carrola et al., 2016; Hatcher et al.,

2011; Perkins & Sprang, 2012). One area of potential secondary traumatic stress for counselors working in corrections is a new awareness that many people in the counselor's life, and perhaps even the counselor, live inside a mental prison of their own without being "in prison" at all. Although this may aid the counselor's ability to empathize with prisoners, for the counselor walking into prison daily, it can be a constant reminder of their own psychological work they need to engage in to avoid countertransference, boundary violations, secondary traumatic stress, or compassion fatigue.

The multiple traumas many inmates experience over their lifetimes are further compounded by the unjust sentencing guidelines that helped create a system where marginalized populations (e.g., racial/ethnic minorities, impoverished persons, and women), particularly those convicted of drug-related offenses, are disproportionately negatively impacted (Ostrom et al., 2004). In fact, the U.S. Justice Department determined there were 10% fewer violent offenders and 15% more drug offenders sentenced to prison between 1980 and 2000, most of these being people of color, poor people, and women (Ostrom et al., 2004). For these inmates who may have always experienced life as a prison, being "in prison" does not necessarily present a new reality. Understanding their experiences of family, friends, and what parts of life they are missing most while being locked up is important to understand what losing their freedom may represent.

Additionally, it is important to consider there are prisoners who do not fit the typical description conjured by the word "inmate." There are people in prison who are not minorities. There are middle-class and wealthy people in prison. "Normal" on the outside is quite different from "normal" on the inside. Being a middle class, suburban, college-educated White man or woman with a career and family who is now imprisoned can be a completely different reality that results in different expressions of grief related to the loss of freedom. In the author's observations over time, some counselors assume that because these individuals had privileges on the outside afforded by their gender, class, or race, they do not need counseling support around multiple traumas that are easily identifiable with racial/ethnic minority, poor, or uneducated inmates. So, understanding the way these inmates experience loss of freedom can be tricky because the counselor's perception may be impacted by implicit biases about who "needs" their services and who does not based on beliefs about each prisoner's sociocultural situation. Counselors, therefore, must continually scan for their own biases in clinical decision-making.

When counselors consider how being sent to prison might be experienced differently by different inmates depending upon their individual sociocultural backgrounds, the counselors are better able to facilitate each inmate's grieving process. For instance, consider what prison might be like for a middle-class man who got into gambling debt and ended up embezzling money to cover his losses, thus landing him in prison. How might this experience be unique from a 25-year-old male who grew up in and out of foster care because his parents were incarcerated, going to inner city schools with few resources and little time or attention for his psychological needs, and who began using and selling drugs as a way to "hustle" and make a living? Conversely, how might the loss of freedom be experienced by a 32-year-old Latina mother of four who was physically and sexually abused most of her life, first by adults in her family and then by her boyfriends and spouse, leading her to use pills to numb the pain of the abuse she has felt her entire life. Take a moment to contemplate each of these questions: How might each of these inmates experience freedom on the outside? How might that affect their perception of the loss of freedom when they are imprisoned? Finally, how might this awareness impact your approach when working with them in counseling? Understanding these individual differences is important for counselors working with the diversity of people with whom they will interact within prison.

However, regardless of race, ethnicity, or socioeconomic status, prisoners often share multiple experiences of relational trauma leading them to their addictions or offending behaviors (Brady et al., 2015; Bronson & Berzofsky, 2017; Green et al., 2016; Johnson & Lynch, 2013; Lynch et al., 2012; Nowotny et al., 2014). In this way, White middle-class or wealthy prisoners share a similar experience with many impoverished inmates or incarcerated racial/ ethnic minorities. The truth is that due to their complex trauma experiences and addictions and/or offending behaviors, all prisoners are at risk for unique mental health challenges (Brady et al., 2015; Green et al., 2016; Lynch et al., 2012; Nowotny et al., 2014). In fact, multiple researchers have documented a commonly experienced constellation of mental health symptoms they call *post-incarceration syndrome*, which can affect any inmate. This syndrome is commonly experienced by those with overlapping complex trauma associated with chronic and repeated exposure to abuse, violence, or other trauma (Herman, 2005; Liem & Kunst, 2013). Post-incarceration syndrome manifests with post-traumatic stress symptoms of persistent reexperiencing, hypervigilance, avoidance, and emotional numbing (Herman, 2005; Liem & Kunst, 2013). Understanding this layer of complexity is important for counselors working with inmates and those who have served time.

Although inmates may have access to counseling in prison, it is generally focused on controlling or changing their offending behaviors rather than focused on the underlying trauma and associated emotional and mental health issues they experience (Bronson & Berzofsky, 2017; Hester & Taylor, 2011; Schetky, 1998) This is true even though these trauma experiences contributed to the behaviors that led to their imprisonment. Because trauma and associated grief and loss are not systematically addressed in prison, counselors must be intentional in addressing these issues with inmates. However, some researchers question whether it is even possible to mourn in prison, due to the limitations around common grieving behaviors (Schetky, 1998). In part, this is because correctional officers have tremendous leeway regarding how and when they restrict movements and activities of prisoners, including often restricting inmate's emotional expression necessary for therapeutic work. Counselors must understand that correctional officers generally have little to no training in mental health, so they frequently act out of their own experiences and/or biases when managing inmates who may be grieving. This circumstance provides an opportunity for counselors to offer some education to correctional staff when they are aware this is happening on a prison unit.

Counselors should look for teachable moments to provide information or training about common issues of mental health/illness, feelings of guilt versus feelings of shame, and grief or loss among inmates. Informal training opportunities are presented daily as counselors interact with correctional colleagues. In these moments, a counselor can offer a reframe of the colleague's uninformed perception of an inmate's behavior or provide information based in the research about a different way to understand the prisoner's emotions or behavior exhibited on the unit. Doing so with a tone of respect is important so that correctional officers do not feel the counselor is being condescending. Building respectful relationships with correctional officers over time can aid their receptiveness to this type of interaction. Prison counselors can also work within the system to offer formal training opportunities, such as developing workshops for continuing education on research-based topics relevant to the behavioral and psychological management of inmates, as well as information on the impact of different interventions, including interpersonal or milieu interventions, as they may affect future relapse or recidivism.

Guilt, Shame, and Social Stigma of Crime: Intrapsychic Loss

As previously identified, one way correctional officers may impede the grieving process for prisoners is to punish them for emotional processing. Officers frequently misinterpret crying or any show of emotion as a loss of behavioral control and therefore follow their training and primary mission to control the inmate's behavior. Consequently, they punish or restrict movement of inmates who are grieving. Some officers even mock inmates who are grieving, in a show of their own machismo, and thus shame the inmate's grieving process. Other inmates may target a vulnerable inmate because the social stigma associated with sadness, loneliness, fear, or other emotions associated with loss are considered socially unacceptable in a prison setting. The grieving inmate may be perceived to be weak and thus become a target. For these reasons, it is common for inmates to feel shamed and stifle their emotions whether grieving for past traumas that led to their using addictive substances or behaviors to cope or grieving for new losses suffered within prison. This can lead to a form of *intrapsychic loss*, where the prisoner's experience results in their "los[ing] an important image of themselves" (Leach et al., 2008, p. 108). This can complicate their ability to reach resolution in the grieving process.

Morse (2001) hypothesized that people must experience emotional suffering until they have "suffered enough" (p. 51) to have resolution of grief around losses. However, when a person is unable to fully and freely experience and work through their grief, they may engage in two types of enduring grief behaviors. The first involves suppressing emotions and focusing on their current circumstances in life. The second is enduring life to just getting through the day. Each of these types of coping further complicates the grieving process.

Further, when the grief experienced is related to the prisoner's behaviors that brought them to prison, the cognitive attribution prisoners give the experience can have an impact on risks associated with relapse and recidivism. When inmates attribute the feeling to doing something wrong for which they are being punished, they have feelings of guilt, which correlate with lower rates of recidivism (Hosser et al., 2008). However, when the inmate's attribution is "I am wrong or bad," they experience feelings of shame, similar to what they may experience from the ways correctional officers manage them in times of grief. This may result in an inability to ever feel as though they have "suffered enough," thus blocking their ability to move through the grief. Shame also correlates with higher incidences of relapse and recidivism upon release (Hosser et al., 2008). This is particularly true if the feelings of shame are associated with losing face or feeling rejected, injuring the prisoner's sense of dominance that is valued in a machismo culture like prison (Muris & Meesters, 2011). For this reason shaming, coupled with targeted violence for being vulnerable in processing "soft" emotions, may increase relapse and recidivism, which is something counselors must guard against when working inside a prison unit. However, it is also important for prison counselors to help inmates work through their complicated feelings of shame associated with their own behaviors that led them to prison and any replicated feelings of shame associated with other traumatic losses, particularly those that are relational in nature. Helping the inmate work through shame is more likely to bring them to a point of resolution from which they can move forward and ultimately reduce the likelihood they relapse or recidivate.

Relational Connection: Attachment Loss

Another significant loss is the loss of relational connection that many prisoners have when they are incarcerated. Their connections to significant people on the outside is severely limited, resulting in *attachment loss*, which is the "experience of separation distress where the [inmate] is searching and longing for [the absent] person" (Leach et al., 2008, p. 108). For some, the burdens of travel and expense are prohibitive, so they do not visit often or ever. Therefore, some prisoners rarely have visitors from the outside. Thus, they may become completely emotionally isolated from a world outside the prison walls.

> There is limited opportunity for contact with family, for intimacy and almost no opportunity to invest in new relationships, either within the prison or with people from the outside. Caution is the norm when it comes to getting close to others.
>
> (Hendry, 2009, p. 274)

This is even more significant for those who have longer sentences or are housed in prisons far from their homes. They may find that even calls or letters become scarce and that life outside moves forward, while their lives virtually stop. In fact, it is not uncommon for family and friends to say that they experience the imprisonment of their loved one as a death.

Attachment

Attachment relationships are probably the most significant motivator of human behavior at its essence, according to much of the research we now have (Siegel, 2020). The lack of attachment is so significant it can lead to failure to thrive in infants. Therefore, it is reasonable to view attachment or relational connection as a survival need. For this reason, addiction and offender counselors often work from the hypothesis that the development of addictions or offending behaviors starts at the door of disrupted early attachments. There is an extensive research base on attachment, which aids our understanding of the significant impact of these early childhood attachments and relationship ruptures from relational trauma (Ainsworth, 1979; Ainsworth & Bell, 1970; Ainsworth et al., 1978; Behrens et al., 2007; Bowlby, 1968, 1973, 1980; Siegel, 2020). In fact, the earliest observations forming the basis of attachment theory were recorded in a systematic manner by John Bowlby at a juvenile detention facility (Bretherton, 1992). More recently, clinicians and researchers have applied attachment theory to explore the impact of relational *dis*connection on individuals who end up using addictive substances or behaviors or who find themselves in prison, finding a predictable developmental trajectory from early unresolved trauma to later development of addictions and offending behaviors (Flores, 2011; Gill, 2014; Morse, 2001).

However, it would be easy to create a caricature of a prisoner's experience that did not fully embrace the diversity of life experiences prisoners represent. With little exposure to prisoners other than on TV or in movies, we often picture a specific image of a prisoner. However, as previously discussed, there is great variability in the backgrounds of individuals who find themselves in prison, so it is important not to assume you can know their attachment histories. Thus, it is crucial that prison counselors take the time to explore the significant relational connections and traumas individual offenders have experienced. This can provide a window into our understanding of the human beings with whom we are working, as unique individuals. By doing so, counselors may find they understand the unique developmental trajectory that led each addict or offender to their current place in time. Further, it may explain their interpersonal maneuvering with staff, other prisoners, and with you as their counselor, in such a way that you better understand how to intervene in an individualized, therapeutic manner.

Prisoners as Significant Others

You may find some prisoners experience relational losses of parents, a spouse, or other family members. Prisoners are often significant in the lives of their own family and friends and often have quite complicated attachment relationships with their own families of origin; their families of choice, including gangs or other criminal groups with whom they are close; and their families of creation, including their romantic partners. There is tremendous variability from prisoner to prisoner regarding how these relationships continue or how they are interrupted or cut off completely while imprisoned. For those who have significant relationship losses, a counselor may need to help them process through their feelings about the others' reactions to their incarceration and their own contribution to the events leading to the relational disconnection and loss.

Prisoners as Parents

Some prisoners tragically experience the loss of their own children while they are locked up. This is a common issue of unresolved loss and ongoing fear for many women in prison whose children have been placed in foster care. It is important to note that in many jurisdictions, women can have their parental rights permanently terminated by the state, if their children are in foster care for more than one year, even if the parent is incarcerated. Additionally, when children are placed with family members, they continue to grow and go through significant milestones while a parent is in prison. This relational disconnection can result in additional points of loss for both male and female parents.

The loss of attachments to children can be among the most heartbreaking to bear witness to for prison counselors. There is a sense of despair and helplessness that inmates experience when losing children that is only comparable to the actual death of a child, yet more complicated in that the child continues to live and becomes attached to others who replace the inmate as parent. This adds to the complex psychological interventions necessary to help the inmate process the loss. Frequently, these losses trigger unresolved grief among other inmates in trans-crisis (James & Gilliland, 2016), which the counselor must be attendant to and manage, particularly if discussions occur within group settings. The prison counselor can help assist the prisoner and other inmates with whom they are close to have a ceremony honoring the relationship and mourning the losses experienced as a result of incarceration; however, it is crucial to adequately prepare the prison director/warden and correctional staff for any such ceremony so that it is properly supported.

Death

While imprisoned, many inmates also experience the loss of a significant person in their lives through death. Sometimes these are their own parents, siblings, spouses, or children. One study estimated that half of prisoners reported losing a family member while incarcerated (Harner et al., 2011). A complication for many prisoners who experience the death of a loved is that the most significant relationships in their lives may not be with people considered traditionally as "family." For those in gangs, their fellow gang members often are identified as family, and it is unacceptable in correctional settings to acknowledge these affiliations, much less grieve the loss of them as part of a healing process. Correctional staff may perceive this process as supporting their gang affiliation. However, regardless of the relationship, inmates are unlikely to be allowed to attend a memorial service, resulting in unresolved loss.

When it is a parent or a child, an inmate may receive a special dispensation to go to a funeral. However, "for those who go to a funeral, the experience is often difficult and intensely painful, especially if they are handcuffed, in prison attire and accompanied by corrections officers" (Hendry, 2009, p. 273). Researchers have documented the prisoner's experience of attending a funeral as degrading, humiliating, dehumanizing, and an embarrassment to others (Ferszt, 2002; Schetky, 1998; Young, 2003). Further, they are not able to share memories of the deceased with other family members through recounting stories together, because if they are allowed to attend the service, they are often severely restricted in their communications or ability to hug or comfort others or receive such comfort themselves (Hendry, 2009). Ferszt (2002) described the prisoner's experience of loss as lacking support or counseling, a loss of time spent with the deceased because of incarceration, and an inability to attend the funeral as significant markers of the complications prisoners experience when they lose a family member.

Inmates also experience death of fellow prisoners while they are incarcerated (Allen et al., 2008; Depner et al., 2018; Maschi et al., 2011). At times, death follows a long illness resulting in the inmates caring for other prisoners in an unusual type of palliative care. Doing so allows the surviving inmates to empathically care for another in a similar situation they are in. On one level, they may experience this as a way to care for themselves in a disembodied fashion, thus leading to a healing experience of self-compassion. On another level, the inmate may experience further trauma and existential angst associated with death and dying and the meaning of a life lived inside prison walls. Some prisoners find meaning and healing in this self-reflection, and others experience further unresolved grief.

Counselors can be helpful in these situations by being aware of when inmates have life-threatening illness on the unit and providing space for prisoners to talk about their experiences. Counselors can facilitate inmates' processing their thoughts and feelings when reflecting on their own lives, as an outgrowth of caring for a fellow inmate who is dying. Additionally, if another inmate dies on the unit, it may be helpful to provide a space for some memorial of the individual's life and a group setting for fellow inmates to process their thoughts and feelings about the loss. Some correctional staff may fear this will glorify the dead inmate's problematic behavior, but by making space to honor the loss, inmates may find some sense of self-worth in knowing that even in prison their lives can positively impact others. In this, they may find meaning that motivates a change in the inmate.

Unresolved Grief in Prison

As illustrated, counselors have an important role in prisons when it comes to processing grief and loss. This unresolved grief can lead to increased risk of recidivism, so it is important counselors proactively process and provide opportunities for ceremony, honoring of the loss, and closure activities or re-storying that may provide healing for inmates so that they do not experience further unresolved grief. However, counselors must remember they are usually hired into prison units that are offering very specific mental health services like 12-step groups, addiction services, or other groups that focus on the offending behaviors. Therefore, any proactive approach to providing space for process-ing and grieving loss, in general, will be the responsibility of each individual counselor.

When grief continues unresolved, it can take one of three forms. The first is *disenfranchised grief*, which is "grief not recognized and supported by soci-ety" or considered insignificant (Leach et al., 2008, p. 108). This can include grief associated with losses related to being in prison or having an addiction. The second is *chronic or pathological grief*, in which the "intensity of the loss becomes an exaggerated magnification of grief, which continues with-out subsiding" (Leach et al., 2008, p. 108). These individuals are likely to self-isolate into a type of post-traumatic reliving of the grief. The final type of unresolved grief is *complicated or traumatic grief*, in which the "intensity of the loss remains high and the grieving process is blocked. Grief remains frozen" (Leach et al., 2008, p. 108). Individuals experiencing this type of grief often have separation loss and traumatic loss that leads to despair similar to, yet distinct from, bereavement-related depression or anxiety.

Interventions

Because of the complexities of grieving in a correctional context, there is a delicate dance of timing and choice of intervention, pacing of the process, and a continuum of therapeutic relational connection or rupture, which counse-lors must negotiate. In this process, counselors continually measure the risks associated with the prisoner's exposed vulnerability and the growth and long-term healing that may come from processing through these experiences. Com-pounding these complex clinical decisions is the fact that, like the prisoners themselves, counselors also may not experience the environment as psycho-logically safe. Therefore, the co-construction of relationship building, process-ing challenging thoughts and feelings about life experiences, and meaning making is quite complicated. Yet it is a crucial foundational part of facilitating the grieving process for incarcerated individuals. This interpersonal process that utilizes the therapeutic relationship as a primary intervention aids the heal-ing of relational disconnections and attachment losses, in particular (Lionells et al., 2014; Teyber & Teyber, 2016).

Intrapsychic losses can often be addressed through use of cognitive interventions. Counselors may use cognitive restructuring techniques that identify the client's distorted thinking patterns associated with self-messages that are destructive. Identifying cognitive schema related to shame-based or hubristic, prideful thinking patterns and addressing these can be helpful in processing intrapsychic losses where the inmate's sense of self is altered by the losses associated with their offending or addictive behaviors. Thought journals, thought stopping, and other similar cognitive behavioral interventions are commonly used in correctional settings and can easily be applied to intrapsychic losses as well.

Finally, counselors can aid inmates with attachment losses through providing space for verbal and emotional processing, use of visualizations around psychological safety to manage vulnerability associated with emotional processing, and use of creative interventions to help prisoners process grief associated with these relational disconnections. Gorle (2008) described the importance of ceremonies or rituals as a vehicle to process feelings of loss, which help individuals navigate the grieving process. Ceremonies or rituals that honor the lost relationship can be quite powerful, but they need to be managed in the prison system. Counselors need to ensure that any ceremonial activities or use of props are approved by the appropriate director or warden and that correctional staff are adequately prepared on how to address the ceremony or ritual and are given specific instructions on how to manage any resulting emotional or behavioral concerns.

Tasks of Grieving

Worden (2018) described the grief process as a series of tasks including acceptance of the loss, working through the pain, learning to adjust after loss, and emotionally relocating the deceased and integrating their new reality into the "here and now." The first task of accepting the loss as a reality is necessary to move forward through the grief process. Having the process interrupted here may result in the loss feeling unreal, so that it is experienced as an ambiguous loss that preempts the individual from completing other tasks of grieving. This is a primary concern for grieving inmates who often stifle their emotions or are unable to connect with the reality of losses experienced outside the walls of the prison (e.g., death of a loved one).

Fully experiencing and working through the emotional pain experienced from the loss is another task of grieving that can be complicated if the individual does not have a supportive social system for the mourning process, which is common in prison. "This acknowledgement is manifested through crying, anger and guilt, anxiety, helplessness and loneliness, and through behaviours such as sleep disturbance and intolerance of others" (Hendry, 2009, p. 273). However, "the unwritten code of behaviour in prison, with its cultural mandate for toughness and for the traditional male stereotype of not showing emotions, is not conducive to these manifestations" (Hendry, 2009, p. 273). So this is another potential challenge to facilitating the grief process in prison.

Inmates must also learn to cope or adjust to the world with the reality of the loss. This could be the loss of a significant person in one's life, the loss of freedom experienced in correctional settings, the loss of a sense of self or identity unmarked by the double stigma of addiction and criminality, or even the loss of the substance or behaviors they utilized to emotionally regulate prior to incarceration. Prisoners also must adjust to the loss of connection to their lives on the outside. Their family's and friends' lives go on. Their children grow and have significant life events, and the prisoner is absent during these. Thus, each significant life event may be felt as a new loss, as may each missed visitation with someone from their life prior to incarceration. In this manner, the losses compile, complicating the grieving process. Therefore, to resolve this task of grieving, it is common for prisoners to ask family not to visit or not to write. However, this act often is impacted by the shame they may feel because of their new identity as "addict" and "offender." If observed, this is something for counselors to process with the inmate.

Finally, emotionally relocating the deceased or the lost part of self, freedom, and so forth into the past and integrating their new reality into the here and now must be done. This involves committing to their new lives moving forward and negotiating a place for important memories of the lost relationship(s), identity, or behaviors while moving forward with a new sense of their life. Ultimately, if an inmate is able to successfully navigate this task, they are able to resolve their grief and create a new life. This resolution will reduce their likelihood of relapse or recidivism in the future. Therefore, although facilitating the grieving process may not be a primary goal for counselors in correctional settings, it is worthy of the counselor's time. It can, in fact, positively impact even the "bottom line" that correctional staff are most concerned with, which is keeping the inmate out of prison after release, or at the least reducing the inmate's triggers for emotional dysregulation that can manifest in additional behavioral issues on the unit.

References

Afuape, T. (2020). Radical systemic intervention that goes to the root: Working alongside inner-city school children, linking trauma with oppression and consciousness with action. *Journal of Family Therapy, 42*(3). https://doi.org/10.1111/1467-6427.12304.

Ainsworth, M. D. S. (1979). Attachment as related to mother-infant interaction. *Advances in the Study of Behavior, 9*, 1–51. Academic Press.

Ainsworth, M. D. S., & Bell, S. M. (1970). Attachment, exploration, and separation: Illustrated by the behavior of one-year-olds in a strange situation. *Child Development, 41*, 49–67.

Ainsworth, M. D. S., Blehar, M. C., Waters, E., & Wall, S. (1978). *Patterns of attachment: A psychological study of the strange situation.* Erlbaum.

Allen, R. S., Phillips, L. L., Roff, L. L., Cavanaugh, R., & Day, L. (2008). Religiousness/spirituality and mental health among older male inmates. *Gerontologist, 48*(5), 692–697. https://doi.org/10.1093/geront/48.5.692

Behrens, K. Y., Hesse, E., & Main, M. (2007). Mothers' attachment status as determined by the adult attachment Interview predicts their 6-year-olds' reunion responses: A study conducted in Japan. *Developmental Psychology, 43*(6), 1553.

Bowlby, J. (1968). *Attachment and loss, vol. 1: Attachment.* Basic Books.

Bowlby, J. (1973). *Attachment and loss, vol. 2: Separation, anxiety, and anger.* Basic Books.

Bowlby, J. (1980). *Attachment and loss, vol. 3: Sadness and depression.* Basic Books.

Brady, K., McCauley, J., & Back, S. (2015). The comorbidity of post-traumatic stress disorder (PTSD) and substance use disorders. In N. El-Guebaly, G. Carra, & M. Galanter (Eds.), *Textbook of addiction treatment: International perspectives* (pp. 1985–2004). Springer.

Bretherton, I. (1992). The origins of Attachment Theory: John Bowlby & Mary Ainsworth. *Developmental Psychology, 28*(5), 759–775.

Bronson, J., & Berzofsky, M. (2017, June). *Indicators of mental health problems reported by prisoners and jail inmates, 2011–2012* (NCJ 250612). U.S. Department of Justice, Bureau of Justice Statistics Website. www.bjs.gov/content/pub/pdf/imhprpji1112.pdf

Carrola, P. A., Olivarez, A., & Karcher, M. J. (2016). Correctional counselor burnout: Examining burnout rates using the Counselor Burnout Inventory. *Journal of Offender Rehabilitation, 55*(3), 195–212. https://DOI.org/10.1080/10509674.2016.1149134.

Chandler, R. K., Fletcher, B. W., & Volkow, N. D. (2008). Treating drug abuse and addiction in the criminal justice system: Improving public health and safety. *Journal of the American Medical Association, 301*(2), 183–190. https:/doi.org/10.1001/jama.2008.976.

Depner, R. M., Grant, P. C., Byrwa, D. J., Breier, J. M., Lodi-Smith, J., Luczkiewicz, D. L., & Kerr, C. W. (2018). People don't understand what goes on in her: A consensual qualitative research analysis of inmate-caregiver perspectives on prison-based end-of-life care. *Palliative Medicine, 32*(5), 969–979. https://doi.org/10.1177/0269216318755624.

Ferszt, G. G. (2002). Grief experiences of women in prison following the death of a loved one. *Illness, Crisis & Loss, 10*(3), 242–254. https://doi.org/10.1177/1054137302010003005.

Field, G. (2004). Continuity of offender treatment: From the institution to the community. In K. Knight & D. Farabee (Eds.), *Treating addicted offenders: A Continuum of effective practices.* Civic Research Institute, 33-1-33-9.

Finlay, I. G., & Jones, N. K. (2000). Unresolved grief in young offenders in prison. *British Journal of General Practice, 35*, 35–42. PMID: 10954941.

Flores, P. J. (2011). *Addiction as an attachment disorder.* Jason Aronson.

Gilbert, K. R. (2007). *Unit 9—Ambiguous loss and disenfranchised grief: Grief in a family context.* http://www.indiana.edu/~famlygrf/units/ambiguous.html

Gill, R. (2014). *Addictions from an attachment perspective: Do broken bonds and early trauma lead to addictive behaviours?* The Bowlby Centre Monograph Series. Routledge.

Gorle, H. (2008). *Unit 14—Ceremonies and rituals for connection and change: Grief in a family context.* www.indiana.edu/~famlygrf/units/ceremonies.html

Green, B. L., Dass-Brailsford, P., De Mendoza, H. A., Mette, M., Lynch, S. M., DeHart, D. D., & Belknap, J. (2016). Trauma experiences and mental health among incarcerated women. *Psychological Trauma: Theory, Research, and Policy*, *8*, 455–463. https://doi.org/10.1037/tra0000113.

Harner, H. M., Hentz, P. M., & Evangelista, M. C. (2011). Grief interrupted: The experience of loss among incarcerated women. *Qualitative Health Research*, *21*(4), 454–464. https://doi.org/10.1177/1049732310373257.

Hatcher, S. S., Bride, B., Oh, H., King, D. M., & Catrett, J. F. (2011). An assessment of secondary traumatic stress in juvenile justice education workers. *Journal of Correctional Health Care*, *17*(3), 208–217. https://doi.org/10.1177/1078345811401509.

Hendry, C. (2009). Incarceration and the tasks of grief: A narrative review. *Journal of AdvancedNursing*,*65*(2),270–278.https://doi.org/10.1111/j.1365-2648.2008.04890.x

Herman, J. (2005). *Trauma and recovery*. Basic Books.

Hester, R., & Taylor, W. (2011). Responding to bereavement, grief and loss: Charting the troubled relationship between research and practice in youth offending services. *Mortality*, *16*(3), 191–203.

Hosser, D. A., Windzio, M., & Greve, W. (2008). Guilt and shame as predictors of recidivism. *Criminal Justice and Behavior*, *35*(1), 138–152.

James, R. K., & Gilliland, B. E. (2016). *Crisis intervention strategies* (8th ed.). Cengage Learning.

Jensen, E. L., Gerber, J., & Mosher, C. (2004). Social consequences of the War on Drugs: The legacy of failed policy. *Criminal Justice Policy Review*, *15*(1), 100–121. https://doi.org/10.1177/0887403403255315

Johnson, K. A., & Lynch, S. M. (2013). Predictors of maladaptive coping in incarcerated women who are survivors of child sexual abuse. *Journal of Family Violence*, *28*, 43–52. https://doi.org/10.1007/s10896-012-94888-3

Karberg, J. C., & James, D. J. (2005). *Substance dependence, abuse & treatment of jail inmates*. Office of Justice Programs, Bureau of Justice Statistics; 2002. Department of Justice publication NCJ 209588. www.bjs.gov/content/pub/pdf/sdatji02.pdf

Lansing, A. E., Plante, W. Y., Beck, A. N., & Ellenberg, M. (2018). Loss and grief among persistently delinquent youth: The contribution of adversity indicators and psychopathy-spectrum traits to broadband internalizing and externalizing psychopathology. *Journal of Child and Adolescent Trauma*, *11*, 375–389. https://doi.org/10.1007/s40653-018-0209-9

Leach, R. M., Burgess, T., & Holmwood, C. (2008). Could recidivism in prisoners be linked to traumatic grief? A review of the evidence. *International Journal of Prisoner Health*, *4*(2), 104–119. https://doi.org/10.1080/17449200802038249

Liem, M., & Kunst, M. (2013). Is there a recognizable post-incarceration syndrome among released "lifers"? *International Journal of Law and Psychiatry*, 1–5. https://doi.org/10.1016/j.ijlp.2013.04.012

Lionells, M., Fiscalini, J., Mann, C., & Stern, D. B. (2014). *Handbook of interpersonal psychoanalysis*. Routledge.

Lynch, S. M., Fritch, A. M., & Heath, N. M. (2012). Looking beneath the surface: The nature of incarcerated women's experiences of interpersonal violence, mental health, and treatment needs. *Feminist Criminology*, *7*, 381–400. https://doi.org/10.1177/1557084112439224

Maschi, T., Dennis, K. S., Gibson, S., MacMillan, T., Sternberg, S., & Hom, M. (2010). Trauma and stress among older adults in the criminal justice system: A review of the literature with implications for social work. *Journal of Gerontological Social Work*, *54*(4), 390–424. https://doi.org/10.1080/01634372.2011.552099

Morse, J. M. (2001). Toward a praxis theory of suffering. *Advances in Nursing Science*, *24*(1), 47–59. https://doi.org/10.1097/000122272-200109000-00007

Mumola, C. J., & Karberg, J. C. (2006). Drug use and dependence, state and federal prisoners, 2004. Office of Justice Programs, Bureau of Justice Statistics; 2004. Department of Justice publication NCJ 213530.

Muris, P., & Meesters, C. (2014). Small or big in the eyes of the other: On the developmental psychopathology of self-conscious emotions as shame, guilt, and pride. *Clinical Child and Family Psychological Review*, *17*, 19–40. https://doi.org/10.1007/s10567-013-0137-z

Nowotny, K. M., Belknap, J., Lynch, S., & DeHart, D. (2014). Risk profile and treatment needs of women in jail with co-occurring serious mental illness and substance use disorders. *Women & Health*, *54*, 781–795. https://doi.org/10.1080/03630242.2014.932892

Ostrom, C. W., Ostrom, B. J., & Kleinman, M. (2004, February). *Judges & discrimination: Assessing the theory and practice of criminal sentencing*. U.S. Department of Justice.

Parkes, C. M. (1998). Coping with loss: Bereavement in adult life. *British Medical Journal*, *316*, 856–859. https://doi.org/10.1136/bmj.316.7134.856

Perkins, E. B., & Sprang, G. (2012). Results from the Pro-QOL-IV for substance abuse counselors working with offenders. *International Journal of Mental Health and Addiction*, *11*(2), 199–213. https://doi.org/10.1007/s004400050120

Root, M. P. P. (2000). Rethinking racial identity development: An ecological framework. In P. Spickard & J. Burroughs (Eds.), *We are a people: Narrative and multiplicity in constructing ethnic identity* (pp. 205–220). Temple University Press.

Sabo, D., Kupers, T. A., & London, W. (2001). *Prison masculinities*. Temple University Press.

Schetky, D. (1998). Mourning in prison: Mission impossible? *Journal of the American Academy of Psychiatry and the Law*, *26*(3), 383–391.

Shivy, V. A., Wu, J. J., Moon, A. E., Mann, S. C., Holland, J. G., & Eacho, C. (2007). Ex-offenders reentering the workforce. *Journal of Counseling Psychology*, *54*(4), 466–473.

Siegel, D. J. (2020). *The developing mind* (3rd ed.). Guilford Press.

Stohr, M. K., & Hemmens, C. (2004). *The inmate prison experience*. Pearson Prentice Hall.

Taxman, F. S., Perdoni, M. L., & Harrison, L. D. (2007). Drug treatment services for adult offenders: The state of the state. *Journal of Substance Abuse Treatment*, *32*(3), 239 254.

Teyber, E., & Teyber, F. (2016). *Interpersonal process in therapy: An Integrative model* (7th ed.). Cengage Learning.

Worden, J. W. (2018). *Grief counseling and grief therapy: A handbook for the mental health practitioner*. Springer.

Young, V. C. (2003). Helping female inmates cope with grief and loss. *Corrections Today*, *65*(3), 76–79.

16 Addiction and Grief in Christianity

John C. Nance

Grief and loss are common experiences for all people, and religious faith does not prevent these experiences. Yet religion has also been identified as a protective factor in helping people live through challenging experiences (Marsiglia et al., 2005). But there are times when even those in a faith community may turn to substance use to deal with trauma. This section will describe the use of faith and religion in the therapeutic process; specifically, Christianity will be described as both faith and religion and how practitioners might utilize the beliefs of an individual in the recovery process. Every individual who has a lived experience relative to Christianity arrives in therapeutic conversation with an experience unique to their own interpretation. This section will explore the definition of Christianity and will describe the varying traditions of Christian teachings relative to substance use and grief. In addition to highlighting the protective factors for some Christians, we will also work to understand how Christian faith can negatively influence individuals as they seek comfort and peace during difficult grieving processes.

As stated, individuals come into treatment for substance use disorders (SUDs) with hugely varying differences relative to concepts of spirituality, faith, and specifically Christian faith. This section will explore how to investigate a client's experience and attitudes toward Christianity. Religion, faith, and faith communities have the capacity to assist individuals in recovery and through grief processes (Muselman & Wiggins, 2012) while they might also contribute to the pain of the grieving and torment. Therefore, we will approach the conversation around Christianity with a lens of curiosity and exploration rather than of certainty and resolve.

Christianity is the largest religion in membership around the world (Hackett & McClendon, 2017). The variances of beliefs and practices within the religion are more than a continuum or dichotomy. The faith and impact of the faith are so varying in nature, counselors must challenge their own reflex reactions charged with personal biases. The righting reflex, often described in motivational interviewing training, highlights the attempt by counselors to quickly fix client problems, which in turn inhibits client change (Rosengren, 2018). Though well intended, counselors in applying their faith perspectives may drive a wedge between the client and the help they seek. The American

DOI: 10.4324/9781003106906-16

Counseling Association code of ethics clearly states that "counselors must be aware of, and avoid imposing their own values, attitudes, beliefs, and behaviors" (American Counseling Association, 2014). This mandate highlights the need for empathic understanding relative to client religious experiences.

Basic Christian Faith Tenets

For this conversation, we will briefly and selectively describe the Christian religion. One or two paragraphs certainly will not provide enough information for practitioners to understand Christianity. As with any religion, centuries, cultures, and personal experiences impact all aspects of religious interpretation and teaching. Sects and denominations arise out of disagreement. With each group, rites, rituals, and traditions hold varying importance. Beyond this overview, further understanding will be left for the development of the therapist.

Practitioners will be challenged to explore with clients their perspectives of the faith. For practitioners who hold a Christian belief perspective, the cautions will be focused on understanding any personal biases and assumptions carried into the therapeutic relationship, remembering our perspectives are our perspectives and not those of our clients. This section will present an integral practice or ideology in the Christian faith, followed by counselor considerations and cautions. Several questions will also be presented for exploration with clients. Practitioners are encouraged to tailor the questions to their needs and client presentations.

Christianity is monotheistic in the core belief of God, meaning the focus is on one god, supreme being, or higher power. The God of Christianity is a triune god composed of God as heavenly father, God as incarnate Son (Jesus), and God as ever-present Holy Spirit. The greatest focus in Christian tenets is based on the belief in the life and teachings of Jesus of Nazareth (God as incarnate Son). His life and divinity was predicted in the Hebrew Bible and further described in later chapters of the Bible by his followers in the earliest years of the first century. Jesus's life was filled with great miracles and a path to the afterlife through believing in him as the resurrected Christ. According to the earliest accounts, Jesus led a perfect life without sin, was pursued by government and religious authorities, demonstrated complete forgiveness, and was killed as a result of supposed radical teachings. The accounts of the early Christian church describe the resurrection of Jesus from the dead, witnessed by his followers of the time.

The Bible, considered the Holy Scripture and foundational text, contains two sections, the Old and New Testaments. The Old Testament, also known as the Hebrew Bible, contains oral tradition accounts of the history of the world and the lineage of Jesus. It is filled with laws and regulations for pure and holy living in community with other believers who are instructed how to remain holy separated from the negative impacts of society. The New Testament is perceived to be the introduction to the life and teachings of Jesus as well as an account of the early Christian church. It portrays Jesus as the savior of the world with new directives for his followers to a separate life of purity while also spreading his teachings.

Accounts of Jesus's teachings and ministry involved miracles and extraordinary acts of healing, provision, and resurrection from the dead. As mentioned, the most defining miracle of note is described as Jesus's resurrection from the dead and ascension into the heavens. These descriptions are very limited and inadequate in conceptualizing the Christian religion. However, they do provide a base for understanding the importance of rites and rituals that may impact clients' perspectives and emotional experiencing relative to their faith history.

Initial Assumptions

Given the wide range of Christian beliefs, determining the client's view on the role of faith, belief, and personal responsibility in guiding their life is important. This faith brings with it varying understandings of how much God intervenes in daily life. Often the phrase "It must be God's will" is used as a reason or divine intention for a negative event. Belief that God is in control of all things often indicates a client who maintains an external locus of control, which may leave them feeling helpless and devoid of responsibility for what happened and future outcomes. The client may believe they must then trust God to take away their pain or intervene in the situation. This perspective may be expressed as "putting it in God's hands" or "turning over to God." Support groups and even ministers may support this view by encouraging the individual to "pray harder" or believe more strongly as a way of solving the issue. While prayer provides great comfort and encouragement for many, others may leave feeling abandoned by their faith.

Faith is one component of intersectional identity and unique to each individual. Faith and religion are powerful motivators throughout life for many individuals. Each Christian believer is unique and holds their own understanding of the religion, faith, and application of the faith. Many hold their Christian faith close throughout life, whereas others experience Christianity as judgmental and a source of pain. Because the Christian church is extremely diverse in belief and approach to the tenets of the faith, practitioners can aid their clients in describing each individual perspective—even as far as how the client perceives the gender of God. Some view God as very gender specific: Father, Heavenly Father, Loving Father, and male in all forms. Although the believer may not describe God as male, it might be helpful to listen for the perspective of the client as they describe their higher power. Practitioners are cautioned to explore their own biases and assumptions relative to their faith and spiritual perspective, being careful not to project into the client's faith world an image of God that we as clinicians create.

Initial Intake and Assessment

Because of vast differences among Christian beliefs, intentional focus must be placed on intake and assessment. As clients enter into therapy for grief and substance use concerns, it is critical for counselors to understand client perspectives on faith and spirituality. Most wellness models incorporate spirituality as a key component among areas of focus. Faith and spirituality are often utilized in coping as well as an integral part of personal identity. A time line of faith development might be useful in understanding a client's view regarding positive or negative faith histories.

For many, concepts of faith, religion, and Christian beliefs may hold deeply painful histories. For the marginalized, the messages of repentance, turning from sin, and righteous living are sources of shame, guilt, and negative self-talk. Throughout this section on Christian perspective of grief and addiction, one must approach clients through a trauma-informed lens, believing the client at some point may have been exposed to distortions of control through faith and beliefs. Clients may push conversations of faith away as a result. This does not necessarily mean they will not return to the conversation in their own healing process. However, clients may need to identify and challenge the early messages and understand the implications on current life.

Christianity, like many faiths, can be very helpful for individuals' healthy living. Spirituality is a critical component of the wellness models. However, clinicians should hold a discerning stance, listening for differences between spirituality, faith, religion, and religiosity. Although Christianity may be helpful or hurtful, counselors may benefit the client by discovering the positive and negative aspects of their faith and faith journey. This will allow clients to retain and incorporate aspects of faith useful in their recovery. It will also provide potential abilities to discern and explore faith in new, autonomous ways.

Grief, Loss, and Christianity

Descriptions of loss are found throughout the Bible as well as solace for the dying and those in bereavement. The book of Ecclesiastes describes how everything has a season and includes a time to weep and a time to mourn (English Standard Version Bible, 2001, Ecclesiastes 3). Christians believe in an afterlife positioned and inhabited by God, offered to those who identify as followers of Jesus the Christ. Grieving clients often present with questions relative to the future and afterlife. Language may reflect ideas of passing over and into the afterlife with hope to reunite someday. Specific scriptures carry with them the opportunity for solace. Scripture passages like "Fear not, for I am with you; be not dismayed, for I am your God" (English Standard Version Bible, 2001, Isaiah 41:10), "Be still and know that I am God" (English Standard Version Bible, 2001, Psalm 46:10), along with many others may be comforting for many believers.

Counselors are encouraged to approach use of scripture with caution and discernment, as the messages also bear the potential for retraumatization. Scripture passages used to console individuals may contain mixed messages. For individuals with traumatic experiences, the passage might carry with it a foreign concept. Peacefulness and calmness may never be perceived options.

With trauma, the activated brain may perceive quiet reflection as dangerous and foreboding.

Types of losses are critical to consider, as clients present with different faith histories and different emotional experiences. There are too many types and specific losses to address in this short section relative to Christianity, substance abuse, and grief. However, a few notable losses relative to faith practices might include divorce, death of a loved one (specifically a child), natural disasters, previous disavowing faith and faith communities, moral injury (i.e., military combat veterans), survivors and loss of abusers, or rejection by faith communities (i.e., LGBTQII individuals). Even the loss of substance use can cause distress and be treatable through faith considerations. Clients who work to make meaning of their losses may seek to understand the loss relative to their faith. This search can involve a crisis of faith filled with questions of "Why?" and "Where is God in all of this?" All of these losses and others are very complex in nature and cannot necessarily be treated easily and rapidly with faith practices.

Alcohol Use in the Christian Community

Christian teachings regarding consumption of alcohol and substances vary greatly with confusing messages, which range from supporting moderate consumption to requiring complete abstinence. Based upon the interpretation of the messages, clients are likely to hear opposing perspectives. Reportedly, Jesus's first miracle was performed at a wedding where he turned water into wine. There are many interpretations regarding consumption of alcohol through Christian communities and are often confusing to individual believers. The New Testament describes consuming alcohol within limits. Many times, the instruction and application of church teachings places extreme judgment and negative messages on consuming alcohol in any amount.

Concepts for Exploration

One of the drivers for substance use and abuse is the concept of shame and guilt (Dearling et al., 2005). How one perceives their role in relation to others is often laced with motivations built on shaming and guilting messages (Lund, 2017). The cognitive distortions of shoulds, oughts, and musts are examples of the guilting reflexes we feel through our own self-talk. The interpretation of scripture and the application of those teachings often lend to this type of negative self-talk. Within Christian faith-based treatment for SUD is a sin model, which emphasizes moral and personal responsibility for disobeying God. This type of cognitive processing has the potential to add to distorted thinking based in shame, guilt, and self-loathing (Sneed et al., 2019).

Several faith expressions are important to note when working with Christian clients. Throughout the teachings of the Bible as well as in current church teachings, forgiveness, sin, repentance, and trust are notable ideas utilized to bring individuals into a closer relationship with God. These concepts are introduced to individuals in order to assist them in an understanding of why Jesus would live among people, die, and then miraculously resurrect from the dead. These basic principles will be briefly described below.

Once again, the Christian church holds widely varying beliefs about the nature of people. Many believe people are "born into sin" based upon the original sin of the earliest of earth's inhabitants and therefore sin is generational and inescapable. Without believing in God, Jesus, and the Holy Spirit, this tenet holds individuals in an inescapable trajectory toward an eternal damnation in the afterlife. Though harsh, this concept permeates the Christian church and regular teachings and interpretations.

Therefore, repentance and trust are important concepts for Christians. The process of acknowledging sin and turning life over to the care of God is critical in the health of a Christian life. Most 12-step programs involve repentance and trust in some form: with that, trust in God and the teachings of the Bible are critical concepts for Christians as they approach life, healing, and restoration. Christians believe in trusting God and turning their lives over to the care of God. Often Christians daily practice the admission of sins and the desire for a life that is more representative of the life lived by Jesus. This desire assists the believer in challenging their hurt and pain to become more whole and healthy in perspective and actions.

Many times, shame and guilt accompany believers as they believe they fail on many fronts. The internal processing of each individual may hold lifelong distortions, which permeate old understandings introduced early in life, or they may be new understandings provided by well-intended believers. Helpful interventions would focus on distorted thought processes characterized by overemphasis on external locus of control as well as those distortions that expose the negative self-talk. Christian clients benefit by learning new areas in which they have control and autonomy.

Another potentially difficult concept for recovering Christian clients is that of forgiveness. Found throughout Christian teachings, the concept of forgiveness carries weight that can be healing and useful. The idea is for individuals to understand the pain they experienced from others or caused for other people and move toward absolving or pardoning the offenses. Many treatment processes and especially 12-step programs hold forgiveness in high importance. Making amends involves taking inventory and, for many, the action of forgiving.

Careful and intentional introduction of the concept is encouraged. As forgiveness may benefit recovery, there exists the potential for intense negative ramifications for trauma survivors. Forgiveness may be a very painful process, which may lead to traumatic reexperiencing or abreaction. To imagine forgiving an abuser or multiple abusers is a concept we as practitioners should use with extreme caution. Clients with trauma histories will need to process through their histories in some way at their pace without the expectation of a perfect and immediate forgiving expression. Conceptually, clients may benefit from the concept of self-forgiveness before wrestling with the idea and task of forgiving others (Hall et al., 2005).

Christians are encouraged to approach God through prayer and meditation. As with many religions, prayer is a means of communication with the Higher Power. Christians differ in their concepts regarding prayer. Some believe they must approach their Higher Power in a repentant mindset with humility and fear. Others approach prayer with confident assurance that their higher power is approachable, gentle, and deeply compassionate.

Prayer may be introduced as mindfulness or meditation practices. Clients are often encouraged to practice mindfulness and centering as they work through emotional awareness. Grounding exercises are central to many therapeutic interventions. Prayer may be particularly useful for Christians as they learn to process through grief and loss.

Prayer can be a difficult concept as clients bring into the therapeutic relationship an array of potentially negative concepts. Critical to working with Christian clients is the exploration of prayer as useful or prayer as a negative imposition in their past. Practitioners are encouraged to understand their concepts and specific wording in prayer with caution relative to the use of "Father" and the phrase "In the name of Jesus Christ." Again, because the Christian faith is so diverse, what is practiced in one Christian circle is not necessarily how others view the faith. Some Christians may view concepts of meditation as originating in other faith communities and will steer clear of the practice and find offense in the concept.

Often the concept of miracles permeates client faith expectations as they pray for healing and health. Because the entire premise of the Christian faith relies on the concept of miracles, believers often hope in miracles throughout their faith practices. Many Christian communities pray for miraculous healing. However, most individuals in recovery with SUDs and grief processes find miracles evasive. Prayers of the recovering Christian may reflect hope and reliance on God to provide the miracle of healthy living. The external locus of control is often evident in relinquishing individual responsibility in sober living and memorializing practices through grief. Processing through grief without evidence of miracles might include self-shame, as historical religious practices and teachings would lay blame on the believer as a lack of faith or strong adherence to rites and rituals.

Reconceptualizing or reframing the client's understanding of miracles might be a helpful process. Miracles may be perceived from a dichotomous perspective—either there is a perfect miracle of healing and restoration, or there is no miracle and the client is left wondering what has happened. Counselors can help clients look toward their abilities and growth processes as miraculous in their own right. The same as the development of a child is perceived as miraculous by many Christians, the growth of the client through the grief, loss, and addiction may be viewed similarly.

Throughout this section, counselors are continuously cautioned to approach clients with discernment from an empathic and exploratory perspective.

Counselors are encouraged to understand their own beliefs, assumptions, and faith perspectives. The American Counseling Association code of ethics mandates that counselors know and avoid imposing their own values, attitudes, beliefs, and behaviors (American Counseling Association, 2014). The following section provides sample questions to assist clinicians in their approach to concepts of Christianity, religion, and faith as they work with grieving clients. These examples are guides meant to steer clinicians as they broach a very complicated part of client identity.

Sample Questions

Intake Questions

Initially, how does faith and religion play out in your world?

Do you find comfort or discomfort when you think about religion and spirituality?

Tell me about your faith history.

Is faith something that would help you as we talk about coping strategies?

Perspectives on Substance Use Questions

What have you believed about alcohol and other substances throughout your life?

How do shame and guilt influence the client's experience with substances?

If shaming and guilt are part of the client's internal processing, what messages from faith communities impact their emotions and their understanding of God?

Questions Regarding Client's Perspective of God

What do you believe about God?

What do you believe related to how God works in the world and specifically in your life?

Does the client demonstrate an internal or external locus of control? To what extent does the client take responsibility for recovery, healing, and well-being? Does the client express their own need for action and work or are they relying on God to take control over all aspects of their situations?

Questions of Practice and Spiritual Expression

Have you ever used prayer as a part of your faith practices?

What has been useful for you as you think about prayer and your faith?

I wonder if prayer and meditation might be a part of your recovery and how we might use the practice to assist your healing.

References

American Counseling Association. (2014). *2014 ACA code of ethics*. www.counseling. org/docs/default-source/default-document-library/2014-code-of-ethics-finaladdress. pdf

Dearling, R. L., Stuewig, J., & Tangney, J. P. (2005). On the importance of distinguishing shame from guilt: Relations to problematic alcohol and drug use. *Addictive Behaviors, 30*(7), 1392–1404. https://https://doi.org/10.1016/j.addbeh.2005.02.002

English Standard Version Bible. (2001). ESV online. https://esv.literalword.com/

Hackett, C., & McClendon, D. (2017). Christians remain world's largest religious group, but they are declining in Europe. *Pew Research Center*. www.pewresearch.org/fact-tank/2017/04/05/christians-remain-worlds-largest-religious-group-but-they-are-declining-in-europe/

Hall, J. H., & Fincham, F. D. (2005). Self-forgiveness: The stepchild of forgiveness research. *Journal of Social and Clinical Psychology, 24*(5), 621–637. https://https://doi.org/10.1521/jscp.2005.24.5.621

Lund, P. (2017). Christian faith and recovery from substance abuse, guilt, and shame. *Journal of Religion & Spirituality in Social Work: Social Thought, 36*(3), 346–366.

Marsiglia, F., Parsai, M., Kulis, S., & Nieri, T. (2005). God Forbid! Substance use among religious and nonreligious youth. *American Journal of Orthopsychiatry, 75*(4), 585–598. https://doi.org/10.1037/0002-9432.75.4.585

Muselman, D., & Wiggins, M. (2012). Spirituality and loss: Approaches for counseling grieving adolescents. *Counseling and Values, 57*(2), 229–240. https://doi.org/10.1002/j.2161-007X.2012.00019.x

Rosengren, D. B. (2018). *Building motivational interviewing skills: A practitioner workbook* (2nd ed.). Guilford Press.

Sneed, K. J., Pittman, J., & Jaillet Keane, D. L. (2019). Social work, Christianity, and addictions: Relationships with God, others, and ourselves. *Social Work & Christianity, 46*(3), 3–6.

17 Grief and Substance Use in Hindu Communities

Sejal Foxx

The 1965 Immigration and Nationality Act invited immigrants with professional backgrounds into the United States. This act opened the doors for those from India to enter into the country. Their arrival brought diverse Hindu rituals, traditions, temples, and religious altars (Harvard University, n.d.). There are about 1.2 billion Hindus worldwide and, although the Census Bureau does not collect data on religion, there are an estimated 1.8 million Hindus living in the United States. That number is expected to increase to 4.8 million by 2050, making the United States the fifth-largest Hindu population in the world (Pew Research Center, 2021). The increase in the U.S. Hindu population has implications for counselors to understand the background of the religion, particularly as it pertains to grief and substance use.

Background of Hinduism

Hinduism predates recorded history and is the oldest practiced religion in the world. It is important to note that Hinduism does not have one core doctrine. Rather, is it about morals, ethics, and a way of life (Radhakrishnan, 1922). It is described more as an ethos than a set of beliefs, thus making it difficult to view the Hindu religion through a monolithic lens (Gupta, 2011). For example, the diversity and plurality within Hinduism can manifest through the worship of deities such as Krishna, Rama, Sita, Vishnu, Shiva, and Ganesh. Although there are many representations, there is only one Reality, *Brahman*, which is infinite and takes multiple forms (Gupta, 2011; Harvard University, n.d.). This one Reality is guided by the Vedas, which are the most ancient scriptures in the world. The Vedas are the wisdom of the ancient sages passed down orally and over generations by Brahmin priests (B. Parikh, personal communication, May 17, 2021).

Hindus are guided by four aims of human life. The first is *Dharma*, or moral law and duty. It is about virtuous and ideal behavior. It is one's purpose in life and being awake to the divine existence within oneself. This is the spiritual path the leads to God. The second is *Artha*, which is wealth and prosperity. It includes everything that allows you to live a fulfilling life and have the means to achieve it. However, one must not stray from *Dharma* to obtain material

DOI: 10.4324/9781003106906-17

things. The third is *Kama*, or experiencing the pleasures of life. Again, *Kama* should not be pursued without the presence of *Dharma*. The fourth and final meaning of life is *Moksha*, or nirvana. It is emancipation, enlightenment, freedom from reincarnation, self-realization, and, at last, unity with God. Hindus believe that *Moksha* may take several lifetimes, or reincarnations, before being achieved (B. Parikh, personal communication, May 17, 2021).

One common Hindu belief that is found in mainstream Western culture is the idea of *Karma*. However, it is often misused or misinterpreted, as it is usually viewed in the context of luck. However, *Karma* is action or work on behalf of others. It is the idea that past and present actions will determine the future. This future may not be in the current lifetime but in future reincarnations as well. Those who live by *Dharma*, a truthful and ethical life, are rewarded and those who do not live life by those principles will receive the opposite (Gupta, 2011). Thus, *Karma* is understanding that actions have consequences and that one has the ability to shape their destiny. It provides for human agency, free will, and hope for a better future.

These ideas are only a fraction of what encompasses Hinduism. Like other religions, there are rituals, ways of prayer and worship, and each is experienced uniquely based on the region of India where one is from, one's village, one's family, and one's own personal beliefs and relationship with God. Therefore, readers of this chapter are asked to do more research and gain deeper knowledge of Hinduism and its plurality to have a better understanding of application with clients. Unfortunately, counseling research and literature related to mental health and Hindus is sparse. Thus, the information related to substance abuse and grief presented in this chapter is adapted from other disciplines and should be used as an overview highlighting considerations rather than a defined set of practices that are directly applied.

Grief, Beliefs, and Rituals

Most Hindus choose cremation for their deceased, and it is completed within 24 hours of death (Gupta, 2011). Prior to cremation, there are rituals that are followed. First, when possible, the body is washed using holy water. This is typically from the Ganges River. After cremation, rituals related to mourning take anywhere from 10 days to two weeks. The house is cleansed and social visits are avoided. During the period of mourning, overexpression of grief is appropriate. However, it is not uncommon for loved ones to express happy emotions in efforts to celebrate one's life. Once the funeral and cremation are complete, ashes are gathered and spread in a body of water, with the preference being the Ganges River. Anniversaries are marked one month and each year after one's death. Long-term bereavement is acceptable in Hinduism; however, excessive displays of grief are not encouraged, as the religion has an acceptance of death (Bhuvaneswar & Stern, 2012).

There are common beliefs related to death that have an impact on the grief process. First, Hindus believe that death is a part of life, and that after death the body serves no purpose. Rather, *Atman*, or the soul, changes bodies through reincarnation. There are "good" and "bad" deaths. Good deaths are when loved ones are prepared, the individual has not suffered, and goodbyes are able to be shared. Bad deaths are suicide, sudden, or traumatic. The "good" or "bad" death is related to *Karma* (Gupta, 2011).

Rituals

Studies have shown that rituals have been associated with positive outcomes such as resilience and coping (Hodge, 2004). There are post-death rituals that families may follow. First, after the death of a loved one, the family will enter into 10–13 days of mourning. During this period, an oil lamp is lit and it is a time is for prayer and meditation, which facilitates the soul's departure from this world to the next. On the 13th day of mourning, it is common for the grieving family to hold a ceremony to help release the soul of the deceased for reincarnation. This period of mourning may be less in the United States, and it is important to note that rituals such as eulogies, embalming, and use of funeral homes are also a variation from the traditional rituals in India (Gupta, 2011). Finally, on the first anniversary of the death, the family will host a memorial event that honors the life of their loved one.

Integration in Counseling

In terms of factors to include for counseling, one may need to consider if the client is a first- or second-generation American to get a sense of the level of acculturation. Gupta's (2011) qualitative study exploring Asian Indian Americans' perspectives on death yielded varied ideas based on generational differences. The differences highlight the need for counselors to ascertain the family's rituals that are most salient. Gupta (2011) also recommends that service providers consider the collectivist nature of the Indian culture. It is not uncommon for family and friends to want to say goodbye to the dying. There is also an interconnectedness between generations, and the elderly often rely on the eldest male adult in the family to lead the ceremonies and rituals. Service providers should also explore to what extent those grieving believe in *Dharma* and *Atman*. These laws of life may be used to help clients process what happens after death and progress through the grief stages.

Substance Use Disorder Among Hindus

Similar to research related to grief processing among Hindus, research is also lacking regarding substance use. This section draws from the limited research and literature that does exist as well and personal experiences from the author. Thus, readers are cautioned not to apply blanket assumptions, given the Hindu population is very diverse in beliefs and adherence to religious guidance and principles.

In a quantitative study of 16,596 respondents of a Canadian survey regarding drinking and religion, researchers found religious beliefs influence attitudes toward alcohol. "Christian denominations for the most part drink at similar nonsignificantly different rates from the non-religious/Atheist, while minority religions and those who prohibit or generally suggest abstention are less likely to report risk drinking" (Tuck et al., 2017, p. 2031). However, factors such as acculturation, migration, and social status can shape drinking behavior. For example, a study exploring immigration and ethnicity indicated populations with traditionally low-risk drinkers began to see heavier drinking the longer one resided in the Canada (Agic et al., 2016). Thus, for this chapter, counselors ought to consider the extent that one is acculturated to U.S. culture.

From a historical perspective, Hinduism has had an ancient history with the association of drugs, likely plants, to create hallucinations. The drug known as *Soma*, according to the Vedas, was used to bring visions, to alleviate physical pain, and to heal disease. However, in modern times, the use of *Soma* has greatly declined and abstinence is preached. Most Hindus are vegetarian and abstain from alcohol and drugs. However, similar to other religions, there is a variation as to the extent to which individuals adhere to a strict way of life. Just as some Hindus eat meat, others partake in alcohol consumption. However, the extent to one consumes alcohol may be too indulgent, thus impeding the process to achieve *Moksha*.

Integration in Counseling

In a qualitative study comparing recovery from drinking among South Asian men and White members of Alcoholics Anonymous (AA), findings indicated that spirituality and religion played an important role. Specifically, South Asian men viewed recovery as a dimension of their spirituality. *Karma* was also a salient concept, however, it was viewed more as fatalistic rather than a source of hope for the future. Overall, recovery for the South Asian men was based on more religious concepts than those attending AA. The authors noted that the participants relied heavily on the temple for a source of support (Morjaria & Orford, 2009).

First, as noted previously, one should consider the level of acculturation and ethnic and religious identity of the client. As many Hindus have a collectivist identity, theories that integrate family systems may be useful in treatment. Use of substances may bring shame and guilt to the family and could cause further anxiety, depression, or feelings of isolation (Rastogi & Wadhwa, 2006). With permission of the client, counselors may seek consultation from priests of Hindu temples to consider systems of support and strategies for intervention. South Asians are more likely to be in recovery when reaffiliated with the religion. The following sections highlight Hindu beliefs that may impede or support addicted clients.

First, most Hindus believe in *Karma* and reincarnation. Through the accumulation of good *Karma*, Hindus seek to transcend to *Moksha*. Although

Hinduism does not speak directly to the use of substances, the laws of life need to be considered, as individuals seek to obtain eventual transcendence or freedom. Thus, counselors should consider to which extent clients and their families believe in the four aims of life: *Dharma, Atma, Kama*, and *Moksha*. These laws give guidance as to how one should live their life. If one is abusing substances, and that use creates negative actions to self and/or others, there will be negative *Karma*.

As a case illustration, if a Hindu individual entered counseling for the abuse of alcohol, drugs, or gambling, then the counselor might want to consider many factors. First, to what extent does the client practice and believe in the Hindu religion? Second, to what extent is the individual acculturated to the American culture? Are collectivist values central to the client? If so, the family should be included to help support the path to healing. It would be prudent to get a sense of how much one is connected to the religion before using strategies for intervention.

Meditation and yoga could also be used to support Hindu clients. The ancient Hindu philosophy of yoga is based on ethical disciplines, individual observances, posture, breath control, withdrawal of senses, concentration, meditation, and enlightenment. Contrary to Western views of yoga, it is more than posing and meditation. The eight practices are principles for living a meaningful life that is based on morals, ethics, and self-discipline. Practicing yoga has been shown to support treatment, recovery, and prevention (Khanna & Greeson, 2013). Counselors are encouraged to research the true origins and practices of yoga before implementing it in practice.

References

Agic, B., Mann, R. E., Tuck, A., Ialomiteanu, A., Bondy, S., Simich, L., et al. (2016). Alcohol use among immigrants in Ontario, Canada. *Drug and Alcohol Review, 35*(2), 163–205. https://doi.org/10.1111/dar.12250

Bhuvaneswar, C. G., & Stern, T. A. (2012). Teaching cross-cultural aspects of mourning: A Hindu perspective on death and dying. *Palliative & Supportive Care, 11*(1), 79–84. https://doi.org/10.1017/S1478951512000946

Gupta, R. (2011). Death beliefs and practices from an Asian Indian American Hindu perspective. *Death Studies, 35*(3), 244–266. https://doi.org/10.1080/07481187.2010.518420

Harvard University. (n.d.). *The pluralism project*. https://pluralism.org/hinduism

Hodge, D. R. (2004). Working with Hindu clients in a spiritually sensitive manner. *Social Work, 49*(1), 27–38. https://doi.org/10.1093/sw/49.1.27

Khanna, S., & Greeson, J. (2013). A narrative review of yoga and mindfulness as complementary therapies for addiction. *Complementary Therapies in Medicine, 21*(3), 244–252. https://doi.org/10.1016/j.ctim.2013.01.008

Morjaria, A., & Orford, J. (2009). The role of religion and spirituality in recovery from drink problems: A qualitative study of alcoholics anonymous members and South Asian men. *Addiction Research & Theory, 10*, 225–256.

Pew Research Center. (2021). *The future of world religions: Population growth projections, 2010–2050*. www.pewforum.org/2015/04/02/religious-projections-2010-2050/

Radhakrishnan, S. (1922). The Hindu dharma. *International Journal of Ethics*, *33*(1), 1–22. www.jstor.org/stable/2377174

Rastogi, M., & Wadhwa, S. (2006). Substance abuse among Asian Indians in the United States: A consideration of cultural factors in etiology and Treatment. *Substance Use & Misuse*, *41*(9), 1239–1249. https://doi.org/10.1080/10826080600754470

Tuck, A., Robinson, M., Agic, B., Ialomiteanu, A., & Mann, R. (2017). Religion, alcohol use and risk drinking among Canadian adults living in Ontario. *Journal of Religion and Health*, *56*(6), 2023–2038. https://doi.org/10.1007/s10943-016-0339-z

18 Addiction and Grief in Islam

Tahsin Ilhan

Loss and grief are among the most painful experiences for all people. Loss is a multidimensional phenomenon that occurs not only with the death of a loved one but also when people are deprived of their possessions or things they have been looking forward to having. We also can see it as a loss in individuals when one has to leave their home country and experiences loss of identity or loss of face due to the effect of acculturation while living as a minority in another country (Arredondo-Dowd, 1981; Leong et al., 2011).

In addition, the exclusion of a person by the community due to substance abuse and loss of reputation often occurs when social norms are intertwined with a community's religious beliefs. This situation is particularly common in Muslim societies where alcohol and drugs are forbidden in the Quran, and using them is considered a sin. For this reason, people who abuse substances in Muslim societies may face different types of losses, such as social exclusion, stigma, and loss of identity.

In this chapter, I provide an overview of the demographic structure of Muslims, the prevalence of substance abuse among them, and the risks and protective factors affecting substance abuse. Then, I focus on what we need to consider when working with clients of Muslim origin who are substance abusers. Having this understanding can help clinicians provide culturally sensitive resources.

Overview of Muslim Populations

Islam is the second-largest religion in the world after Christianity, with approximately 1.8 billion believers. Although Islam, like Christianity and Judaism, emerged in the Middle East, today the population of Muslims living in this region and North Africa makes up approximately 20% of the total Muslim population. The majority of the remaining population (about 62%) lives in countries such as Indonesia, India, Pakistan, Bangladesh, Iran, and Turkey in the Asia-Pacific region, while 15% live in sub-Saharan Africa, 2.7% in Europe, and 0.3% in the North and South American continent (Pew Research Center, 2019). However, the demographic structure changes frequently due to globalization and unemployment, inequality of opportunity, war, and political reasons.

DOI: 10.4324/9781003106906-18

As a result of immigration to the West from regions where Muslims are densely populated, the Muslim population has been increasing dramatically, especially in the United States, Canada, Australia, and Europe. From this movement, Islam has become the second-largest religion in many countries of Europe and ranks third in the United States. It is estimated the Muslim population of 3.45 million people living in the United States will reach 8.1 million in 2050 and therefore be the second-largest religious group, thereby making up 2.1% of the total population of the country (Pew Research Center, 2018).

In fact, all these numbers tell us something important: if the estimates about population statistics are correct, the weight of Muslims in the multicultural structure of the Western world will increase and become a permanent part of the West. Of course, we know based on years of experience this integration will not be easy for both cultures. However, we need to develop more effective methods to solve the escalating psychological problems that arise as a reflection of the adaptation problems of second- and third-generation Muslims. For this reason, it becomes even more important for mental health professionals to take into account their culture-specific dynamics and protective factors in addition to universal intervention methods when working with clients from the Muslim culture and their families.

Substance Abuse

Substance abuse is one of the most important problems threatening the future of societies. According to the United Nations Office on Drugs and Crime (UNODC) World Drug Report (2020), the number of people using illicit drugs increased from 210 million to 260 million between 2009 and 2018. Approximately 35.6 million of these people (0.7% of the adult population) suffer from substance use disorders. Cannabis is the most commonly abused illicit drug (about 192 million people), followed by opioids, amphetamines, prescription stimulants, ecstasy, and cocaine, respectively. Alcohol consumption is also on the increase. According to the World Health Organization's (WHO) Global Status Report on Alcohol and Health (2019), in the last 12 months, 43% (2.348 billion) of the population aged 15 and over were current drinkers; the highest rates were found in the European region (59.9%), the region of the Americas (54.1%), and the Western Pacific region (53.8%). The amount of pure alcohol consumption per capita increased from 5.5 liters in 2005 to 6.4 liters in 2016. In the same report, it was stated the highest alcohol consumption was in Europe (with 9.8 liters), and the population "with the lowest per capita consumption (less than 2.5 liters) lives in the WHO Eastern Mediterranean Region or in other Muslim-majority countries" (WHO, 2019, p. 41).

Perspectives on Alcohol and Drug Addiction in Islam

The prohibition on alcohol in Islam took place in three stages and within 17 years due to the educational background and deep-rooted customs of the

Arab society at that time. In the first verse about alcohol, the harms of alcohol are mentioned (verse 219 of Surah Al-Baqara), and the second verse orders not to approach prayer until one is conscious enough to know what one is saying while drunk (verse 43 of Surah An-Nisa). With the following verses in the 17th year following the birth of Islam, alcohol was completely prohibited:

> You who believe, intoxicants (khamr) and gambling, idolatrous practices, and (divining with) arrows are repugnant acts—Satan's doing—shun them so that you may prosper. With intoxicants and gambling, Satan seeks only to incite enmity and hatred among you, and to prevent you from remembering God and prayer. Will you not give them up?
>
> ([Abdel Haleem, 2005] Maida, 90–91)

Because substances such as drugs were not used in the early periods of Islam and in the geography where Arabs lived, it is accepted that the verses in the Surah al-Maida are only about alcohol. However, later on, it was debated among Islamic scholars of the period whether the similar ban included drugs and their derivatives together with the abuse of these substances in Muslims. As a result, the idea that the word intoxicant (*khamr*) mentioned in the verses 90–91 of the Surah Al-Maida is an umbrella concept that includes all kinds of intoxicating substances, and using drugs should therefore be considered *haram* (forbidden; Ali, 2014). On the other hand, there are those who argue that smoking and chewing khat (the leaves of *Catha edulis* Forsk) are in a similar category and should be regarded as haram (Juni, 2014), and there are those who argue that they are halal (permissible) or detested or discouraged (Douglas & Hersi, 2010). Therefore, sensitivity to alcohol and drugs among Muslims does not apply to smoking and khat. This is especially evident in smoking rates (World Health Organization, 2019).

Prevalence of Substance Abuse Among Muslim Populations

According to the WHO's *Global Status Reports on Alcohol* (2019), the consumption of pure alcohol per capita in 2016 in 40 majority Muslim countries, which are also members of the Organization of Islamic Cooperation, is 1.73 liters, which is well below the world average. In addition, the alcohol consumption rate of individuals over the age of 15 was also very low in these countries. For example, the rate of alcohol use in the past 12 months was 22.7% in Indonesia, 6.9% in Turkey, 2.8% in Egypt, 1.2% in Pakistan, and 0.9% in Algeria. On the other hand, although these figures look very promising at first glance, it would not be fair to reach a conclusion by just looking at the total alcohol consumption rates in Muslim-majority countries. The rate of individuals who have never consumed alcohol in these countries reaches up to 97% because the Quran strictly prohibits alcohol (Peacock et al., 2018). Therefore, it would be more appropriate to focus individual consumption of alcohol by those who do drink alcohol. Otherwise, the fact that alcohol is a risk factor for individuals living in these countries would be ignored. Those who do drink alcohol are consuming at levels similar or higher to Western countries. For example, in Turkey, per capita alcohol consumption is 2 liters, but with over 89% of the population abstaining from alcohol use, per capita consumption is 28.5 liters for those who do drink alcohol (WHO, 2019).

It is important to look at the data of three countries for a better understanding of the subject. According to the WHO Global Status Report on Alcohol and Health (2019), although the percentage of current drinkers in Indonesia is considerably higher than the percentage of current users in Algeria and Turkey, pure alcohol consumption per capita is 3.4 liters in Indonesia, 29.1 liters in Algeria, and 28.5 liters in Turkey. The prevalence of alcohol use disorders and alcohol addiction is 0.8% in Indonesia and Algeria and 8.1% in Turkey, which is almost the average of the European region, which is 8.8%. Of the three countries compared, the status of Algeria is quite interesting, because alcohol consumption per capita is less than 1 liter, but for those who drink, they consume an average of 29.1 liters; however, only 0.8% report an alcohol use disorder. The two most important reasons for this discrepancy may be (a) hesitation to seek for treatment for alcohol addiction due to concerns for stigma and social exclusion and (b) the low reliability of statistics on alcohol addiction. Obviously, this discrepancy in numbers applies to many Muslim-majority countries, such as Iran, Afghanistan, Pakistan, and Morocco.

So far, the focus has been on the prevalence of substance abuse in predominantly Muslim countries. Now we will look at the situation of Muslims living as a minority in Western countries regarding substance abuse. In a study conducted to compare the prevalence of substance abuse in the general Finnish population with the immigrant (Russian, Kurdish, Somali) population that came to Finland, the lowest rate of binge drinking ($\geq$5 drinks on one occasion) was found in Muslim-origin Somali and Kurdish populations (Salama et al., 2018). The study also reported the prevalence of cannabis use in the Kurdish population was very low compared to the Russian population, while there was no cannabis use in the Somali and Finnish populations. In a study conducted in Ontario, Canada (Tuck et al., 2017), it was found that 95% of the participants belonging to different faith groups (e.g., Lutheran, Anglican, Presbyterian, no religion/atheist, United Church of Canada, Roman Catholic, and Jewish) drank alcohol at least once in their lifetime, but this rate was 42.6% among Muslims. A similar situation applies to current drinking and binge drinking rates, as well. Of the Muslim participants, 27.42% stated that they consumed alcohol in the last 12 months, and 11.8% reported they consumed alcohol at a risky rate. Similar findings regarding substance abuse rates apply to Arab Americans living in the United States. According to the 2002–2008 data of the National Survey on drug use (cited in Arfken et al., 2011), lifetime alcohol use by Arab Americans was 50.8%, alcohol use in the last month was 26.4%, and binge drinking in the last month was 10%. Although these rates were considerably higher compared to countries with predominantly Muslim populations, they are lower compared to the rates of the general U.S. population.

In studies conducted with samples of Muslim adolescents and emerging adults, it has been found that although the rates of substance abuse among them are lower than other reference groups, they use substances more than adults do. This applies to countries where Muslims live as a minority or a majority. On the other hand, it has been reported in comparative studies (Badr et al., 2014; Helmer et al., 2014) that adolescents of Muslim origin use substances less than similar age groups of other ethnicities. In a study of a large population ($n = 44,610$) of ninth-grade students from 21 different ethnic backgrounds in Germany (Donath et al., 2011), the prevalence of lifetime alcohol use was lower in those with Muslim origin than adolescents of other backgrounds except for Iran; yet, these rates were found to vary between 60% and 33.5%. Similarly, binge drinking rates in the last 30 days were lower in adolescents of Islamic origin compared to adolescents of North American and Western European descent, with rates ranging from 40.8% (Iran) to 11.3% (Lebanon). In another study (Bradby & Williams, 2006) comparing the substance abuse prevalence of Asian and non-Asian high school students in Glasgow and Scotland, it was found Muslim students used substances less than other students (e.g., Sikh, Hindu, Christian).

A limited number of studies conducted among a minority population of Muslim-origin university students living in Western countries has shown the prevalence of substance abuse is lower than that of other students. In a study using the 2001 database of Harvard School of Public Health College Alcohol Study (CAS; Ahmed et al., 2014), the prevalence of substance abuse among Muslim students in the last year was reported to be 46.6% for alcohol and 24.6% for illicit drugs. In another study covering only one university, much lower rates of alcohol use (9%) among Muslim students were reported (Arfken et al., 2013). This surprising finding is quite unexpected, because it is lower than or close to the rates of use among university students in Muslim-majority countries.

Risk and Protective Factors of Substance Abuse Among Muslim Populations

Risk Factors

The lower prevalence of substance abuse among Muslims compared to different religious groups as reported in many comparative studies, especially the reports of the WHO and the United Nations on substance abuse, can be explained by many reasons. First, it is necessary to discuss how much the data reflect the truth. Because substance abuse statistics are largely based on self-report questionnaires, it is assumed participants will give correct answers in these studies. However, in Muslim societies where substance abuse (alcohol and drugs) is accepted as a sin and therefore not welcomed, the anxiety about being stigmatized reduces the reliability of the answers given to the question-naires, and sometimes substance abusers (especially women) do not want to participate in surveys (AlMarri & Oei, 2009). In addition, people who abuse substances either rarely present to substance abuse treatment centers or go to other countries for treatment for fear of stigmatization (Al-Ansari et al., 2020; Khampang et al., 2015).

Another statistical risk factor is the ban on the sale of alcohol in some Mus-lim-majority countries or the high cost of alcohol products, which results in illegal supply and consumption of alcohol, thereby making it difficult to obtain real data. For example, according to the WHO's Global Status Report on Alco-hol and Health (2019), two-thirds of pure alcohol consumption per capita in the Eastern Mediterranean region (where the majority of the population is Mus-lim) and half of the consumption in the Southeast Asia region is unrecorded. As a result, the figures emerging in studies do not reflect the truth, and drug addiction is seen as if it were only a problem of Western societies.

Studies on substance abuse emphasize that acculturation (Abuelezam et al., 2018; Arfken et al., 2009; Salama et al., 2018) has an important role among risk factors, especially for Muslims living as a minority in West-ern countries. In other words, the rate of substance abuse is higher among Muslims who abandon their cultural identity and assimilate into the culture of the country in which they live (Arfken et al., 2009). Another important risk factor for substance abuse is discrimination, especially Islamophobia, which has escalated since 9/11; exposure to more discrimination as a result of Islamophobia is a stressor in itself (Dotinga et al., 2006; Hassouneh & Kulwicki, 2007). For this reason, Muslims who are exposed to discrimina-tion, especially adolescents, may abuse substances to cope with stressful situations and mental problems that develop due to these conditions, such as anxiety, depression, and post-traumatic stress disorder (PTSD; Amri et al., 2013). Apart from acculturation and discrimination, many factors are asso-ciated with substance abuse in Muslim societies as well as other cultures, including insecure attachment to parents (Koçhan & Ilhan, 2015), insuffi-cient parental control, substance abuse by one or both parents (Taremian et al., 2018), substance abuse among peers, low socioeconomic status (Badr et al., 2014), adolescence and emerging adulthood (Stone et al., 2012), low academic performance (Cox et al., 2007), and loss/grief. On the other hand, sex is both a risk and a protective factor in terms of substance abuse. For example, as in any society, men use drugs more than women among Mus-lims. In this respect, male sex is a risk factor for substance abuse. However, especially in Muslim societies, women are shown less tolerance of substance abuse than men, and therefore women are more subjected to stigma (Hasan et al., 2009; Khoei et al., 2018). On the one hand, this is a protective factor, as it causes women to use substances less frequently; on the other hand, it is considered a risk factor because it causes women who abuse substances to seek help less frequently.

Protective Factors

Studies have shown substance abuse is the lowest among Muslim communities compared to many religious and ethnic groups. The most important reason for this situation is the strict prohibition of alcohol and other narcotic substances in the Quran (verses 90–91 of Surah Al-Maida) and their acceptance as unclean. In addition, the hadiths of Prophet Muhammed, such as "Of that which intoxicates in a large amount, a small amount is haram, too" and "Alcohol is the mother of every evil," are a source of protective reference relating to both substance abuse and substance use. According to the Islamic belief, to worship appropriately, one should be aware of what one is doing during worshipping and keep one's body (physically and spiritually) away from unclean things. For this reason, Muslims pay attention to being clean while praying five times a day, reading the Quran, fasting, or performing pilgrimage. For example, in a study conducted on Turkish and Moroccan Muslim immigrants in the Netherlands (Dotinga et al., 2006), it was reported that the rate of substance abuse was lower among those who prayed five times a day compared to those who prayed less often and among those who performed Ramadan fasting compared to those who did not. In a study involving Muslim college students in the United States, it was reported that faith was an important factor in terms of substance use, and students who participated in religious activities used substances less than others (Abu-Ras et al., 2010).

In addition to believing in God and fulfilling religious practices, living in a religious social environment is an important protective factor in terms of substance abuse (Unlu & Sahin, 2016). Another protective factor is Muslims who live in another country as a minority and adhere to their own cultural roots and values without being exposed to acculturation (Abuelezam et al., 2018; Khawaja, 2016).

Recovery from Substance Abuse in Muslim Populations and Implications for Mental Health Professionals

As in many countries, there are various centers/clinics to serve recovering substance abusers in Muslim-majority countries. However, as stated in the risk factors section of this chapter, some of those who abuse substances are reluctant to apply to such centers especially due to concerns for stigmatization; if possible, they prefer receiving treatment in places farther from their own circles (Al-Ansari et al., 2020). For example, Arfken and Ahmed (2016) stated that Muslim Americans, especially women, who abused substances preferred treatment centers that are farther away from their communities. Obviously, the main reason for this situation stems from the lack of knowledge about substance addiction and mental health among Muslims rather than Islam's ban on alcohol and drugs. For this reason, preventive psychoeducational studies have been conducted recently on the recovery processes of Muslims regarding substance addiction and mental health. For example, in a study conducted in Canada (Hassan et al., 2020), Muslims were given 90-minute seminars; as a result of these training programs, the attitudes of the participants to get help from professionals increased significantly.

Another issue related to centers for substance addiction treatment is the intervention approaches used in treatment. There are some claims the protective/healing factors of culture and religion are not taken into account enough in these centers, and therefore the treatment protocols used are ineffective in preventing relapse (Adam et al., 2011; Gunsu, 2018). Religion is not only a protective factor but also plays an important role in the treatment process (Morjaria & Orford, 2009). It has been observed that spiritual and cultural dynamics have been integrated into standard treatment protocols or, alternatively, religious-based modalities have been developed when working with clients of Islamic origin who attach particular importance to religious values (Akter, 2020; Al-Omari et al., 2015; Jazaeri et al., 2010). For example, there are eight modalities as an alternative to government-supported rehabilitation centers in Malaysia, and most of them use Islamic approaches that include practices such as worshipping, prayer, repentance, and Quran lessons (Adam et al., 2011).

In addition to treatment approaches for drug addiction in Muslim-majority countries, there are some services for the Muslim minority in Western countries, though in limited numbers. For example, Millati Islami, which was founded in the United States in 1989 for Muslims suffering from addiction, has been implementing a 12-step intervention program for many years. While developing this program, Millati Islami based the program on the 12-step program of Alcoholics Anonymous but also made some additions by rejecting some content that is not suitable for Islam (see Table 18.1). However, the lack of controlled studies to demonstrate the effectiveness of spiritual interventions added to standard treatment protocols or developed as an alternative is one of the weaknesses of such promising interventions. Therefore, controlled and independent studies are needed to reveal the effectiveness of such programs, which involve the protective factors of the religion of Islam.

In addition, it will be useful to develop modalities that take into account the loss-grief models in the treatment process of Muslims who abuse substances and to test their effectiveness. As far as it is known, loss and grief models were not taken into account in the intervention modalities for substance addiction, which were developed as sensitive to culture. However, one of the reactions individuals show at the beginning of substance addiction is *denial*, and this reaction is quite compatible with Kübler Ross's (1969) model. Individuals using substances feel *anger* when they begin to be deprived of the substance at the beginning of the treatment, and they can *barter* with God or someone else and give some promises to themselves so that the recovery process will be successful. For example, the client may have a motivation such as, "I promise, now I will be better than before, and I will get back what I have lost." Also, clients may fall into *depression* thinking about what they have lost due to past

Table 18.1 A Comparison Between the Millati Islami and Alcoholics Anonymous 12-Step Programs

Millati Islami 12 Steps		Alcoholics Anonymous 12 Steps	
1	We admitted that we were neglectful of our higher selves and that our lives have become unmanageable.	1	We admitted we were powerless over Alcohol—that our lives had become unmanageable.
2	We came to believe that Allah could and would restore us to sanity.	2	Came to believe that a Power greater than ourselves could restore us to sanity.
3	We made a decision to submit our will to the will of Allah.	3	Made a decision to turn our will and our lives over to the care of God as we understood Him.
4	We made a searching and fearless moral inventory of ourselves.	4	Made a searching and fearless moral inventory of ourselves.
5	We admitted to Allah and to ourselves the exact nature of our wrongs.	5	Admitted to God, to ourselves and to another human being the exact nature of our wrongs.
6	Asking Allah for right guidance, we became willing and open for change, ready to have Allah remove our defects of character.	6	Were entirely ready to have God remove all these defects of character.
7	We humbly ask Allah to remove our shortcomings.	7	Humbly asked Him to remove our shortcomings.
8	We made a list of persons we have harmed and became willing to make amends to them all.	8	Made a list of all persons we had harmed, and became willing to make amends to them all.
9	We made direct amends to such people wherever possible, except when to do so would injure them or others.	9	Made direct amends to such people wherever possible, except when to do so would injure them or others.
10	We continued to take personal inventory and when we were wrong promptly admitted it.	10	Continued to take personal inventory and when we were wrong promptly admitted it.
11	We sought through *Salaat* and *Iqraa* to improve our understanding of *Taqwa* and *Ihsan*. *Salaat*: Prayer service in Islam *Iqraa*: Reading and studying *Taqwa*: God consciousness; proper Love and respect for Allah *Ihsan*: Though we cannot see Allah, He does see us.	11	Sought through prayer and meditation to improve our conscious contact with God as we understood Him, praying only for knowledge of His will for us and the power to carry that out.
12	Having increased our level of *Iman* (faith) and *Taqwa*, as a result of applying these steps, we carried this message to humanity and began practicing these principles in all our affairs.	12	Having had a spiritual awakening as the result of these steps, we tried to carry this message to alcoholics and to practice these principles in all our affairs.

Source: Ali, M. (2014). Perspectives on drug addiction in Islamic history and theology. *Religions,* 5(3), 912–928.

substance addiction. Sometimes, clients may come to the phase of *acceptance* with effective alliance without fully experiencing all these processes. To do this, as stated by Amri and Bemak (2013), mental health professionals working with Muslim immigrants can use culture-sensitive approaches such as the multiphase model of psychotherapy (MPM) to better benefit their clients in the recovery process. In this way, the therapeutic alliance between the therapist and the client can be established faster and stronger.

References

Abdel Haleem, M. A. S. (2005). *The Qur'an: A new translation*. Oxford University Press.

Abuelezam, N. N., El-Sayed, A. M., & Galea, S. (2018). The health of Arab Americans in the United States: An updated comprehensive literature review. *Frontiers in Public Health, 6*, 262. https://doi.org/10.3389/fpubh.2018.00262

Abu-Ras, W., Ahmed, S., & Arfken, C. L. (2010). Alcohol use among US Muslim college students: Risk and protective factors. *Journal of Ethnicity in Substance Abuse, 9*(3), 206–220.

Adam, F., Ahmad, W. I. W., & Fatah, S. A. (2011). Spiritual and traditional rehabilitation modality of drug addiction in Malaysia. *International Journal of Humanities and Social Science, 1*(14), 175–181.

Ahmed, S., Abu-Ras, W., & Arfken, C. L. (2014). Prevalence of risk behaviors among US Muslim college students. *Journal of Muslim Mental Health, 8*(1), 5–19. https://doi.org/10.3998/jmmh.10381607.0008.101

Akter, N. (2020). *Acceptance and commitment therapy protocol for the treatment of substance abuse among Muslims* (Doctoral dissertation). Widener University.

AlMarri, T. S. K., & Oei, T. P. S. (2009). Alcohol and substance use in the Arabian Gulf region: A review. *International Journal of Psychology, 44*, 222–233. https://doi.org/10.1080/00207590801888752.

Al-Ansari, B., Noroozi, A., Thow, A. M., Day, C. A., Mirzaie, M., & Conigrave, K. M. (2020). Alcohol treatment systems in Muslim majority countries: Case study of alcohol treatment policy in Iran. *International Journal of Drug Policy, 80*, 102753. https://doi.org/10.1016/j.drugpo.2020.102753

Al-Omari, H., Hamed, R., & Tariah, H. A. (2015). The role of religion in the recovery from alcohol and substance abuse among Jordanian adults. *Journal of Religion and Health, 54*(4), 1268–1277.

Ali, M. (2014). Perspectives on drug addiction in Islamic history and theology. *Religions, 5*(3), 912–928.

Amri, S., & Bemak, F. (2013). Mental health help-seeking behaviors of Muslim immigrants in the United States: Overcoming social stigma and cultural mistrust. *Journal of Muslim Mental Health, 7*(1), 43–62.

Amri, S., Nassar-McMillan, S., Amen-Bryan, S., & Misenhimer, M. M. (2013). Counseling Arab Americans. In C. C. Lee (Ed.), *Multicultural issues in counseling: New approaches to diversity* (pp. 87–104). American Counseling Association.

Arfken, C. L., & Ahmed, S. (2016). Ten years of substance use research in Muslim populations: Where do we go from here? *Journal of Muslim Health, 10*(1), 13–24. https://doi.org/10.3998/jmmh.10381607.0010.103

Arfken, C. L., Ahmed, S., & Abu-Ras, W. (2013). Respondent-driven sampling of Muslim undergraduate US college students and alcohol use: Pilot study. *Social Psychiatry and Psychiatric Epidemiology, 48*(6), 945–953.

Arfken, C. L., Arnetz, B. B., Fakhouri, M., Ventimiglia, M. J., & Jamil, H. (2011). Alcohol use among Arab Americans: What is the prevalence? *Journal of Immigrant and Minority Health, 13*(4), 713–718.

Arfken, C. L., Kubiak, S. P., & Farrag, M. (2009). Acculturation and polysubstance abuse in Arab-American treatment clients. *Transcultural Psychiatry, 46*(4), 608–622.

Arredondo-Dowd, P. M. (1981). Personal loss and grief as a result of immigration. *Personnel & Guidance Journal, 59*(6), 376–378.

Badr, L. K., Taha, A., & Dee, V. (2014). Substance abuse in Middle Eastern adolescents living in two different countries: Spiritual, cultural, family and personal factors. *Journal of Religion and Health, 53*(4), 1060–1074.

Bradby, H., & Williams, R. (2006). Is religion or culture the key feature in changes in substance use after leaving school? Young Punjabis and a comparison group in Glasgow. *Ethnicity and Health, 11*(3), 307–324.

Cox, R. G., Zhang, L., Johnson, W. D., & Bender, D. R. (2007). Academic performance and substance use: Findings from a state survey of public high school students. *Journal of School Health, 77*(3), 109–115.

Donath, C., Gräßel, E., Baier, D., Pfeiffer, C., Karagülle, D., Bleich, S., & Hillemacher, T. (2011). Alcohol consumption and binge drinking in adolescents: Comparison of different migration backgrounds and rural vs. urban residence-a representative study. *BMC Public Health, 11*(1), 1–14.

Dotinga, A., van den Eijnden, R., Bosveld, W., & Garretsen, H. (2006). Religious, cultural and social cognitive correlates of alcohol use among Turks and Moroccans in The Netherlands. *Addiction Research & Theory, 14*(4), 413–431. https://doi. org/10.1080/16066350600609925

Douglas, H., & Hersi, A. (2010). Khat and Islamic legal perspectives: Issues for consideration. *Journal of Legal Pluralism and Unofficial Law, 42*(62), 95–114.

Gunsu, O. (2018). Drug addiction and religion: HIGED example. *Addicta: The Turkish Journal on Addictions, 5*, 37–54. http://doi.org/10.15805/addicta.2018.5.1.0006

Hasan, N. M., Loza, N., El-Dosoky, A., Hamdi, N., Rawson, R., Hasson, A. L., & Shawky, M. M. (2009). Characteristics of clients with substance abuse disorders in a private hospital in Cairo, Egypt. *Journal of Muslim Mental Health, 4*(1), 9–15.

Hassan, A. N., Ragheb, H., Malick, A., Abdullah, Z., Ahmad, Y., Sunderji, N., & Islam, F. (2020). Inspiring Muslim minds: Evaluating a spiritually adapted psycho-educational program on addiction to overcome stigma in Canadian Muslim communities. *Community Mental Health Journal*, 1–11. https://doi.org/10.1007/s10597-020-00699-0

Hassouneh, D. M., & Kulwicki, A. (2007). Mental health, discrimination, and trauma in Arab Muslim women living in the U.S.: A pilot study. *Mental Health, Religion, and Culture, 10*, 257–262. https://doi.org/10.1080/13694670600630556

Helmer, S. M., Mikolajczyk, R. T., McAlaney, J., Vriesacker, B., Van Hal, G., Akvardar, Y., . . . Zeeb, H. (2014). Illicit substance use among university students from seven European countries: A comparison of personal and perceived peer use and attitudes towards illicit substance use. *Preventive Medicine, 67*, 204–209.

Jazaeri, S. A., Habil, H. B., Rashid, R., Siddiq, A., Zahari, M. M., & Peters, H. (2010). Islamic treatment/approach to drug addiction treatment in Malaysia. *Asian Journal of Development Matters, 4*(2), 154–167.

Juni, M. H. (2014). Tobacco use is prohibited (Haram) in Islam. *International Journal of Public Health and Clinical Sciences, 1*(2), 19–28.

Khampang, R., Assanangkornchai, S., & Teerawattananon, Y. (2015). Perceived barriers to utilise methadone maintenance therapy among male injection drug users in rural areas of southern Thailand. *Drug and Alcohol Review, 34*(6), 645–653.

Khawaja, N. G. (2016). Acculturation of the Muslims Settled in the West. *Journal of Muslim Mental Health, 10*(1), 1–7.

Khoei, E. M., Jamshidimanesh, M., Emamian, M. H., Sheikhan, F., Dolan, K., & Brady, K. T. (2018). Veiled truths: Iranian women and risky sexual behavior in the context of substance use. *Journal of Reproduction & Infertility, 19*(4), 237–246.

Koçhan, K., & Ilhan, T. (2015). Examining of the attachment style to parents, depression levels, and stress management styles of private soldiers in terms of substance abuse. *Addicta: The Turkish Journal on Addictions, 2*(2), 61, 109.

Kübler-Ross, E. (1969). *On death and dying.* Macmillan.

Leong, F. T., Kim, H. H., & Gupta, A. (2011). Attitudes toward professional counseling among Asian-American college students: Acculturation, conceptions of mental illness, and loss of face. *Asian American Journal of Psychology, 2*(2), 140–153. https://doi.org/10.1037/a0024172

Morjaria, A., & Orford, J. (2009). The role of religion and spirituality in recovery from drink problems: A qualitative study of Alcoholics Anonymous members and South Asian men. *Addiction Research and Theory, 10,* 225–256.

Peacock, A., Leung, J., Larney, S., Colledge, S., Hickman, M., Rehm, J., . . . Ali, R. (2018). Global statistics on alcohol, tobacco and illicit drug use: 2017 status report. *Addiction, 113*(10), 1905–1926.

Pew Research Center. (2018). *New estimates show US Muslim population continues to grow.* www.pewresearch.org/fact-tank/2018/01/03/new-estimates-show-u-s-muslim-population-continues-to-grow/

Pew Research Center. (2019). *The countries with the 10 largest Christian populations and the 10 largest Muslim populations.* www.pewresearch.org/fact-tank/2019/04/01/the-countries-with-the-10-largest-christian-populations-and-the-10-largest-muslim-populations/

Salama, E., Niemelä, S., Suvisaari, J., Laatikainen, T., Koponen, P., & Castaneda, A. E. (2018). The prevalence of substance use among Russian, Somali and Kurdish migrants in Finland: A population-based study. *BMC Public Health, 18*(1), 651. https://doi.org/10.1186/s12889-018-5564-9

Stone, A. L., Becker, L. G., Huber, A. M., & Catalano, R. F. (2012). Review of risk and protective factors of substance use and problem use in emerging adulthood. *Addictive Behaviors, 37*(7), 747–775.

Taremian, F., Yaghubi, H., Pairavi, H., Hosseini, S. R., Zafar, M., & Moloodi, R. (2018). Risk and protective factors for substance use among Iranian university students: A national study. *Substance Abuse Treatment, Prevention, and Policy, 13*(1), 46.

Tuck, A., Robinson, M., Agic, B., Ialomiteanu, A. R., & Mann, R. E. (2017). Religion, alcohol use and risk drinking among Canadian adults living in Ontario. *Journal of Religion and Health, 56*(6), 2023–2038.

Unlu, A., & Sahin, I. (2016). Religiosity and youth substance use in a Muslim context. *Journal of Ethnicity in Substance Abuse, 15*(3), 287–309.

UNODC. (2020). *World drug report.* Drug Use and Health Consequences. https://wdr.unodc.org/wdr2020/

WHO. (2019). *Global status report on alcohol and health 2018.* www.who.int/publications/i/item/9789241565639

19 A Buddhist Perspective on Loss Due to Addiction

Christie Nelson

The experience of loss is inevitable and at some point, we all face the pain and ensuing grief inherent in this human condition. Some forms of loss are temporary and easily disregarded, whereas others are more enduring and not necessarily quick to resolve. Other forms of loss are not readily apparent or widely accepted as legitimate. The grief associated with loss due to addiction can be considered a special type of loss, a disenfranchised loss that can lead to grief that may be complicated by deep levels of guilt and shame. This grief may go unrecognized and thus unresolved, which might threaten the long-term sobriety of clients in recovery from addiction.

The grieving process can be considered an important aspect of treatment for clients in recovery. Helping professionals may consider addressing unresolved grief that might have preceded the addiction, along with losses sustained during the active phase of addiction and the losses incurred due to giving up the substance or addictive process itself (Furr et al., 2015). While there may be any number of unique losses associated with addiction, research has shown that common areas of loss reported by individuals receiving treatment may include those related to finances, loss of a particular way of life, loss of relationships, lost access to places associated with the addiction, the inability to self-medicate or escape from feelings through using, and loss of or damage to spiritual connections (Furr et al., 2015).

As a helping professional, it is likely that you will encounter clients from myriad religious and spiritual backgrounds. Buddhism may be one such tradition, considered by some a religion and by others a way of life. Although not a common practice in the United States, it is estimated that by 2050 the United States will be home to 5.5 million Buddhists, becoming the tenth-most practiced faith (Connor et al., 2015). As with any cultural, religious, or spiritual group, individuals within these groups are diverse. Self-reported Buddhists can include immigrants to the United States whose religious observance follows carefully prescribed rituals emphasizing strong connections to family traditions and honoring ancestors (Feuerherd, 2018). Then, there are those individuals who have converted to Buddhism, or who may be second-generation, U.S.-born Buddhists. An estimated quarter of American Buddhists are considered converts, described as aspirants seeking spiritual awakening who tend

DOI: 10.4324/9781003106906-19

to be attracted by meditation practices (Feuerherd, 2018). Within this diverse group of American Buddhists, there may be differences between the Western Buddhism pursued by converts and the ethnic Buddhism of Asian immigrants, with the role of the latter meeting both social and spiritual needs within Asian communities, providing a sense of comfort and connection to their native lands (Coleman, 2002).

Traditionally, lay Buddhists follow five precepts of conduct, which include (a) refraining from killing any living being, (b) not stealing, (c) avoiding sexual misconduct, (d) speaking the truth, and (e) abstaining from taking intoxicants that will cloud the mind. In certain settings, there is some debate over the interpretation of the precept involving intoxicants and whether this means total abstinence or avoiding excessive use (Newman et al., 2006). However, research has shown that practicing Buddhists were less likely to drink than nonpracticing Buddhists (Newman et al., 2006). In Buddhist countries such as Thailand, substance abuse treatment programs have been developed around Buddhist principles and often utilize monk healers (Pengpid & Peltzer, 2021). Buddhist principles such as mindfulness have been integrated into many Western psychotherapeutic programs focused on the treatment of substance use disorders (Nelson & Gutierrez, 2019) and have been found to have positive results (Montero, 2017). The effectiveness of these treatment protocols provide an avenue to providing meaningful treatment to those whose backgrounds include Buddhist principles and linking these principles to the 12 steps (Groves, 2014).

Since its inception, Buddhism has been influenced by the culture in which it exists. Early Buddhist practice in India was informed by Hinduism, and as it spread to China, Tibet, Japan, Korea, and Southeast Asia, it melded with and subsumed other Eastern practices such as Confucianism, Taoism, Shintoism, and indigenous shamanic practices. Japanese Zen and Tibetan Buddhist traditions were brought to the West by Asian teachers, while Vipassana teachings of the Theravada tradition were carried back by Westerners who went to Southeast Asia to seek them out (Coleman, 2002). Although Buddhists have been in America since about 1850, Buddhism has gained wider appeal over the last 70 years and has once again been transformed as it continues to merge with American culture and Westernized worldviews. As culture plays a significant role in both addiction and grief, the culturally aware clinician will consider the uniqueness of each client and the intersectionality of Buddhist thought with other salient cultural characteristics when attempting to understand the nature of loss due to addiction through a Buddhist lens.

Historical Context

All forms of Buddhism share a common goal: liberation from craving, clinging, and the delusion and suffering they cause. The word *buddha* is derived from the root *budh*, which means "to wake"; it is a title given to a person who has awakened to the highest knowledge of reality (Humphreys, 2005). Commonly, a buddha is someone who has achieved supreme enlightenment (*nirvāṇa* in Sanskrit or *nibbāna* in Pali) and has transcended the karmic cycle of suffering and aimless drifting through mundane existence.

Although little factual information is known about the individual who set the wheel of Buddhism in motion, it has been noted that before he was a buddha, he was a prince named Siddhārtha Gautama born in Northern India in Lumbini around 563 BC, in what is now modern-day Nepal. As the story goes, Siddhārtha lived a lavish and cloistered existence, sheltered from the outside world, until he glimpsed four sights that changed the course of his life: old age, sickness, a corpse, and a wandering ascetic. These sights affected Siddhārtha so profoundly that he renounced his worldly life and at age 35 took up the path of a mendicant to discover the true nature of reality and to find an end to suffering. For six years Siddhārtha practiced strict austerity and meditated until he realized that the path to enlightenment could not be achieved through self-mortification. His realization hinged on the understanding that the cessation of suffering and the liberating path could be found neither in overindulgence nor deprivation of the human faculties but in a middle way between the two. It was upon this middle way that Siddhārtha ultimately achieved liberation.

The Middle Way

The teaching (*Dharma* in Sanskrit) advocated by the Buddha over 2,500 years ago was originally directed to his fellow ascetics and was then passed down orally, through many generations of teacher and pupil, before being written down (Allen, 2008). The discourses of the Buddha, known as the Triple Basket (*Tipiṭaka* in Pāli), were collected in the first century and organized into three parts: sermons, monastic law, and Buddhist psychology. The first exposition of the Buddha's teaching was the sermon on the Middle Way, also referred to as the Buddha's First Discourse, where he "set in motion the wheel of the law" (Allen, 2008).

The Middle Way awakened to by the Buddha "gives rise to vision, which gives rise to knowledge, which leads to peace, to direct knowledge, to enlightenment, to Nibbāna" (Bodhi, 2000, p. 1843). The Middle Way, also known as the Noble Eightfold Path, along with the Four Noble Truths constitute the essential elements of all subsequent teachings within the various schools of Buddhism. Although a thorough explication of the Four Noble Truths and the Noble Eightfold Path would require a much deeper investigation than what can be provided here, it seems important for a clinician to have at least a basic understanding of these two Buddhist doctrines. For the reader interested in learning more about Buddhist doctrines and practices, see *Tricycle: The Buddhist Review* at www.tricycle.org, an online resource dedicated to all things Buddhist.

The Four Noble Truths

Pāli is one of the languages in which Buddhist scriptures are preserved. The English word suffering is typically used to denote, what in Pāli, is known as *dukkha*. However, no word in English captures its full essence. *Dukkha* can also be described as unsatisfactoriness, dis-ease, discomfort, frustration, or disharmony with the environment (Humphreys, 2005). Through the teaching of the Four Noble Truths, the Buddha described the nature of *dukkha* and offered a way to transcend the cycles of suffering. The Four Noble Truths are as follows:

1   The noble truth of suffering: Birth is suffering, aging is suffering, illness is suffering, death is suffering; union with what is displeasing is suffering; separation from what is pleasing is suffering; not to get what one wants is suffering; in brief, the five aggregates subject to clinging are suffering.

2   The noble truth of the origin of suffering: It is this craving that leads to renewed existence, accompanied by delight and lust, seeking delight here and there; that is, craving for sensual pleasures, craving for existence, craving for extermination.

3   The noble truth of the cessation of suffering: It is the remainderless fading away and cessation of that same craving, the giving up and relinquishing of it, freedom from it, nonreliance on it.

4   The noble truth of the way leading to the cessation of suffering: It is this noble eightfold path; that is, right view . . . right concentration. (Bodhi, 2000, p. 1844)

The Noble Eightfold Path

The Noble Eightfold Path is the fourth noble truth and contains the eight elements of right view or understanding, right intention or thought, right speech, right action, right livelihood, right effort, right mindfulness, and right concentration. This path, which ultimately leads to liberation from all unsatisfactoriness, dis-ease, discomfort, frustration, and disharmony, is a way of life to be practiced daily. The eight factors are commonly grouped together into three fundamentals of Buddhist training: moral conduct, mental discipline, and wisdom. Moral conduct is practiced through right speech, right action, and right livelihood. Mental discipline is achieved through right effort, right mindfulness, and right concentration. Wisdom is embodied through right understanding and right thought. It is important to note that the path factors are to be considered as a whole, like spokes supporting the smooth functioning of a wheel.

While entire texts have been dedicated to the explication of the Noble Eightfold Path, the Venerable Walpola Sri Rahula (n.d.) provides a concise and easy to comprehend starting point. Ethical conduct is built upon universal love and compassion for all living beings and is exemplified through (a) right speech (avoiding harmful speech and using words that are true, friendly, benevolent, gentle, meaningful, and useful); (b) right action (cultivation of moral, honorable, and peaceful conduct); and (c) right livelihood (abstaining from making a living through a profession that brings harm to others). Mental discipline is achieved by training the mind through the meditative practices of (a) right effort (the energetic will to cultivate and bring to perfection wholesome states of mind); (b) right mindfulness (diligent awareness of the body, feelings, activities of the mind, and conceptions of things); and (c) right concentration (single-pointed contemplation leading to equanimity). Within the wisdom branch, (a) right thought embodies selfless detachment and thoughts of love and non-violence for all beings and (b) right understanding is clarity of the Four Noble Truths (understanding of things as they really are), which are fully developed through meditation.

Applying Buddhist Practices to Addiction Loss

Grief theory reminds us that we are hardwired for attachment in a world that, according to Buddhist thought, is subject to ceaseless change and impermanence, so it is no wonder that loss is accompanied by great suffering (Neimeyer & Young-Eisendrath, 2015). The ability to express and tolerate intense feelings is necessary for grief to be resolved, which may be a challenging process for individuals in recovery (Furr et al., 2015). However, conscious exploration of losses can provide the lessons most needed to learn to help individuals become wiser and more spiritually evolved (Das, 2004). In this sense, Buddhist teaching is as impactful today as it was over 2,500 years ago and offers a relevant way to view loss related to addiction in the context of modern helping relationships and clinical practice.

With an understanding of both the Four Noble Truths and the Noble Eightfold Path, helping professionals have the foundation upon which to undertake the practice of engaging clients in their losses associated with addiction. From a modern cognitive behavioral perspective, Huxter (2015) has suggested the Four Noble Truths might be described as (a) there are presenting problems (*dukkha*), (b) there are causative factors leading to the development of issues and psychological patterns maintaining them (the causes of *dukkha*), (c) reduction of the level of suffering or a complete resolution of the problem is possible (freedom from *dukkha*), and (d) there are treatments using cognitive, behavioral, and affective strategies that address both the causative and maintaining factors (the causes for freedom from *dukkha*).

Relating to Loss With Wisdom

At this point, a case example may be helpful. Meet Jack, a 35-year-old male who had begun practicing Buddhism as a late adolescent. He enjoyed a deep faith and committed practice through regular meetings with a *sangha* (Buddhist community) and had participated in numerous meditation retreats. In his late twenties Jack sustained a serious leg injury from a near-fatal car accident that required several surgeries. During his convalescence, Jack was prescribed pain medication and although he took them as indicated at first, his usage became uncontrolled and ultimately led to an opioid addiction. Now with six months of sobriety behind him and trying to put the pieces of his life back together, he is seeking help from you. With palpable shame in his voice, Jack recounted various losses, including turning his back on his Buddhist practice, loss of his home and career, and loss of many friendships. Among his presenting issues, he also reported damaged relationships with his parents, siblings, and former partner. The biggest regret shared by Jack was being absent from the life of his 9-year-old-daughter.

The Buddha noted that it is easy to become distracted and fall off the path, especially for laypeople (those not protected by monastic life). In Jack's case, the accident and introduction of prescription pain medication contributed to a downward cascade of subsequent consequences that can be looked at through the Four Noble Truths, namely, the law of dependent origination, also referred to as conditioned arising, which details the causal links involved in the creation and maintenance of suffering. This teaching states that all phenomena arise from an endless chain of past causes that generate outcomes with infinite consequences. The second Noble Truth asserts that craving (the striving for things to exist according to what we desire and for the ending of that which we no longer desire) leads to endless renewal and rebirth. In other words, everything is connected to and dependent upon everything else. Past actions lead to future actions in an ongoing stream of experience. This can also be thought of in terms of *karma*, which is a Sanskrit word denoting "action and the corresponding result of action" (Humphreys, 2005).

By engaging in the Noble Path, Jack can create the conditions in which to relate to himself, his experiences, and to others with a deeper and more compassionate understanding of the nature of reality. In this way, he can use the power of the present moment and his ability to make wise choices to generate positive *karma*. Using the Four Noble Truths, Jack can contemplate his losses and through wisdom generate self-love and kindness for the person he was, the person he is now, and for the person he has yet to become. Through the application of right view and right understanding (Eightfold Path items one and two), Jack can begin to process his losses and the underlying shame without attaching unproductive self-blame. As described in the Noble Path, right view embodies selfless detachment and thoughts of love for all beings (including self), and right understanding is holding an intention to see things as they really are (clarity of the Four Noble Truths). The Eightfold Path outlines a process for changing and releasing unhelpful habits and behaviors and developing what is helpful to reach desired goals that are beneficial for self and others (Huxter, 2015).

Addressing Jack's shame and guilt in relation to his losses would also be essential for the maintenance of his sobriety and sustained wellness. Snoek and colleagues (2021) suggested that the quality of one's self-blame has been shown to impact a recovering individual's attitude toward their personal agency, either deeming themself as someone with a fixed and unchanging disposition (destructive shame and guilt) or as someone capable of changing themself (productive shame and guilt). For those with destructive shame and guilt, interventions are needed to help them move away from fixed negative appraisals of self (Snoek et al., 2021). From the Buddhist point of view, nothing remains the same, and it is through clinging to what "seems to be real" and the aversion to necessary change that causes suffering. However, even suffering is impermanent and subject to change. In a practical sense, Jack's shame and guilt can serve as a means to wisely contemplate the suffering that he has caused others, as well as himself, which might then be used as motivation to employ the additional path factors and to mourn his losses with wise compassion.

The Buddha delineated an ethical code of conduct built upon universal love and compassion for all living beings as demonstrated through right speech, right action, and right livelihood (Eightfold Path items three, four, and five). By cultivating an honorable and peaceful way of life and speaking to others with words that are meaningful and true, Jack could act upon his desire to put the pieces of his life back together and start rebuilding his career and relationships with friends and family, while addressing his losses. Grief is not about forgetting or severing ties with the past, rather it is about recognizing and honoring a changing relationship with that which is no more, while staying mindfully present to the ebbs and flows of the grief experience (Wada & Park, 2009). Using a "middle-way" approach to working with grief, Wada and Park (2009) suggest that recognizing the transitory nature of suffering may give the grief-stricken strength to endure the pain of loss. With a deeper understanding of its impermanence, Jack might be more inclined to relate to his pain and grief with less attachment to it.

In fact, meditating on impermanence is an integral part of Buddhism, essential to nurturing a full awareness and appreciation for the transitory nature of life and all things (Das, 2004). Meditation itself is important in Buddhist practice as a means of attaining the mental discipline outlined in the Eightfold Path (items six, seven, and eight) to cultivate and bring to perfection wholesome states of mind and equanimity. In turn, mental training bolsters all other elements of the Noble Path. While there are many forms of meditative practices in Buddhism, such as walking meditation, chanting, mindfulness, and *zazen*, any of which would be applicable to aid in the grieving process, *Metta*, also known as loving-kindness meditation, may be especially helpful in Jack's case. *Metta* is a practice that fosters compassion and love for ourselves and generates loving intentions for others and the world, qualities that would be beneficial to process the grief accompanying losses due to addiction.

In Closing

The nature of change and loss are the most basic and essential teachings to those walking the path of the Buddha (Das, 2004). While numerous losses may result from addiction, including losing one's way spiritually, a place from which to begin the grieving process might be to honor the loss of connection with Buddhism itself, as in Jack's story. Fortunately, the Buddhist path toward liberation relies on a system rooted in the compassion that is ever-present in each moment and accessible to all beings. Reentry is as simple as setting the right intention to do so.

References

Allen, G. F. (2008). *The Buddha's philosophy: Selections from the Pāli canon and an introductory essay*. Routledge.

Bodhi, B. (2000). *The connected discourses of the Buddha: A new translation of the Samyutta Nikaya*. Wisdom.

Coleman, J. W. (2002). *The new Buddhism: The western transformation of an ancient tradition*. Oxford University Press.

Connor, P., Hackett, C. P., Skirbekk, V., & Stonawski, M. (2015). *The future of world religions: Population growth projections, 2010–2050*. Pew Research Center.

Das, L. S. (2004). *Letting go of the person you used to be: Lessons on change, loss, and spiritual transformation*. Harmony.

Feuerherd, P. (2018, April 10). How American Buddhism is like an elephant. *JSTOR Daily*. https://daily.jstor.org

Furr, S., Johnson, W., & Goodall, C. (2015). Grief and recovery: The prevalence of grief and loss in substance abuse treatment. *Journal of Addictions & Offender Counseling*, *36*(1), 43–56. https://doi.org/10.1002/j.2161-1874.2015.00034.x

Groves, P. (2014). Buddhist approaches to addiction recovery. *Religions*, *5*(4), 985–1000. https://doi.org/10.3390/rel5040985

Humphreys, C. (2005). *A popular dictionary of Buddhism*. Routledge.

Huxter, M. (2015). Mindfulness and the Buddha's Noble Eightfold path. In E. Shonin, W. Van Gordon, & N. Singh (Eds.), *Buddhist foundations of mindfulness* (pp. 29–53). Springer International. https://doi.org/10.1007/978-3-319-18591-0

Montero, R. (2017). The value of mindfulness practice for people with substance use problems. *Journal of Social Work Practice in the Addictions*, *17*(4), 433–441. https://doi.org/10.1080/1533256X.2017.1358993

Neimeyer, R., & Young-Eisendrath, P. (2015). Assessing a Buddhist treatment for bereavement and loss: The mustard seed project. *Death Studies*, *39*(5), 263–273. https://doi.org/10.1080/07481187.2014.937973

Nelson, C., & Gutierrez, D. (2019). Mindfulness- and acceptance-based intervention for opioid dependence in groups with open enrollment. In T. J. Buser, P. S Lassiter, & K. Brown-Rice (Eds.), *Annual review of addictions and offender counseling, volume IV: Best practices* (pp. 29–45). Wipf and Stock.

Newman, I., Shell, D., Li, T., & Innadda, S. (2006). Buddhism and adolescent alcohol use in Thailand. *Substance Use & Misuse*, *41*(13), 1789–1800. https://doi.org/10.1080/10826080601006490

Pengpid, S., & Peltzer, K. (2021). The prevalence and correlates of substance use disorders among patients of two different Treatment settings in Thailand. *Substance Abuse Treatment, Prevention and Policy*, *16*(1), 1–10. https://doi.org/10.1186/s13011-021-00345-2

Rahula, W. (n.d.). The noble eightfold path: The Buddha's practical instructions to reach the end of suffering. *Tricycle: The Buddhist Review*. https://tricycle.org

Snoek, A., McGeer, V., Brandenburg, D., & Kennett, J. (2021). Managing shame and guilt in addiction: A pathway to recovery. *Addictive Behaviors*. https://doi.org/10.1016/j.addbeh.2021.106954

Wada, K., & Park, J. (2009). Integrating Buddhist psychology into grief counseling. *Death Studies*, *33*(7), 657–683. https://doi.org/10.1080/07481180903012006

20 Counseling Activities to Address Grief and Substance Use

Kathryn Hunsucker and Susan R. Furr

Engaging clients through activities enriches their knowledge about recovery and can help them connect emotionally with the recovery journey. For activities to have a successful outcome, there must first be a therapeutic relationship between the client and counselor that takes place in a safe environment. Some guidelines to create this safety include always asking permission before asking a client to disclose, being careful to respect personal space, and acknowledge boundaries around activities that may involve touch. Be mindful of not conducting emotionally provocative activities at the end of the treatment week, as clients will need space to process the emotions that arise. Being alone on a weekend without having processed the powerful emotions these activities may evoke may lead to relapse.

Grief/Loss Inventory

Understanding the connection between substance use and grief and loss may be a new concept for many people in treatment. The following inventory provides an extensive look at losses clients may not have considered in relation to their substance use. This inventory developed by Furr et al. (2015) examines losses from three time periods: early life losses, losses while using, and losses upon entering treatment. As the clinician, you will need to assess your client's emotional strength to examine these losses. For someone just entering treatment, you may choose to have them complete the first column, "Entering Recovery," as the initial focus on loss. Clients have a host of feelings about giving up their substance, but they may not have thought of the decision to enter treatment as one connected with grief and loss. This focus may help clients normalize some of the feelings they are experiencing. They may wonder how making such a positive decision to stop using has so many difficult feelings.

The column of the table labeled "While Abusing" may be more beneficial as a client is beginning to recognize the consequences of their substance use. Because clients may feel guilt and shame over these actions, they may engage in a lot of self-blame, so it may be helpful for them to reframe some of their feelings in terms of the losses they have experienced. Just because their actions led to the losses does not mean they do not grieve what they lost. It is only by facing the

DOI: 10.4324/9781003106906-20

pain of grief that emotional energy can be freed from the past and used for engaging in positive actions. Acknowledging these losses can align with 12-step work.

However, for many clients, understanding the impact of earlier life losses may be key to long-term abstinence. The third column provides the option of identifying losses prior to addiction. Clients will need to develop some emotional resiliency in order to delve into early life traumas but may benefit from understanding how substance use has been a way of coping with these losses. Making peace with the past assists them with moving out of the loss–addiction cycle. Clients need to have built coping skills to deal with painful feelings that emerge. If you find a client is not ready for this in-depth work, it may be better to have them "bookmark" these life events, knowing they can get to them later after having more recovery time.

Instructions for Client

Loss is a part of life for everyone. For those who have experience addiction, loss may be found throughout your life experiences. Below are listed different types of losses you might have experienced at different times in your life. I am going to ask you to identify losses at three different times in your life. We are going to begin with (a) losses that you have experienced during the time you entered recovery; (b) losses during the time you were actively abusing your substance(s); and (c) losses prior to the time you began abusing your substance(s). Recalling these losses may trigger feelings you may not have considered associated with your substance use. Please know that it is up to you how much you want to share at any point in time.

Loss and Substance Use

Experience	Entering Recovery	While Abusing	Prior to Abusing
1. Parents' divorce or separation			
2. Physical abuse			
3. Sexual abuse			
4. Verbal abuse			
5. Witnessed violence			
6. Self-esteem damaged			
7. Someone special died			
8. Loss of support from others			
9. Child(ren) lost through divorce or separation			
10. Your child died			
11. Marriage ended			
12. Romantic relationship ended			

(Continued)

Experience	Entering Recovery	While Abusing	Prior to Abusing
13. Friendship(s) ended			
14. You lost your independence			
15. Social life suffered			
16. You lost your job			
17. Loss of material possessions			
18. Decrease in status			
19. Serious health problems			
20. Loss of goal or dream			
21. Financial problems			
22. Poor academic performance			
23. Homelessness			
24. Memory problems			
25. Loss of ability to think clearly and logically			
26. Driver's license revoked			
27. Spiritual connections lost or damaged			
28. No longer have meaning in life			
29. Victim of crime			
30. Committed crime			
31. Diagnosed with HIV			
32. Gave up use of substance			
33. Gave up way of life			
34. Loss of friendship with those who use			
35. Lost places where used			
36. No longer could escape feelings through using			

Processing Questions

Losses From Entering Treatment

What has surprised you most about what you have to give up to enter treatment?
What did your substance do for you that you are going to miss?
How have your relationships changed since entering treatment?
Who do you turn to now for support? How different is support since entering treatment?

Losses While Using

As you begin looking back on your days of using, how did your life change?
What were the benefits you found from using? What were the costs?

What would you most like to regain from your past, prior to when your substance became a problem? What steps do you have to take to get there?

How do you seek forgiveness for the past? How do you forgive yourself?

Losses Prior to Using

How have you dealt with early life losses? What was the most difficult loss you faced?

What coping skills did you use that were helpful?

Who was there for support for you during these losses?

How did you express your feelings of hurt, sadness, or anger over the losses?

What role did your substance begin to play in how you addressed these losses?

Life Events Bingo

Life Events Bingo can be used as an icebreaker when beginning a new recovery group as a way of introducing the concept of change and loss related to substance use.

Instructions: Move around the group, introducing yourself and searching for individuals who have experienced each life event within the past year. When you find someone who has experienced a particular event, interview him or her to find out what coping techniques were most useful in dealing with that change.

Depending on the time available, play "5-in-a-row" or "full card" bingo. Remind participants that their emphasis should be on making contact with others in the group and learning about the variety of coping skills people use in response to stressful situations. Filling out the bingo card is only a secondary goal.

After the group activity is completed, the group leader reconvenes the group to come back as a large group to have a group discussion about the activity. The leader will start by asking what they learned about loss and coping. The leader will ask members to volunteer to share their experiences of this activity with the group. Some possible processing questions include:

- What changes did you find you had in common with others? What change that you experienced was unique?
- What changes created a sense of loss? How did you cope with that loss? Was substance use a part of that coping?
- What coping skills did you find that someone used that you also used? How healthy was this skill?
- What coping skills were used that you want to learn about?

Life Event Bingo

Find someone here who has experienced these life events during the past year. Introduce yourself and ask that person to describe the coping technique that worked best for them in that situation and write the coping technique or the person's name in the appropriate box. Try to find a different person for each event.

Addiction	Been Involved in Accident	Moved	Education Change	Disagreements with Others
Given Up Something	Trust from Others	Money	Employment Change	Something New in Your Life
Freedom Taken Away	Abuse	Self-Esteem Loss	Dreams Changed	Death of Loved One
Lost Possessions	Injury	Loss of Goals	Changes in Responsibilities	Lost Friend
Legal Issues	Health Problems	Missed Something Important	Lifestyle Changed	Relationship Changed

Source: Hunsucker (2000).

Seasons of Grief and Loss

The group leader will create a handout that displays pictures of trees that reflect different seasons (Fall, Winter, Spring, Summer) as a visual illustration of seasons of grief and loss. The handout should include space for members to respond to the following questions. According to Joyce Berger (1993), grief is a season's cycle. Distribute worksheets for members to use for reflection.

Fall: Ask members about the characteristics of fall. What is happening to the tree? How does this relate to your substance use? What were the warning signs that problems were ahead?

Key points: Rich colors occur; values and meaning surface as the potential loss is signaled. The loss occurs (gradual or sudden). Visible reminders are strewn around. Everyone's colors come out. The leaves falling are a fresh reminder of a lived past. Time sense is disrupted; the present is no longer a continuation of the past; a significant "marker event" has occurred.

Winter: Ask members about what winter represents. What does the change in weather mean to them? How does the tree losing its leaves relate to giving up one's substance?

Key points: Empty, cold darkness. You want out and the season to be over, but you cannot get out. Deep, reflective time is needed to prepare for spring. This is the searching time and time of isolation (often a major trigger for relapse). You may be continually looking for what was lost and recalling memories of your other life. Yet you may experience shock each time you face the reality of your loss of your substance.

Spring: Ask members about the meaning of spring. What are the possibilities that new "buds" or growth represent? What is needed for growth (sun, rain, nourishment, protection from harmful insects)? What makes new growth vulnerable (late freeze)? What protections need to be put in place?

Key points: Cleaning away the dead branches and leaves; planting for the new. Spring harvest is planted from last year's seeds. By letting the natural process just occur, trees will bud again. Time to let go of the "deadwood" so sunlight can nourish the new buds. This is a time for closure about events of the past. Holding on to old memories prevents making new ones.

Summer: Ask members about what summer means to them. What do they look forward to in summer? What does the tree in full canopy provide (shade, home for birds, clean air)? How does summer apply to your recovery?

Key points: Summer is a time busy with new experiences and spending time with people; yet it can also be a slow time that opens the door to risks. It is often a time of exploration and making new memories and a time for fun.

Adapted from: Berger, J. S. (1993). Seasons metaphor, music as a catalyst for pastoral care within the remembering tasks of grief, D.M.A. dissertation. Kentucky: Southern Baptist Theological Seminary.

Financial Cost of Substance Use

Financial losses are a major part of substance abuse. How much have you lost during your time of letting substances control your life?

1 Average amount spent on your substance on a typical day/night's use: $_____

2 Add in additional costs (tips, gas $; pool/games; drinks for others;

   cab fare; hotel; ATM fees; extra cigarettes) $_____

3 Number of days/nights per week you usually used: X_____

4 Subtotal for weekly usage: $_____

5 Subtotal for monthly average: X_____

                                                                            $_____

6   Subtotal for yearly use: X12

                                                                        $_____

7   Multiply by number of years spent using: X_____
8   Subtotal estimated cost of use: $_____
9   Estimate amount spend on legal fees (court costs, bonds, fines; probation
     fees; assessments/treatment; lawyers) $_____
10 Multiply by the number of times involved in legal systems:

                                                                        X_____
11 Subtotal of legal cost: $_____
12 Add subtotal from line 8:   +$_____
13 Total estimated costs of substance use to date $_____

- Are you surprised by how much you have spent?
- What life events did you avoid or miss because of financial difficulties?
- What goals would you like to achieve as you move forward?

Writing a Good-Bye Letter to Your Addiction

This activity often takes place early in recovery treatment as clients are confronting loss of their substances. Research has shown that similar brain reactions occur with addiction and falling in love (Chambers & Wallingford, 2017), so the idea of a good-bye letter to one's substance of addiction is one way of addressing the sense of loss and yearning the client encounters when giving up the substance. Saying good-bye in this manner will help clients hold themselves accountable for future actions and provide encouragement to maintain abstinence in the future. Clients may think this is an unusual request at first or may even find it daunting. Prepare them for the fact that strong emotions may arise, but they will find benefit in getting these feelings out in the open. This activity can also be used when a client is addressing unresolved grief. There are three parts to this activity: writing a good-bye letter to the substance, writing a letter in return from the substance, and reflecting on the handout, "*I am your disease.*"

Instructions: Saying good-bye is never easy. However, before you can open new doors in your life, you have to close the ones that are now in the past. It is an act of love to release a part of your life that will always remain important to you in memory but which you must now live without. Your first task is to write a good-bye letter to your substance. Express your thoughts and feelings as openly as possible as you are writing.

A couple of key points are as follows (leader uses these as needed):

1   Focus on the "why" you need to end this relationship. What brought you
     to this point?
2   Recall what you believed this relationship would give you and how that
     has let you down.

3   Write about what you have lost due to this relationship.
4   Discuss the benefits of ending this relationship.
5   Explain the importance of your new relationship with not using.
6   Let addiction know your relapse plan in case you come back to your substance.
7   Discuss your new strengths to live without your substance.
8   Say good-bye.

It is important for the client to share this letter by reading it out loud either to the counselor or to the group. These letters can be very powerful in the group setting where others may gain new insights into their own "breakups" with addiction. Be sure to attend to the emotions expressed by each individual before moving on to another letter.

In the next step, clients should write a response to the letter they have written to their addiction. Have them write from the perspective of what their addiction would say in response to the first letter. After writing this letter, share the handout, "I am your disease."

Possible processing questions:

What surprised you about your reactions to writing this letter? What was difficult about it?
What did you say that empowered you to continue writing?
What did you discover that you may miss about your substance?
When you listened to other members' letters, what similarities did you discover?
How can you use this letter in the future to gain strength in your recovery?
Are you surprised by what your addiction said back to you?
Based on the letter from your addiction, how is your addiction still waiting for you?

Chambers, R., & Wallingford, S. (2017). On mourning and recovery: Integrating stages of grief and change toward a neuroscience-based model of attachment adaptation in addiction treatment. *Psychodynamic Psychiatry*, *45*(4), 451–473. https://doi.org/10.1521/pdps.2017.45.4.451

I Am Your Disease

I hate meetings. I hate higher power. I hate anyone who has a program. To all who come in contact with me, I wish you death and I wish you suffering.

Allow me to introduce myself. I am the disease of addiction. Cunning, baffling, and powerful—that's me. I have killed millions and I am pleased. I love to catch you with the element of surprise. I love pretending I am your friend and lover. I have given you comfort, have I not? Wasn't I there when you were lonely? When you wanted to die, didn't you call me? I was there. I love to make you hurt. I love to make you cry. Better yet, I love when I make you so numb you can neither hurt or cry. You can't feel anything at all. This is true glory. I will give you instant gratification and all I ask of you is long-term suffering. I've been there for you always. When things were going right in your life, you invited me. You said you didn't deserve these good things; I was the only one who would agree with you. Together we were able to destroy all things good in your life.

People don't take me seriously. They take strokes seriously, heart attacks seriously, even diabetes they take seriously. Fools that they are, they don't know that without my help these things would not be made possible. I am such a hated disease and yet I do not come uninvited. You choose to have me. So many have chosen me over reality and peace.

More than you hate me, I hate all of you who have a 12-step program. Your program, your meetings, your higher power all weaken me, and I can't function in the manner I am accustomed to.

Now I must lie here quietly. You don't see me, but I am growing bigger than ever. When you only exist, I may live. When you live, I only exist. But I am here . . . and until we meet again, if we meet again, I wish you death and suffering.

What Baggage Do You Carry?

Instructions: People who develop issues around substance use often have internalized a number of negative messages about themselves. Some of these messages may have come from childhood while other messages may have been based on behaviors while using. In addition, our culture gives many messages around grief and loss that interfere with processing the feelings that accompany loss. Messages such as "take it like a man" or "tears are a sign of weakness" may have prevented you from grieving some of the losses you have experienced.

Create a sheet with pictures of different types of bags under the question, "What baggage do you carry with you when you think about grief, loss, and addiction?" On the bags, identify messages you may have received about your worth or about how to express your feelings. Any messages you have received that have made your feel worthless, incapable, unlovable, or not valued are important to identify, as these messages interfere with your ability to build the confidence needed for your recovery.

Processing questions:

- How easy was it to recall negative messages from your past? How surprised were you by how strong these messages still are?
- What role (if any) did these messages play in your use of substances?
- How did messages about grief and loss affect the ways in which you addressed your grief? Were you given permission to grieve losses, particularly non-death losses?
- How have your life choices been affected by the negative messages you received?

- How have you passed these negative messages on to others in your family?
- How do you feel when you repeat these messages to yourself?

Circle of Grief

Anniversaries of our significant losses, both positive and negative, often serve as triggers for relapse. The pain of remembering may be more than we want to experience. By identifying those times that may stir up thoughts and emotions you are not aware of, we can be prepared to address these emotions as they arise. In the space below, list your significant losses in the months when they occurred.

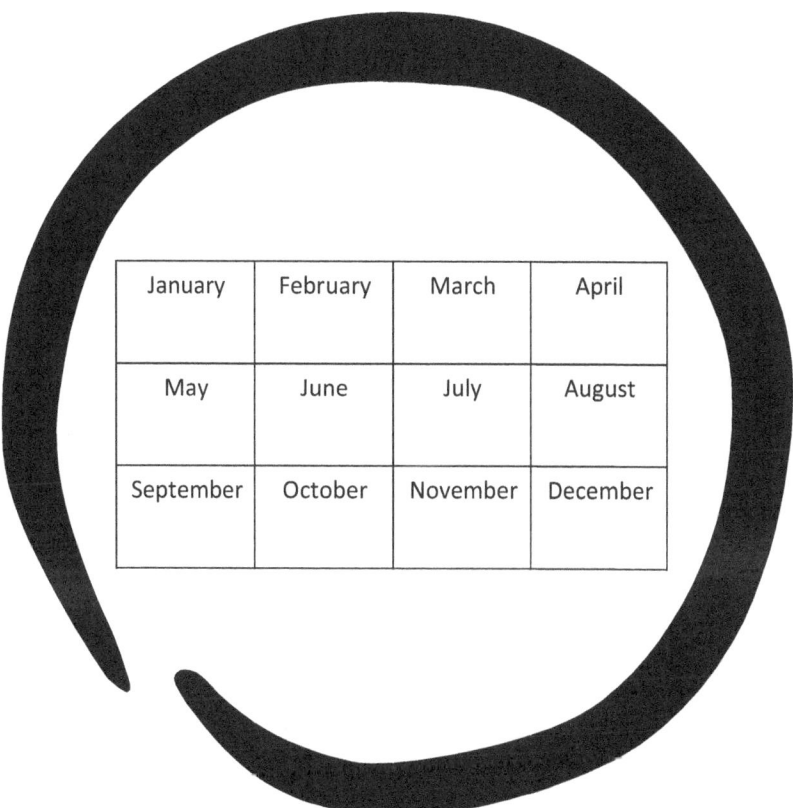

January	February	March	April
May	June	July	August
September	October	November	December

- What can you do to prepare for the emotions evoked by your loss anniversary?
- What rituals can you create to give meaning to your loss?
- Who can you invite to help you process your loss?
- How do you honor the memory and meaning of your loss?

Your Personal Support System

1   Write down those in your support network and others that you can turn to when you experience painful feelings or want to drink or use.
2   Write down what you feel you need to continue working on to understand and accept the grieving process.
3   Write down a situation in your past that caused you pain but eventually got better/healed.
4   Write down areas in your life where you have realized that you are not able to function as you did in the past.
5   Write down ways you are taking care of your own basic needs or how you plan to begin to meet your basic needs.
6   Write down your source of spiritual support.

Flower in My Garden for Grief Recovery

1   Draw five petals (any kind) and when you finish write something about your loss in each petal (examples: Who, What, When, Where, Why).
2   In the center of your flower, write what represents your basis or center or what grounds you.
3   Draw a stem and write on it what holds you up in life and will support you in your grief process.
4   Draw leaves on the stem and write in the names of people who support you.
5   Draw roots that symbolize things you like to do and other internal resources that help ground you.
6   For the ground, draw your environment that provides you with external resources.
7   Draw an object on the ground that represents your memories.
8   Draw an animal that represents you.
9   Draw a blade of grass and write something that holds you back in dealing with your grief.
10 Draw a second blade of grass telling something you need to help you deal with your grief.
11 Draw a third blade of grass, which is a loose end that needs to be tied up.
12 Draw a fourth blade of grass that tells something you should be doing but are not doing.

Lifeline Exercise

On the lifeline provided below, starting at the left side of the page, write down your birthday. On the rest of the line, note your age and any specific important life events to the present. Underneath the life event, note your thoughts and/ or feelings surrounding the event. (Use as many sheets of paper as necessary.)

$$\longleftarrow\!\!\!\!-\!-\!-\!-\!-\!-\!-\!-\!-\!-\!-\!-\!-\!-\!-\!-\!\!\!\!\longrightarrow$$

Once completed, you may want to have your client go back and indicate ages where substance use began or increased significantly, treatment episodes, recovery periods, and relapse periods.

If completing this activity in a group setting, you can have members form dyads or triads and discuss their patterns of loss and substance use.

Processing questions:

- What similarities did you notice among group members in the losses that occurred?
- Were you given permission to grieve your losses?
- What links did you notice (if any) between your losses and your substance use?
- How did you cope with your losses?

Reference

Furr, S. R., Johnson, W. D., & Goodall, C. S. (2015). Grief and recovery: The prevalence of grief and loss in substance abuse treatment. *Journal of Addictions and Offender Counseling*, *36*(1), 43–56. https://doi.org/10.1002/j.2161-1874.2015.00034.x

21 Using Metaphors

An Effective and Person-Centered Approach to Grief and Substance Abuse Counseling

Derrick Johnson and Hannah Glenn

Helping clients make sense of challenging experiences such as loss and addiction involves clients processing both cognitions and emotions (Wagener, 2017), and the use of metaphors has been shown to facilitate the emotional changes expected in the therapeutic relationship (Gelo & Mergenthaler, 2012). Through the exploration of metaphors, clients can gain insight into their emotional reactions and the meaning they create of situations. Metaphors are a perception and a subjective interpretation involving personal meaning making. They host the intersection of senses, feelings, and interpretations that produce an innate and soulful understanding of people and their lived experiences. When a client in treatment for addiction shares "he is drowning his sorrow," the client is not describing a physical action but conveying his helplessness to control his feelings. This imagery is much more powerful than just saying he does not know how to grieve.

According to Kok et al. (2011), metaphors are implicit similes based on the transference of concepts. In psychotherapy, clients share their innermost thoughts, feelings, and fears. Throughout this process, they utilize metaphors to both explain and convey their narrative and share their sense making of the world around them. In this chapter, we will explore the usage of metaphors in counseling as well as meaning making for both the client and counselor.

According to Labov and Fanshel (1977), language plays a central role in the counseling experience, and talk is at the center of understanding and developing unconditional positive regard. In other words, the creation of shared meaning utilizing metaphors by both clients and counselors is a common occurrence and represents not only understanding but provides a mental visualization of the psychological and emotional experience (McMullen, 1989). Research has demonstrated the use of metaphors created a significantly stronger reaction in regions of the brain associated with processing emotions than use of literal expressions (Citron & Goldberg, 2014). Even the use of the less creative expressions of idioms triggered stronger emotional responses compared to literal phrases (Citron et al., 2019). This research supports the concept that metaphoric language may be a gateway to connecting with emotions. While usage of metaphors is gaining ground across many domains, it is important to note

DOI: 10.4324/9781003106906-21

that each realm of usage serves as the connections between the cognitive and the emotional processes of a lived experience (Neimeyer & Mahoney, 1995).

Metaphor utilization in therapy is an indirect way of dealing with content without always bringing it into consciousness (Dwairy, 2002). Grief and loss, for example, encompass areas of direct and passive pain and often are processing events that people both repress and ignore. However, through metaphor utilization, meaning making is "constructed" bit by bit as pieces of loss are confronted and feelings expressed. According to Tay (2016), metaphor is "a strategy to symbolize and communicate difficult-to-describe abstractions" (p. 11). In other words, the objective of utilizing metaphors creates opportunities for clients to restructure deep concepts of thought and to realize different constructs of reality, thus aiding in processing emotional pain in increments or within the client's present sense of emotional safety (Lyddon et al., 2001). Coulson and Van Petten (2002) suggested metaphors help to access and symbolize emotions and uncover and challenge inferred assumptions. In the realm of a counseling or psychotherapy interchange, metaphors reveal meaning and affect. Levitt et al. (2000) asserted a client's speech content and its personal meaning is a measure of in-session experiencing. This is important, because during and through the counseling experience, the patients' inner references become the focus of attention and most importantly imply the person is "actively" participating and implementing exploration. In the example of grief and loss, the process of coping is complex as one moves in and out of different stages or tasks of understanding the loss. This is particularly important because processing loss requires dealing with pain, confusion, and denial, as well as acceptance, all jointly creating a union of meaning and a unique and better understanding for the client (Rowat et al., 2008). In other words, metaphors reveal both meaning and affect for the client experiencing the loss. As an example of metaphoric understanding and meaning, let's use the loss of a 30-year career and a garden hose.

> Clyde and his family worked for a company in a small town and had deep ties regarding their association with the company, which symbolized safety and belonging for not only Clyde the employee but also for Clyde's journey as a young man. Due to the recession, Clyde was terminated without severance pay, medical benefits, or retirement pension plan. Clyde's belonging to company ran deeper than a job; it was something that has given influence to his being over the life span. Clyde was accustomed to this connection not only as a source of economic support but also as part of his social and emotional identity. Suddenly, and in less than one hour, his way of existing and knowing himself no longer existed.

But what does that have to do with a garden hose? In counseling, Clyde shared his frustration with winding up his garden hose. After each watering session, the hose was wound clockwise back onto the hose reel, assuming its regular and consistent hose placement. One day, however, the hose was wound counterclockwise and against its established memory. The hose fought back and would not lay flat, nor would it stay on the hose reel. With each strong attempt to wrap the hose around the reel, the memory of the rubber hose fought back and created a chaotic and disheveled existence, not to mention the feelings of aggravation and impatience experienced by Clyde. This event became symbolic of the job loss that created chaos and a feeling of being turned upside down, without a sense of purpose. In other words, like a garden hose wound in the wrong direction, his feelings of security vanished, and his life was no longer structured in a predictable and organized manner—a complete and total loss of homeostasis. This metaphor became an understanding of meaning as well as an appropriate visualization (Low et al., 2010), as both are relevant in the creation of a stronger meaning of what loss is to this person.

In addition to providing a more accurate and deeper understanding, metaphors provide a means of better expression of a lived experience. Thus, metaphors provide structure for thoughts as well as actions and assist in a client's understanding of the things or the experiences in terms of another (Lakoff & Johnson, 1980). For instance, "in the statement, 'she is sharp as a tack,' not only is the conceptual idea of intelligence expressed, but also a visual and tactile imagery adds a more vivid level of understanding" (Levitt et al., 2000, p. 24). These same researchers asserted that due to the different levels of sensory and informational meanings, metaphors conjure an experiential response in the listener and accurately capture emotion, sometimes better than the use of adjectives or labels. Therefore, the use of metaphors in therapy sessions provides numerous advantages and functions.

Metaphors facilitate insight and provide stronger communication alliances (Angus, 1994), which is observed as clients communicate with a stronger connection and a better means of expressing self and their lived histories. This process aids in reconstructing life narratives and provides clients with a more coherent and encompassing personal/metaphoric experience (Siegelman, 1990). Additionally, Berlin et al. (1991) asserted metaphors provide paths of both self-growth and new solutions for lived experiences. This is specifically beneficial in working with different mental and emotionally based pathologies because it provides opportunities for a counselor to introduce new insights into past behaviors and allows the use of a metaphor to model the new skill of reframing to the client. This intervention modality, for instance, aids in removing feelings of shame and guilt that many clients experience when revealing and sharing painful and personal events of the past. This deletion encourages a more trusting and safer environment for the client, which also encourages a stronger sense of belonging for both the client and the therapist. Incorporating metaphors in the counseling experience increases therapeutic rapport and encourages a more person-centered approach to re-storying the narrative of one's life.

Clients generate metaphors without realizing the content they are conveying. It is up to the counselor to recognize these images as powerful openings into the client's emotional world. When the client generates a metaphor, the counselor can help the client elaborate on the meaning metaphor and the underlying feelings (Wagener, 2017). The use of open-ended questions or reflections can foster increased detail about the metaphor, particularly by exploring emotions connected to the metaphor. Often, metaphors trigger greater recognition of the emotional content beneath the metaphor and allows the client to connect the metaphor with other life experiences. Counselors can also generate metaphors based on past experiences with other clients in similar circumstances. For example, the counselor might share a perception about the client such as "as I listen to you, I get the picture of you being buried under the weight of your substance—that it is so heavy you can hardly breathe. I wonder what you might see in that image."

Metaphoric utilization not only aids in redirecting depressive symptomologies but also is an effective tool when counseling persons living with post-traumatic stress disorder or in traumatic situations. For counselor and clients alike, the pressure to understand and interpret meaning often presents challenges that become an added source of anxiety. According to Angus (1994), successful psychotherapy sessions develop a core metaphorical theme that relates to the main or perceived issue(s). In contrast, this same writer further posits unsuccessful therapeutic relationships utilize figurative language when describing experiences and in many cases are unrelated to the primary theme or reasoning for attending therapy. This research suggests intentionality, structure, and pre-planning regarding word choice and session structure as an essential component of therapeutic engagement. This is also useful in narrative development when working with groups, adolescents, and adults as well as the support systems of those receiving treatment. This is achieved as the application of metaphors encourages a constructivist approach through emphasizing "active meaning making" versus the flatness of straight facts about the client and/or their life realities (Neimeyer & Mahoney, 1995). This is an important factor because clients, especially those in crisis, do not always have the words to express their deepest feelings and emotions. This creates a therapeutic disadvantage because essential meanings are overlooked or not heard by the therapist, and the depth of pain and suffering is therefore marginalized. Encouragement of storytelling or personal narratives utilizing metaphors as communication vehicles promotes a more complete and accurate therapeutic understanding for the therapist as well as the client. These efforts build trust between client and counselor where the patient feels understood and heard, two of the most essential components of therapeutic engagement.

References

Angus, L. E., & Hardtke, K. K. (1994). Narrative processes in psychotherapy. *Canadian Psychology*, *35*, 190–203. https://doi.org/10.1037/0708-5591.35.2.190

Berlin, R. M., Olson, M. E., Cano, C. E., & Engel, S. (1991). Metaphor and psychotherapy. *American Journal of Psychotherapy*, *45*, 359–367. https://doi.org/10.1176/appi.psychotherapy.1991.45.3.359

Citron, F., Cacciari, C., Funcke, J., Hsu, C., & Jacobs, A. (2019). Idiomatic expressions evoke stronger emotional responses in the brain than literal sentences. *Neuropsychologia, 131*, 233–248. https://doi.org/10.1016/j.neuropsychologia.2019.05.020

Citron, F., & Goldberg, A. (2014). Metaphorical sentences are more emotionally engaging than their literal counterparts. *Journal of Cognitive Neuroscience, 26*(11), 2585–2595. https://doi.org/10.1162/jocn_a_00654

Coulson, S., & Van Petten, C. (2002). Conceptual integration and metaphor: An event-related potential study. *Memory and Cognition, 30*(6), 958–968. https://doi.org/10.3758/BF03195780

Dwairy, M. (2002). Foundations of psychosocial dynamic personality theory of collective people. *Clinical Psychology Review, 22*(3), 343–360. https://doi.org/10.1016/S0272-7358(01)00100-3

Gelo, O., & Mergenthaler, E. (2012). Unconventional metaphors and emotional-cognitive regulation in a metacognitive interpersonal therapy. *Psychotherapy Research, 22*(2), 159–175. https://doi.org/10.1080/10503307.2011.629636

Kok. J. K., Lim, C. M., & Low, S. K. (2011). Attending to metaphor in counseling. *International Conference on Social Science and Humanity, IPEDR* (Vol. 5, pp. 54–58). IACSIT Press.

Labov, W., & Fanshel, D. (1977). *Therapeutic discourse: Psychotherapy as conversation*. Academic Press.

Lakoff, G., & Johnson, M. (1980). *Metaphors we live by*. University of Chicago Press.

Levitt, H., Korman, Y., & Angus, L. (2000). A metaphor analysis in treatments of depression: Metaphor as a marker of change. *Counselling Psychology Quarterly, 13*(1), 23–35. https://doi.org/10.1080/09515070050011042

Low, G., Todd, Z., Deignan, A., & Cameron, L. (2010). *Researching and applying metaphor in the real world*. John Benjamins.

Lyddon, W. J., Clay, A. L., & Sparks, C. L. (2001). Metaphor and change in counseling. *Journal of Counseling and Development, 7*(3), 269–274. https://doi.org/10.1002/j.1556-6676.2001.tb01971.x

McMullen, L. M. (1989). Use of figurative language in successful and unsuccessful cases of psychology: Three comparisons. *Metaphor and Symbolic Activity, 4*(4), 203–225. https://doi.org/10.1207/s15327868ms0404_1

Neimeyer, R. A., & Mahoney, M. J. (1995). *Constructivism in psychotherapy*. American Psychological Association.

Rowat, R., De Stefano, J., & Drapeau, M. (2008). The role of patient-generated metaphors on in session therapeutic processes. *Archives of Psychiatry and Psychotherapy, 1*, 21–27.

Siegelman, E. Y. (1990). Metaphors of the therapeutic encounter. *Journal of Analytical Psychology, 35*(2), 175–191.

Tay, D. (2016). Metaphor and psychological transference. *Metaphor and Symbol, 31*(1), 11–30. https://doi.org/10.1080/10926488.2016.1116903

Wagener, A. (2017). Metaphor in professional counseling. *Professional Counselor, 7*(2), 144–154. https://doi.org/10.15241/aew.7.2.144

Metaphor Examples

Client-Generated Metaphors

1. *Client*: While speaking in group, Darren stated, "I cannot believe Jerry did this! Sure, I knew he looked around, we all do, but I never thought he

was cheating on our relationship. Then I caught him. It felt like the impact of a tsunami. One minute it is this little ripple in the ocean and you turn around and a massive wave of water and elements flood over you, obliterating every structure that stood. And then, as if that's not enough, the water reverses and goes back to the sea. The ups and the downs to the 'no he didn't' to 'I'll kill him!' There nothing left but pieces of debris floating around me."

Counselor: Let us stay with that image for a minute. Tell us about your reaction when you saw that wall of water coming at you? What did you do to survive? After the waves receded, what did you see around you? What pieces were left of what you lost? You may have felt great sadness over your loss, what did you do with the pain (pick up pieces or find ways to numb the pain).

2. *Client*: "I remember being in labor with Jeanne, she is my only baby. The contractions were slight but they would build in intensity. Then, I thought I was going to pass out—I remember thinking . . . my God . . . get this child out of me! Then she arrived. I totally forgot about the discomfort—my angel is here, with me, safe. You know, the withdrawals from heroin were kind of the same. Little cravings and then big cravings and then feeling like I was going to go crazy. The intensity of the pain, the withdrawals, it would come and go and come back even worse."

    Counselor: Tell us more about how you got through the pains of labor; I bet it felt like it would never end. How is this similar to withdrawal?
    Client: When I am in withdrawal, that's what I think about. Having my little angel, my Jeanne. The pain and cravings are so similar in intensity . . . it's almost like a rhythm . . . if I can make it through right now, I think I'll be ok.

Counselor-Generated Metaphors

1. *Counselor*: "Beginning treatment is may seem like an impossible task where you do not have the skills to get you to the finish line. Think of it this way—you are on a commercial airliner, a 777, and the pilots need you to fly for them. *What would you be feeling?* You take the seat; they tell you step by step exactly what to do. With each maneuver they guide you, and even tell you the physical sensation you are going to feel. *How are you reacting now?* You are flying this plane, and now you have got to land this baby! You are NOT alone, you have the captain, co-captain, and ground control with you, right there, right beside you and over the radio. A team ready to guide you with every maneuver. A hundred feet, 50, 25, 8, 7, 5 feet, . . ., 3, 2 1, you landed it . . . pulling back on the thrusters, you successfully stop the aircraft, you are safe. *What emotions flow over you upon success?* Just as the landing may not have been the smoothest, you

landed it and you are safe." *What parallels might you see to managing your recovery?*

> Think about this when you want to use. Of course, you know how to do that, but to stop using meth isn't easy. It takes skills and it takes the help of others. You are the captain: don't be scared to do your job! Reach out, ask for help!

2. *Counselor*: Dealing with returning home is often a challenge. You have been talking about how to rebuild trust after a long time of not being there for your family. Think of it like this: you look out of your breakfast nook window every morning, and each morning this spring you see that little robin, bit by bit, build her nest, her home. *What does she have to do to build her home?* She brings in one twig one piece of brush at a time. *Does she do this alone?* No, the male also gathers materials, but she does most of the building. *How might this apply to your return?* She stays busy, focused, fulfilling her goal step by step. One hour, one day at a time. Does she get tired? Yes. Does she want to stop? Yes. But she keeps going. Building a safe place, a home. *What are her rewards for taking these small steps?*

3. *Counselor*: In recovery, we often talk about the grief journey, but what does that really mean? Think about planning an adventure that is challenging but would be a real achievement if you plan your trip well. *Where would you like to go?* You goal could be to climb a mountain or navigate a river. *How would you begin your planning?* (need a destination, a timetable). *What would you need to bring with you?* (goods to meet your basic needs: food, appropriate clothing, shelter, gear). *What do you need to keep you safe?* (water, heat for cooking, compass to not get lost, a way to communicate in case you have difficulties). *How do you handle the unexpected, when you run into the path being blocked or rapids that are powerful?* (slow down and regroup, look for other paths, find others to get help with alternatives). *What are your rewards as you achieve your goal?* (can see my achievements, experience something I have not seen before, discover new aspects of myself). *How do these steps relate to your grief journey?*

Index

Page numbers in *italics* indicate a figure and page numbers in **bold** indicate a table on the corresponding page.